T0289658

Airway Management: Techniques and Tools

Airway Management: Techniques and Tools

Edited by Richard Wright

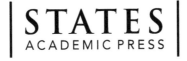

States Academic Press,
109 South 5th Street,
Brooklyn, NY 11249, USA

Visit us on the World Wide Web at:
www.statesacademicpress.com

ISBN: 978-1-63989-781-0

Cataloging-in-Publication Data

Airway management : techniques and tools / edited by Richard Wright.
    p. cm.
Includes bibliographical references and index.
ISBN 978-1-63989-781-0
1. Airway (Medicine). 2. Trachea--Intubation. 3. Artificial respiration.
4. Anesthesiology. I. Wright, Richard.
RC732 .A37 2023
616.2--dc23

Table of Contents

Preface

I am honored to present to you this unique book which encompasses the most up-to-date data in the field. I was extremely pleased to get this opportunity of editing the work of experts from across the globe. I have also written papers in this field and researched the various aspects revolving around the progress of the discipline. I have tried to unify my knowledge along with that of stalwarts from every corner of the world, to produce a text which not only benefits the readers but also facilitates the growth of the field.

Airway management refers to the maneuvers and medical procedures necessary to restore or preserve a person's breathing or ventilation. It is usually classified into two levels, namely, basic and advanced. Basic techniques are typically non-invasive and do not necessitate the use of specialized medical equipment or advanced training. These comprise head and neck maneuvers to improve back blows, ventilation and abdominal thrusts. Advanced techniques necessitate specific medical equipment and training. They are further divided anatomically into supraglottic devices and infraglottic techniques. Airway management can be necessary for individuals in a variety of situations ranging from simple choking to complex airway obstruction. It is a crucial technique for clinicians practicing emergency medicine and providing care to patients in critical circumstances. This book is a detailed explanation of the various techniques and tools used in airway management. It covers in detail some existent theories and innovative concepts related to this domain. The readers would gain knowledge that would broaden their perspective in this area of emergency medicine.

Finally, I would like to thank all the contributing authors for their valuable time and contributions. This book would not have been possible without their efforts. I would also like to thank my friends and family for their constant support.

Editor

Detrimental effects of filling laryngotracheal airways to excessive pressure (DEFLATE-P): A quality improvement initiative

Ashley V. Fritz[*] , Gregory J. Mickus, Michael A. Vega, J. Ross Renew and Sorin J. Brull

Abstract

Background: This quality improvement (QI) project was performed at a single center to determine the incidence of postoperative complications associated with use of cuffed airway devices. An educational program was then completed that involved training our anesthesia providers about complications related to excessive cuff pressure and how to utilize a quantitative cuff pressure measurement device (manometer). The impact of this educational initiative was assessed by comparing the incidence of postoperative complications associated with the use of airway devices before and after the training period.

Methods: After approval by our institution's Institutional Review Board, a pre-intervention (baseline) survey was obtained from 259 adult patients after having undergone surgery with general anesthesia with the use of an endotracheal tube (ETT) or laryngeal mask airway (LMA). Survey responses were used to determine the baseline incidence of sore throat, hoarseness, and dysphagia. Once these results were obtained, education was provided to the anesthesia department members addressing the complications associated with excessive cuff pressures, appropriate cuff pressures based on manufacturer recommendations, and instructions on the use of a quantitative monitor to determine cuff pressure (manometry). Clinical care was then changed by requiring intraoperative cuff pressure monitoring throughout our institution for all surgical patients. After this educational period, 299 patients completed the same survey describing postoperative airway complications.

Results: The use of manometry reduced the incidence of moderate-to-severe postoperative sore throat in the pre- vs. post-intervention groups (35 patients vs 31 patients, $p = 0.045$), moderate to severe hoarseness (30 patients vs 13, patients $p = 0.0001$), and moderate-to-severe dysphagia (13 patients vs 5 patients, $p = 0.03$).

Conclusion: Caring for patients in the perioperative setting frequently entails placement of an airway device. This procedure is associated with several potential complications, including sore throat, coughing, and vocal cord damage. Our quality improvement initiative has shown that intraoperative management of intra-cuff pressure based on manometry is feasible to implement in clinical practice and can reduce postoperative airway complications.

Keywords: Sore throat, Cough, Vocal cord damage, Cuff pressure, Manometry

* Correspondence: Fritz.Ashley@mayo.edu
Department of Anesthesiology and Perioperative Medicine, Mayo Clinic, 4500 San Pablo Road S, Jacksonville, Florida 32224, USA

Background

Sore throat, dysphagia, and hoarseness are multifactorial postoperative complications after general anesthesia in which manipulation of the airway is required. The incidence of post-operative sore throat (POST) has been reported to occur in 17.5–26% of postoperative patients [1, 2] but some studies have reported incidences as high as 50% [3, 4]. The pathologic process has been suggested to involve direct mucosal injury and inflammation related to airway instrumentation and presence of foreign airway objects [5]. Excessive cuff pressures of airway devices have been implicated as a cause of POST [6, 7].

There are reports of mixed efficacy in prevention of POST by pharmacologic modalities, such as topical anesthetics [8]. Moreover, non-pharmacologic modalities, including preoperative licorice water gargling, [9] have also been reviewed, ultimately showing limited impact on complications [5, 7, 9]. Alternatively, Farhang et al. showed that preoperative zinc lozenges were able to reduce the incidence of POST by 24% ($p < .05$) within the first 2 post-operative hours [10].

Chang et al. demonstrated that tapered ETT cuffs, as compared to cylindrical ones, reduce post-operative sore throat by as much as 22% ($p = .003$) [11]. Interestingly, two studies comparing open abdominal surgery to laparoscopic techniques revealed that manometry-measured endotracheal tube (ETT) cuff pressures significantly increased after abdominal insufflation or Trendelenburg positioning, and subsequently resulted in more frequent POST events [12, 13]. Koyama et al. demonstrated that the application of lubricant to the cuff can prevent such increases in pressure via a reduction of gas diffusion into the cuff [14]. Another study compared a novel laryngeal mask airway (LMA) with intra-cuff pressure measurement versus a traditional LMA, finding a significant reduction in postoperative pharyngolaryngeal complications [15]. Interestingly, Corda et al. found that utilizing syringe rebound pressure alone (as a surrogate for measurement of intra-cuff pressure with manometry) was enough to reduce the incidence of POST [16]. In lieu of manometry, it is worthwhile to note two double-blind, randomized controlled trials that have reported success in reducing postoperative respiratory complications by titration of ETT cuff pressure based on the anesthesia machine volume-time curve and minimizing or eliminating the difference between the inspiratory and expiratory volume [17, 18]. None of these interventions, however, completely eliminated POST.

Most clinicians employ subjective measures to mitigate the burden of POST, such as manually palpating the pilot balloon to assess intra-cuff pressure. However, objective measurements of ETT cuff pressures to obtain and maintain recommended ranges provide a more significant reduction in these postoperative complications

[6]. A review of several studies has recently introduced the idea of physical tissue damage as a precursor to postoperative airway complications [5], consistent with other recent studies regarding manometry [6, 7, 13, 19–21]. Minimizing airway cuff pressures may be the key to reducing POST. Although the use of manometry is not commonplace, the availability of new, compact and portable devices allows easy integration into everyday practice and may help reduce the incidence of postoperative complications [8, 19, 20]. We therefore initiated this quality improvement project to determine whether monitoring of cuff pressures (and presumably, preventing intraoperative cuff over inflation) would translate into improved patient care and a lower incidence of complications. We deliberately used a novel, easy to use, and inexpensive manometer (the AG CUFFILL) to facilitate provider acceptance and use. Other pressure monitors (for instance, Cufflator manometer, manufactured by Posey, Sulz, Germany) are much larger and more expensive, and need to be cleaned to prevent vertical bacterial transmission.

One of the most important etiologies of POST is tissue ischemia secondary to cuff over-distension. In our study, we sought to eliminate overinflated cuffs by measuring and ensuring appropriate intraoperative intra-cuff pressure. Our project aimed to determine the incidence of postoperative airway complications at our institution, and inform our anesthesia providers of these patient care concerns. We also sought to educate our department about airway complications that might be due to excessive airway device cuff pressures. Finally, we adjusted clinical practice to incorporate routine measurement of cuff pressures after airway manipulation and then investigated whether this practice change had an impact on the incidence and severity of POST.

Methods

After receiving Institutional Review Board (IRB) approval, a pre-intervention baseline assessment of POST complications was conducted through an originally developed questionnaire (Additional File 1) that documented the airway device utilized, dexamethasone administration, and contained questions delineating the severity of sore throat, hoarseness, coughing, and dysphagia in the postoperative period (Supplemental Material). The symptoms were rated on a 4-point subjective, verbal scale ranging from "none" to "severe." A questionnaire was administered to adult patients (> 18 years old) who had undergone outpatient or inpatient surgery under general anesthesia with ETT or LMA. The questionnaires were completed prior to discharge from Phase 2 recovery. The discharge criteria are based on Aldrete's Modified Phase I Post-anesthesia Recovery Score, as depicted in Table 1 [22]. No patients were excluded from participation in this post-operative

Table 1 Aldrete's Modified Phase I Post Anesthesia Recovery Score

Neurologic	• Fully awake, able to answer questions • Able to move four extremities voluntarily or on command
Respiratory	• Breathing deeply and coughing freely • Able to maintain oxygen saturation > 92% on room air
Cardiovascular	• Blood pressure and heart rate within 20% of pre-anesthetic/sedation level

assessment after the practice change was implemented, and pre-intervention questionnaires were collected over several months at random intervals. A power analysis was performed using the lowest reported incidence of POST (14.4%), considering a 50% reduction in the incidence as significant at $p < 0.05$. To reach statistical significance, a total of 200 patients ($n = 200$) were considered for inclusion. Of note, during the pre-intervention time period, physicians and nurse anesthetists were blinded to the project intent.

An educational module was created and distributed electronically to our anesthesia providers. The module contained pre-test questions and evaluated knowledge of the incidence of POST as well as the recommended ETT and LMA cuff pressures. Information on the reported incidence of POST and recommended cuff pressures was provided, as well as step-by-step text instructions for measurement of cuff pressure with an electronic manometry device (AG CUFFILL™), (Hospitech Respiration, Ltd., Mercury Medical, Clearwater, FL) (Fig. 1). This in-service was followed by a brief instructional video and a link to the manufacturer's instructional video. Changes were made to the electronic medical record (EMR) prompting provider input of ETT and LMA cuff pressures before and after intervention. This built-in

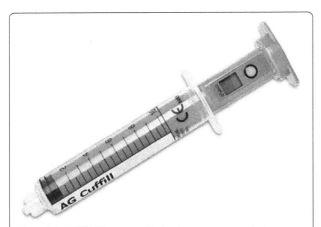

Fig. 1 AG Cuffiill™ Manometry Device. The manometry device (cmH2O) provided for cuff pressure measurement during the post-interventiom phase

visual reminder assisted the transition of objective manometry assessment into everyday practice.

The post-intervention questionnaire was collected over 10 months, and contained questions identical to the pre-intervention questionnaire with additional fields for initial and adjusted cuff pressures, where applicable. Data analysis was performed using a two-tailed Fisher's exact test to determine the impact our educational intervention on initial cuff pressures, adjusted cuff pressures, as well as the frequency of POST, hoarseness, and dysphagia.

Results

A total of 259 pre-intervention and 350 post-intervention questionnaires were collected over 23 months, including 362 ETTs and 152 LMAs (Fig. 2). Subsequently, 95 patients were excluded secondary to undergoing general anesthesia with a natural airway or monitored anesthesia care (MAC). The use of manometry reduced the incidence of moderate-severe postoperative sore throat in the pre- and post-intervention groups (35 patients vs 31 patients, $p = 0.045$, respectively). Moderate to severe hoarseness was also reduced with the application of manometry when comparing pre-intervention (initial pressure) and post-intervention (adjusted pressure) groups (30 patients vs 13 patients, $p = 0.0001$), respectively. Finally, moderate to severe dysphagia was also reduced with the use of manometry when comparing pre- and post- intervention groups (13 patients vs 5 patients, $p = 0.03$, respectively), as identified in Table 2. The use of manometry demonstrated that initial cuff pressures in both airway devices were consistently above recommended values. On average, the initial ETT cuff pressure was 38 ± 18 cm H_2O. Average adjusted pressure for ETTs was 27 ± 4 cm H_2O. Mean initial pressure for LMAs was 66 ± 18 cm H_2O. Mean adjusted pressure for LMAs was 55 ± 8.4 cm H_2O (Table 3).

Discussion

This QI project demonstrated that the utilization of a quantitative device that objectively determines the pressures of ETT and LMA cuffs can reduce the incidence of postoperative airway complications. Specifically, this action led to a significant reduction in the incidence of sore throat ($p = 0.045$), hoarseness ($p = < 0.001$), and dysphagia ($p = 0.03$) (Table 2).

Our findings were in congruence with previous studies. Liu et al. evaluated 509 patients undergoing elective surgery with general anesthesia and endotracheal intubation. These investigators determined that patients who had their cuff pressures adjusted had a lower incidence of post-operative sore throat ($p = < 0.001$) as well as decreased injury to tracheal mucosa as indicated by blood streaked expectoration ($p = 0.089$) [6]. A similar study

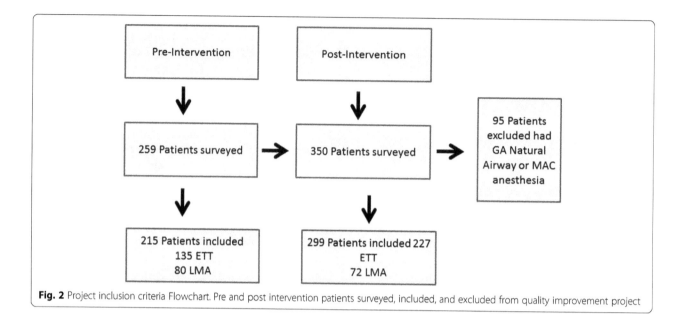

Fig. 2 Project inclusion criteria Flowchart. Pre and post intervention patients surveyed, included, and excluded from quality improvement project

conducted by Li et al. evaluated the incidence of post-operative respiratory complications in patients who underwent general anesthesia with LMAs and demonstrated lower LMA cuff pressures decreased incidence of sore throat ($p = 0.022$), and dysphagia ($p = 0.007$) [23].

While it is difficult to quantify the total cost of postoperative airway complications, the cost of the intervention is minimal. For instance, the AG CUFFILL device can be reused up to 100 times, since measurement of cuff pressures needs not be performed in a sterile fashion. The AG CUFFILL syringe, for instance, has a local cost of $20.00 per unit, resulting in a "cost per use" of only $0.20. The cost of reusable manometers such as the Cufflator™ (VBM Cuff Pressure Gauge, VBM Medizintechnik GmbH, Sulz, Germany) and the Portex Cuff Inflator Pressure Gauge (Smith Medical ASD Inc., Dublin, OH, USA) require a more substantial initial investment of $309.00 and $84.95, respectively. These devices are also larger than the AG CUFFILL syringe, making their use and storage in the limited OR setting much more problematic. These devices also need to be calibrated regularly and require routine maintenance, increasing their cost of use. In comparison, the AG CUFFILL device does not require routine calibration. While it is difficult to quantify the financial burden of postoperative airway

complications, patient safety and satisfaction are universally paramount. Future endeavors describing the effects of confounders may help develop more appropriate and simpler methods to alleviate and prevent postoperative airway complications.

There are several limitations to our project. Manometry represents one objective measure to reduce postoperative respiratory complications; however this is a dilemma with a multitude of variables. Other factors not evaluated in our project that can contribute to POST include preoperative sore throat, trauma during instrumentation of a difficult airway, size of the airway device, the use of neuromuscular blocking agents, presence/absence of cuff lubrication, and length of surgery. Our project may have also been influenced by the Hawthorne Effect as providers knew that cuff pressures were going to be checked after our educational intervention.

As with any new endeavor, there will be challenges to implementation and resistance to alteration of current practice. Our initiative provides insight into such a process, with emphasis on brief, straight-forward education. With the marked reduction in unadjusted and adjusted cuff pressures during the post-intervention phase, our results reinforce how common overinflated cuff

Table 2 Reduction in Postoperative Airway Complications

N = 299 total	Pre-Intervention (n)	Post-Intervention (n)	P-Value
Sore Throat	35	31	0.0457
Hoarseness	30	13	0.0001
Dysphagia	13	5	0.0301

Table 3 Post-intervention initial and adjusted cuff pressures (cm H2O)

N = 299 total	Initial (SD)	Adjusted (SD)	Range Pre-Intervention	Range Post-Intervention
ETT	38 (18)	26.7 (4.3)	9 to OP	17 to 30
LMA	66.1 (17.7)	54.8 (8.4)	20 to OP	22 to 60

OP Over Pressure or beyond 100 cm H2O, *ETT* Endotracheal Tube, *LMA* Laryngeal Mask Airway, *SD* Standard Deviation

pressures are and establishes that utilizing a quantitative device to guide cuff pressure is feasible. In addition, the EMR (electronic medical record) can provide visual cues and reminders to the provider requiring the clinician to measure, adjust, and document the ETT and LMA cuff pressures. The online module, instructional videos, hands-on tutorial, as well as EMR reinforcement solidified the behavioral modification for cuff pressure monitoring. Future investigations are warranted to confirm such findings.

Conclusions

Caring for patients in the perioperative setting often entails placement of an airway device with potential adverse effects and complications that warrant further investigation. Our quality initiative has shown it is feasible to implement manometry into everyday practice, which resulted in a marked reduction in postoperative airway complications. As technology continues to advance, it is imperative for us to utilize the tools provided to our advantage, for the benefit of our patients, and the establishment of a refined standard of care.

Abbreviations
EMR: Electronic Medical Record; ETT: Endotracheal Tube; IRB: Institutional Review Board; LMA: Laryngeal Mask Airway; MAC: Monitored Anesthesia Care; OP: Over Pressure; POST: Post-Operative Sore Throat; QI: Quality Improvement; SD: Standard Deviation

Acknowledgements
We would like to extend our gratitude to all of the Mayo Clinic Florida post-anesthesia care unit staff, especially our nursing team leaders, for their assistance with the questionnaire.

Declarations
1. This paper has not been published or submitted for publication elsewhere.
2. The paper has been read by all co-authors.
3. The paper is being submitted under the category of original research

Authors' contributions
AVF and MAV collected and analyzed patient data, AVF, MAV, and GJM contributed to manuscript preparation, SJB and JRR designed the project and edited the manuscript, All authors approved the final manuscript.

References
1. Higgins PP, Chung F, Mezei G. Postoperative sore throat after ambulatory surgery. Br J Anaesth. 2002;88:582–4.
2. Grady DM, McHardy F, Wong J, Jin F, Tong D, Chung F. Pharyngolaryngeal morbidity with the laryngeal mask airway in spontaneously breathing patients: does size matter? Anesthesiology. 2001;94:760–6.
3. Christensen AM, Willemoes-Larsen H, Lundby L, Jakobsen KB. Postoperative throat complaints after tracheal intubation. Br J Anaesth. 1994;73:786–7.
4. McHardy FE, Chung F. Postoperative sore throat: cause, prevention and treatment. Anaesthesia. 1999;54:444–53.
5. Scuderi PE. Postoperative sore throat: more answers than questions. Anesth Analg. 2010;111:831–2. https://doi.org/10.1213/ANE.0b013e3181ee85c7.
6. Liu J, Zhang X, Gong W, et al. Correlations between controlled endotracheal tube cuff pressure and postprocedural complications: a multicenter study. Anesth Analg. 2010;111:1133–7. https://doi.org/10.1213/ANE.0b013e3181f2ecc7.
7. Tanaka Y, Nakayama T, Nishimori M, Tsujimura Y, Kawaguchi M, Sato Y. Lidocaine for preventing postoperative sore throat. Cochrane Database Syst Rev. 2015;(7):CD004081. https://doi.org/10.1002/14651858.CD004081.pub3.
8. Arts MP, Rettig TC, de Vries J, Wolfs JF, In't Veld BA. Maintaining endotracheal tube cuff pressure at 20 mm Hg to prevent dysphagia after anterior cervical spine surgery; protocol of a double-blind randomised controlled trial. BMC Musculoskelet Disord. 2013;14:280. https://doi.org/10.1186/1471-2474-14-280.
9. Ruetzler K, Fleck M, Nabecker S, et al. A randomized, double-blind comparison of licorice versus sugar-water gargle for prevention of postoperative sore throat and postextubation coughing. Anesth Analg. 2013;117:614–21. https://doi.org/10.1213/ANE.0b013e318299a650.
10. Farhang B, Grondin L. The effect of zinc lozenge on postoperative sore throat: a prospective randomized, double-blinded, placebo-controlled study. Anesth Analg. 2018;126:78–83. https://doi.org/10.1213/ANE.0000000000002494.
11. Chang JE, Kim H, Han SH, Lee JM, Ji S, Hwang JY. Effect of endotracheal tube cuff shape on postoperative sore throat after endotracheal intubation. Anesth Analg. 2017;125:1240–5. https://doi.org/10.1213/ANE.0000000000001933.
12. Yildirim ZB, Uzunkoy A, Cigdem A, Ganidagli S, Ozgonul A. Changes in cuff pressure of endotracheal tube during laparoscopic and open abdominal surgery. Surg Endosc. 2012;26:398–401. https://doi.org/10.1007/s00464-011-1886-8.
13. Geng G, Hu J, Huang S. The effect of endotracheal tube cuff pressure change during gynecological laparoscopic surgery on postoperative sore throat: a control study. J Clin Monit Comput. 2015;29:141–4. https://doi.org/10.1007/s10877-014-9578-2.
14. Koyama Y, Oshika H, Nishioka H, et al. K-Y jelly inhibits increase in endotracheal tube cuff pressure during nitrous oxide exposure in vitro. BMC Anesthesiol. 2018;18:99. https://doi.org/10.1186/s12871-018-0566-9.
15. Wong DT, Tam AD, Mehta V, Raveendran R, Riad W, Chung FF. New supraglottic airway with built-in pressure indicator decreases postoperative pharyngolaryngeal symptoms: a randomized controlled trial. Can J Anaesth. 2013;60:1197–203. https://doi.org/10.1007/s12630-013-0044-2.
16. Corda DM, Robards CB, Rice MJ, et al. Clinical application of limiting laryngeal mask airway cuff pressures utilizing inflating syringe intrinsic recoil. Rom J Anaesth Intensive Care. 2018;25:11–8. https://doi.org/10.21454/rjaic.7518.251.cuf.
17. Bolzan DW, Gomes WJ, Faresin SM, de Camargo Carvalho AC, De Paola AA, Guizilini S. Volume-time curve: an alternative for endotracheal tube cuff management. Respir Care. 2012;57:2039–44. https://doi.org/10.4187/respcare.01812.
18. Bolzan DW, Gomes WJ, Peixoto TC, et al. Clinical use of the volume-time curve for endotracheal tube cuff management. Respir Care. 2014;59:1628–35. https://doi.org/10.4187/respcare.02683.
19. Seet E, Yousaf F, Gupta S, Subramanyam R, Wong DT, Chung F. Use of manometry for laryngeal mask airway reduces postoperative pharyngolaryngeal adverse events: a prospective, randomized trial. Anesthesiology. 2010;112:652–7. https://doi.org/10.1097/ALN.0b013e3181cf4346.
20. Ryu JH, Han SS, Do SH, Lee JM, Lee SC, Choi ES. Effect of adjusted cuff pressure of endotracheal tube during thyroidectomy on postoperative airway complications: prospective, randomized, and controlled trial. World J Surg. 2013;37:786–91. https://doi.org/10.1007/s00268-013-1908-x.
21. Chantzara G, Stroumpoulis K, Alexandrou N, Kokkinos L, Iacovidou N, Xanthos T. Influence of LMA cuff pressure on the incidence of pharyngolaryngeal adverse effects and evaluation of the use of manometry during different ventilation modes: a randomized clinical trial. Minerva Anestesiol. 2014;80(5):547–55.
22. White PF, Song D. New criteria for fast-tracking after outpatient anesthesia: a comparison with the modified Aldrete's scoring system. Anesth Analg. 1999;88:1069–72.
23. Li BB, Yan J, Zhou HG, Hao J, Liu AJ, Ma ZL. Application of minimum effective cuff inflating volume for laryngeal mask airway and its impact on postoperative pharyngeal complications. Chin Med J. 2015;128:2570–6. https://doi.org/10.4103/0366-6999.166034.

2

Airway management in children with hemifacial microsomia: A restropective study of 311 cases

Jin Xu[1], Xiaoming Deng[1*] and Fuxia Yan[2*] (iD)

Abstract

Background: Hemifacial microsomia (HFM) is a congenital craniofacial malformation which is associated with difficult airway. Anesthesiologists may experience difficult intubation in children with HFM. Mandibular distraction could increase the length of the mandible. Theoretically, it should be advantageous to laryngeal view during tracheal intubation. This study reviewed airway management in children with HFM, assessed the efficiency of direct laryngoscopy versus airway-visualizing equipment during the tracheal intubation and determined whether mandibular distraction could improve the laryngoscopic view in children with HFM.

Methods: A retrospective review of cases involving children with HFM aged 5 to 17 years old underwent anesthesia from December 2016 to April 2019 at a single center was performed. The demographic data, preoperative airway assessments, procedure type, anesthetic technique, method of airway management, anesthetists' comments on mask ventilation, laryngoscopy and intubation parameters were collected.

Results: At last, 136 HFM children entered this study, a total of 311 anesthesia procedures were completed during the study period. Face mask ventilation was possible for most of children except 1 child (bilateral involvement) required two practitioners. The success rates of intubation for the primary video laryngoscopy and fibroscopy were both 100%, but 79.5% for direct laryngoscopy ($P < 0.001$). 95 (38.9%) children who had difficult laryngoscopic view (DLV) were significantly correlated with failed direct laryngoscopy ($P < 0.001$). Airway-visualizing equipment (video laryngoscope and Fiberscope) was the primary airway technique in 3 (75%) bilaterally involved children. 60 children underwent both mandibular distraction osteogenesis and the removal of distractor. The laryngoscopic views improved in 26 (43%) children after treatment with mandibular distraction ($P < 0.001$).

Conclusions: Airway-visualizing equipment can be effectively utilized for intubation in HFM children with DLV. Mandibular distraction could improve the laryngeal view effectively.

Keywords: Difficult, Airway, Children, Anesthesia, Hemifacial microsomia

* Correspondence: dengxiaoming2003@sina.com; yanfuxia@163.com
[1]Department of Anesthesiology, Plastic Surgery Hospital, Chinese Academy of Medical Sciences and Peking Union Medical College, No. 33, Ba Da Chu Road, Shi Jing Shan, Beijing 100144, China
[2]Department of Anesthesiology, Fuwai Hospital, National Center for Cardiovascular Diseases, Chinese Academy of Medical Sciences and Peking Union Medical College, 167 North Lishi Road, XiCheng District, Beijing 100037, China

Background

Hemifacial microsomia (HFM) is a congenital craniofacial malformation that features hypoplasia and asymmetry in skeletal tissue as well as in soft tissue [1]. As HFM involves the structure of the first and second pharyngeal arches, it presents across a wide area, which includes the maxilla, mandible, external ear, middle ear ossicles, facial and trigeminal nerves, temporal bone, and muscles of facial expression [2].

As the second most common facial birth defect after cleft and palate deformities, HFM has an estimated incidence ranging from 1:3500 to 1:5600 [3]. Anesthesiologists who anesthetize children are likely to encounter this disorder. Establishing airway management for patients with HFM is a challenge for anesthesiologists. Because HFM is associated with mandibular hypoplasia and temporomandibular joint abnormalities, these malformations can cause difficulties for direct laryngoscopy and endotracheal intubation.

After McCarthy et al. first reported lengthening the human mandible by gradual distraction, mandibular distraction osteogenesis has gradually become the preferred technique to treat HFM because this process allows for a stable expansion of the mandible with concurrent lengthening and expansion of the surrounding muscle and soft tissue [4]. Theoretically, the distraction device could improve mouth opening and alter the laryngoscopic view during tracheal intubation. The current literature on airway management in HFM patients is limited to case reports and very small case series. However, the efficacy of different airway techniques in pediatric airways remains unknown.

The primary objective of the study was to assess the efficiency of direct laryngoscope versus airway-visualizing equipment during the tracheal intubation for children with HFM. The second objective was to determine whether mandibular distraction could improve visualization of the laryngeal structure in HFM children with DLV.

Methods

Patients

Approval for the study was obtained from our institution's Ethics.

Committee (Reference No. ZX2019–21, date of approval 23/5/2019). Data of all intubations for children with HFM (aged 5 to 17 years) performed at the Plastic Surgery Hospital, Chinese Academy of Medical Science, Peking Union Medical College, Beijing, China (Plastic Surgery Hospital, Chinese Academy of Medical Science, Peking Union Medical College) from December 2016 to April 2019 were retrospectively evaluated. The selection period was from the time of establishing an electronic medical records system and integrating the clinical data

in our hospital to the present. The diagnosis of HFM was confirmed by the craniofacial surgery team.

Materials

Using anesthesia records and a difficult airway database, the following data were collected: basic demographics of the patients; preoperative airway assessments (modified Mallampati classification (MMP), thyromental distance (TMD), interincisor gap (IIG), forward protrusion of the mandible (FPM)); reasons for anesthesia according to procedure type; anesthetic technique used; anesthetists' comments on mask ventilation, laryngoscopy, and intubation; the first attempt airway device, rescue device(s) and number of attempts;

A four-point scale, originally described by Han et al. [5], was used to define and classify the face mask ventilation process, as follows:

- Grade I: ventilated by mask;
- Grade II: ventilated by mask with an oropharyngeal airway/adjuvant with or without a muscle relaxant;
- Grade III: difficult ventilation (inadequate, unstable, or requiring two practitioners) with or without a muscle relaxant;

Table 1 The demographics and anesthesia date

Age(years) (n = 311)	
5–8	173(55.6%)
9–13	102(32.8%)
14–17	36(11.6%)
Sex (n = 136)	
Male	84(62%)
Female	52(38%)
Side involved (n = 311)	
Left	157(50.4%)
Right	150(48.2%)
Bilateral	4(1.3%)
Anesthesia (n = 311)	
Endotracheal tube	307(98.7%)
Intubation under spontaneous breathing	1(0.3%)
Intubation with muscle relaxants	306 (99.7%)
LMA	4(1.2%)
Mask ventilation classification (n = 311)	
I	292 (93.8%)
II	18 (5.7%)
III	1 (0.3%)
IV	0 (0%)

Mask ventilation classification, Class I: ventilated by mask; Class II: ventilated by mask with oral airway/adjuvant with or without muscle relaxant; Class III: difficult ventilation (inadequate, unstable, or requiring two providers) with or without muscle relaxant; Class IV: unable to mask ventilate with or without muscle relaxant

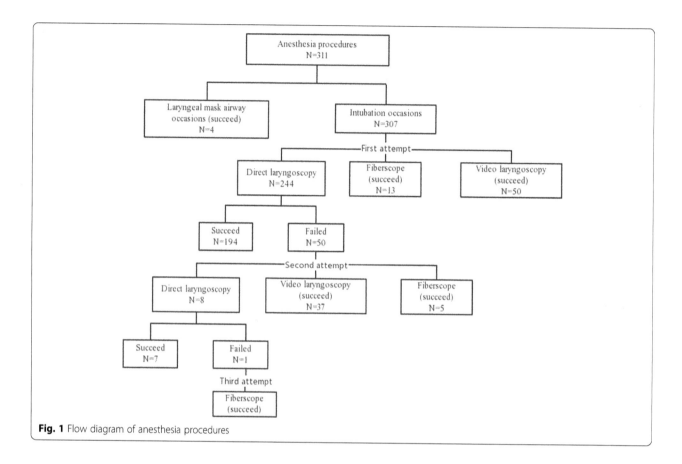

Fig. 1 Flow diagram of anesthesia procedures

- Grade IV: unable to mask ventilate with or without a muscle relaxant.

The recorded description of the direct laryngoscopic view was graded using the Cormack-Lehane (CL) classification [6], as follows:

- Grade I: full view of the glottis;
- Grade II: partial view of the glottis or arytenoids;

- Grade III: partial or full view of the epiglottis;
- Grade IV: no visualization of either the glottis or epiglottis.

Grades I and II were defined as easy laryngoscopic view (ELV), while grades III and IV were defined as DLV.

The MMP was used to evaluate the trachea with the aid of a light; the patient was sitting upright with the

Table 2 Summary of intubation devices (n = 307)

P	Direct laryngoscopy	Video laryngoscopy	Fiberscope	P-value
First attempt airway device(n = 307)	244	50	13	
First pass success(n = 257)	194(79.5%)	50(100%)	13(100%)	P<0.001*
direct laryngoscopy view				
I	63(26.5%)			
II	80(33.6%)			
III	77(32.4%)			
IV	18(7.6%)			
Data missing	6			
Second pass success(n = 49)	7	37	5	
Third pass success(n = 1)			1	

*Fisher's exact test; * Statistically significant difference (P < 0.05)

head in a neutral position, mouth fully opened and tongue fully protruded [7]. The patients were categorized as follows:

- Class I: soft palate, fauces, anterior and posterior tonsillar pillars, and the entire uvula are visible;
- Class II: soft palate, fauces, and uvula are visible;
- Class III: soft palate and base of uvula are visible;
- Class IV: only the hard palate is visible.

The TMD was measured with a rigid rule from the thyroid notch to the lower border of the mandibular mentum while the head was fully extended and the mouth was closed. Considering that TMD does not consider an individual's body proportions, the ratio of height to TMD (RHTMD) [8] was calculated to predict DLV. The RHTMD was calculated as height (in cm)/TMD (in cm).

The IIG was measured between the upper and lower incisors at the midline when the mouth was fully opened.

FPM was assessed as the ability to protrude the mandibular incisors in front of the maxillary incisors and was graded as follows:

- Grade I: the mandibular incisors could protrude in front of the maxillary incisors;
- Grade II: the mandibular incisors could not protrude in front of the maxillary incisors.

All decisions and treatments regarding airway management were at the discretion of the anesthesia provider and were not influenced by the study design.

Statistics

Statistical analyses were performed by using SPSS 23 for Windows (SPSS Inc., Chicago, IL, USA). The data are presented as frequencies (both absolute and percentage). A proportional analysis was performed via Fisher's exact test. The McNemar test was used to test for significance in pass success of first attempt of direct laryngoscopy and DLV changes from mandibular distraction osteogenesis (First-stage) to removal of distractors (Second-stage). Spearman rank correlation was used to test for the relationship between the DLV and failed intubation by direct laryngoscopy.

Airway predictors were entered into a multivariate logistic regression analysis to determine the independent predictors for DLV. It is now believed that microtia is a forme fruste of HFM [2]. Estimating a 30% incidence of difficult intubation in school-aged children with microtia [9], a sample size of 141 patients was calculated to have a power of 0.85 and a significance level of 0.05 to detect a difference in predictors between the ELV and DLV groups with PASS software (version 11; NCSS LLC, Kaysville, UT, USA).

The ability of each independent predictor to predict DLV and the cutoff values for each predictor were evaluated by the receiver operating characteristic (ROC) curve analysis. The sensitivity, specificity, positive predictive value (PPV), negative predictive value (NPV) were calculated for significant variables identified from the ROC curves. Different combinations of predictors were also analyzed. ROC curve analysis was conducted with MedCalc Statistical Software 12.7.7 (MedCalc Software bvba,

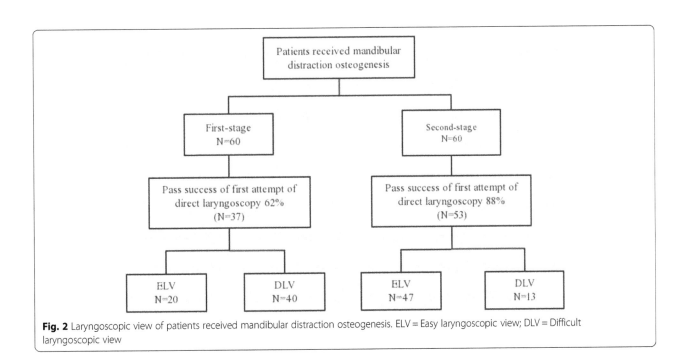

Fig. 2 Laryngoscopic view of patients received mandibular distraction osteogenesis. ELV = Easy laryngoscopic view; DLV = Difficult laryngoscopic view

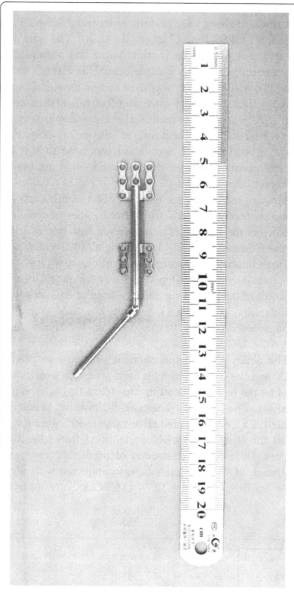

Fig. 3 Mandibular distractor. A semiburied unidirectional distraction device (CIBEI MEDICAL INSTRUMENT CO, LTD, Ning Bo, China) . The distractor activation arm is pointing anteriorly

Ostend, Belgium; http://www.medcalc.org; 2013). $P <$ 0.05 was considered statistically significant.

Result

For the 136 children known to have HFM, a total of 311 general anesthesia procedures were completed during the study period. Of the 105 children who received general anesthesia on at least one occasion, 82 (62%) were males. 4 patients had bilateral involvement. The patients' characteristics and anesthesia data are shown in Table 1.

In total, 62% of the procedures involved the mandible, 32% involved the ear, and 6% involved other structures.

Anesthesia technique

All anesthesia procedures were performed by specialist anesthetists. Inhalation induction was used for 7 procedures (2%) by sevoflurane, and intravenous induction was used for 304 procedures (98%) with 0.2–0.3 µg/kg of sufentanil, propofol 2–3 mg/kg intravenously. Muscle relaxants were administered before intubation and the use of the laryngeal mask airway for 310 procedures with 0.6 mg/kg rocuronium. Only 1 procedure in 1 child with bilateral involved was intubated under spontaneous breathing without muscle relaxants. The children's head was placed in the 'sniffing position'when performing intubation.

Airway management

The anesthetists described the initial face mask ventilation process after administering anesthesia as grade I for 292 procedures (93.8%), grade II for 18 procedures (5.7%, requiring oropharyngeal airway) and grade III for 1 procedure (0.3%, requiring two practitioners). Grade III was found in the children with bilateralinvolvement who required two practitioners. For other anesthesia procedures, mask ventilation was possible.

The methods of airway management for each anesthesia episode were as follows(Fig. 1): laryngeal mask airway was used for 4 anesthesia procedures in 4 children, and all ventilation procedures were successful; tracheal intubation was planned for 307 procedures in 132 children, with 244 procedures in 76 children undergoing direct laryngoscopy, 50 procedures in 44 children undergoing channeled video laryngoscopy(Tosight® TSEL-2000, China) and 13 procedures in 12 children undergoing fibroscopy. The first pass success rates of video laryngoscopy and fibroscopy were both 100%. However, direct laryngoscopy had a lower success rate ($n = 194$, 79.5%) ($P < 0.001$). In 50 cases of first failed intubation, 42 cases were converted to video laryngoscopy ($n = 37$, 74%) or fibroscopy ($n = 5$, 10%), and all procedures were successful. The other 8 cases (16%) underwent a second attempt of intubation by direct laryngoscopy, 7 cases were success, but 1 case failed the procedure twice, and the procedure was converted to fibroscopy, which was finally successful. 4 anesthesia procedures in 4 children were bilateral involvement. Among them, 2 procedures in 2 children were intubated with the assistance of a fiberscopy, 1 procedure underwent video laryngoscopy, 1 child with a grade IV laryngoscopic view underwent a blind intubation by direct laryngoscopy. A description of the laryngoscopic view was recorded for 238 (97.5%) of the 244 procedures intubated by directed laryngoscopy. A total of 95 (38.9%)

procedures had CL grade 3 ($n = 77$) and grade 4 ($n = 18$) laryngeal views, which were significantly correlated with failed intubation ($P < 0.001$). Table 2 summarizes the method of intubation and CL classification.

A total of 60 children underwent both mandibular distraction osteogenesis(first-stage) and removal of distractors(second-stage) (Fig. 2). The distraction (Fig. 3) was started at a rate of 1 mm/day 4 to 7 days after the first-stage operation. The overall distraction distances ranged from 20 to 40 mm. And then the distractors were left in place for 4 to 10 months for consolidation. At last, the distractor was carried out to remove at the second-stage operation (Fig. 4). The laryngoscopic views and first attempt of intubation under direct laryngoscopy during first-stage and second-stage are presented in Table 3. Of these 60 children, only 1 child's laryngoscopic view more difficult during second-stage after the procedures than first-stage undergoing direct laryngoscopy. A total of 26 (43%) children who had DLVs during the first-stage converted to ELVs during the second stage ($P < 0.001$). In total, 16 (27%) children, who failed intubation of the first attempt during the first stage, had a successful direct laryngoscopy after the procedures ($P < 0.001$).

There were no cases of 'can't intubate, can't ventilate' situations, and no emergency cricothyroidotomy or tracheostomy airway management procedures were needed.

Airway prediction

For 238 patients intubated by direct laryngoscopy, there was sufficient information about the airway assessments to predict difficult laryngoscopy. A multivariate logistic regression analysis showed that IIG, RHTMD and FPM were independent predictors of DLV (Table 4).

The ROC analysis to predict DLV (Table 5) revealed that RHTMD was the best predictor, with an AUC of 0.720, a sensitivity of 86.25%, and a specificity of 45.71%.

The combination of RHTMD, FPM, and IIG was the best predictor for DLV, with an AUC of 0.782, a sensitivity of 94.12%, and a specificity of 88.57%.

Discussion

This review of 311 anesthesia procedures of airway management in 136 children with HFM is the largest reported up to now. Our results provide evidence for the effective use of intubation equipment in children with HFM. Although video laryngoscopy and fibroscopy could improve the intubation success rate, direct laryngoscopy is still the first choice and standard technique for tracheal intubation in most cases. Children who presented difficult laryngeal visualization were correlated with failed intubation by direct laryngoscopy.

In the past decade, airway management techniques have changed dramatically. With the development of airway-visualizing devices that are increasingly used today, the selection of the primary airway device has shifted away from conventional direct laryngoscopy to manage difficult intubation. Owing to its portability and easy handling, video laryngoscopes may provide an accessible alternative to fibroscopy. Unsurprisingly, 74% of failed intubations were rescued with video laryngoscopes in our review. Moreover, video laryngoscopy was the primary choice in cases of anticipated difficult intubations. But a meta-analysis demonstrated that while video laryngoscopy improved glottis visualization in children, this device prolonged the intubation time and increased the incidence of failed intubations [10]. A possible explanation may lie in the pediatric endotracheal tube does not always pass straight through the vocal cords when guided by the video laryngoscopy blade. Hence, video laryngoscopy are not recommended in children who may not tolerate long periods of apnea.

In our review, the practice of fiberoptic-assisted tracheal intubation was applied with a low frequency(4.2%, 13/307).

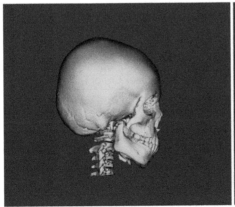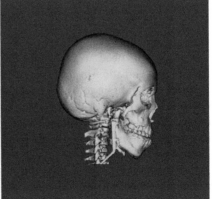

Fig. 4 Preoperative three-digital image demonstrating mandibular distraction osteogenesis expand the mandible. a. Image collected before mandibular distraction osteogenesis. b. Image collected 6 months after mandibular distraction osteogenesis

Table 3 Laryngoscopic view of patients undergoing mandibular distraction osteogenesis(First-stage I) and removal of distractors(Second-stage)

PProcedure		First-stage (n = 60)	Second-stage (n = 60)	P-value
First attempt of direct laryngoscopy(n = 60)		60	60	
Pass success		37(62%)	53(88%)	P<0.001*
Laryngoscopic view				
ELV	I	3	20	P<0.001*
	II	17	27	
DLV	III	32	11	
	IV	8	2	

*McNemar test; *Statistically significant difference (P < 0.05)
ELV Easy laryngoscopic view, DLV Difficult laryngoscopic view

The introduction of the video laryngoscopy might weaken the education of trainees for fiberoptic-assisted tracheal intubation, which is a skill that takes time to master and maintain [9]. Regardless of which airway-visualizing devices is chosen, the primary goal of maintaining the pediatric airway is to ensure oxygenation and ventilation [11]. Both expected and unexpected difficult intubation mean oxygenation impairment, and neither the video laryngoscopy nor the fiberoptic bronchoscope are the solution.

For children who were bilateral HFM, airway management should be approached cautiously. The small mandible and severely limited submandibular space restrict vocal cords exposure during direct laryngoscopy. In the study of Nagorzian et al. [12], the incidence of difficult intubation in bilateral HFM cases was almost threefold higher than that in cases of unilateral HFM. Our review included 4 patients with bilateral involved HFM, 3 patients required airway-visualizing equipment for a successful intubation and 1 patient underwent a blind intubation with a direct laryngoscope. However, our review did not compare the influences of unilateral and bilateral HFM on laryngoscopic view for absence of laryngoscopic view assessment for bilateral HFM absence. Anesthesiologists prefered airway-visualizing equipment for intubation in bilateral HFM impling high risk of difficult intubation by airway assesement. Although airway-visualizing equipment could increase success rate of intubation, it still need to note that the possibility of difficult mask ventilation in bilateral HFM children. Hence, it is rational and safe to intubate under spontaneous breathing.

In this study, the IIG, TMD, and FPM grades were independent predictors of DLV in children with HFM. MMP, the most commonly used airway assessment test for adults, was unable to predict DLV. A possible explanation for this finding is that children with HFM are likely to have a smaller submandibular space than adults, and the MMP does not accurately predict poor visualization of the glottis during direct laryngoscopy.

No predictive test can have 100% sensitivity and specificity for DLV. However, various preoperative tests could reduce the incidence of unanticipated failures in visualizing laryngeal structures and the number of potentially unnecessary interventions required when a difficult airway is not anticipated. In our study, the sensitivity, specificity, and AUC for the combination of TMD, IIG, and FPM were 94.12, 88.57%, and 0.782, respectively. The use of this combination is the best method to predict DLV in HFM children.

Mandibular distraction osteogenesis allows for increasing the vertical length of the mandible, increasing the bone stock, improving soft tissue asymmetry and reducing relapse [13], thereby altering the laryngoscopic view during tracheal intubation. Latency period was allowed for 4 to 7 days before distraction began. The distraction device was initiated at a rate of 1 mm/day. Generally, the overall distraction distances range from 20 to 40 mm, according to the preoperative design. Afterward, the distractor was left in place for 4 to 13 months for consolidation. The distraction device is continuously used until it is removed during the second-stage operation [1]. Our results show that 43% children (26/60) improved laryngeal exposure and decrease intubation difficulty under direct laryngoscopy during the second-stage operation. These results are consistent with those

Table 4 Multivariate logistic regression showing the independent predictors of DLV(n = 238)

Predictors	β	Wald	P-value	OR	95% C.I.for OR	
					Lower	Upper
MMP(≥III)	0.299	0.553	0.457	1.349	0.613	2.967
IIG	−0.707	4.235	0.040*	0.493	0.252	0.967
RHTMD	0.128	15.766	< 0.001*	1.137	1.067	1.211
FPM	−1.450	9.065	0.003*	0.235	0.091	0.603

*Statistically significant difference (P < 0.05)
DLV Difficult laryngoscopic view, MMP Modified Mallampati classification, IIG Interincisor gap, RHTMD Ratio of height to thyromental distance, FPM Forward protrusion of the mandible

Table 5 Statistical results of the predictors for predicting DLV

	AUC	95%CI	cut-off	Sensitivity %	Specificity%	PPV %	NPV %
IIG	0.625	0.543–0.702	≤3.5	55.41	68.35	62.1	62.1
FPM	0.609	0.528–0.687	>1	32.00	89.87	75.0	58.2
RHTMD	0.720	0.650–0.784	>28.83	86.25	45.71	54.8	81.4
RHTMD+FPM	0.755	0.678–0.822	> 0.6211	55.71	85.90	78.0	68.4
RHTMD+IIG	0.741	0.662–0.809	> 0.4073	74.29	62.82	64.2	73.1
IIG + FPM	0.695	0.615–0.767	> 0.3406	70.27	64.56	65.0	69.9
RHTMD+IIG + FPM	0.782	0.707–0.846	> 0.2857	94.12	88.57	62.6	83.7

*Statistically significant difference ($P < 0.05$)
DLV Difficult laryngoscopic view, *MMP* Modified Mallampati classification, *IIG* Interincisor gap, *RHTMD* Ratio of height to thyromental distance, *FPM* Forward protrusion of the mandible

of previous studies that mandibular distraction osteogenesis could improve the laryngeal view, increase the airway volume and mandibular volume [14–16]. However, some complications can occur after surgical correction, such as infection and ankylosis of the temporomandibular joint, which can cause intubation to be more difficult. Hence, for patients who require a procedure after an initial mandibular distraction, the airway should be approached more cautiously.

Our study has some limitations. This is a retrospective study, which has inherent limitations. No prospective standardization in airway management was performed or recorded by the anesthetists. The completeness and accuracy of the data were somewhat limited in the anesthesia records. Future research in airway management for HFM patients should be prospective with standardized protocols for airway management and utilize a survey form. Finally, we do not have detailed information on the airway complications that occurred during anesthesia or in the postanesthesia care unit (PACU). Further research might shed more light on this problem.

Conclusion
Children with HFM have a higher incidence of DLV. Airway-visualizing equipment increases the first pass success rates of intubation compared with direct laryngoscopy, facilitates intubation in children with DLV. A prior mandibular distraction could improve laryngeal views, decrease the degree of intubation difficulty at the second stage of the operation. However, for all patients with HFM, alternative airway equipment should be prepared.

Acknowledgements
None.

Authors' contributions
XD: Designed the study, data extraction, manuscript preparation. JX: Analyzed the data and wrote the manuscript. FY:contributed to review the manuscript. XD and FY takes the full responsibility for the integrity of the work. All authors read and approved the final version of the manuscript.

References
1. Wang X, Feng S, Tang X, Shi L, Yin L, Liu W, et al. Incidents of mandibular distraction Osteogenesis for Hemifacial Microsomia. Plast Reconstr Surg. 2018;142:1002–8.
2. Keogh IJ, Troulis MJ, Monroy AA, Eavey RD, Kaban LB. Isolated microtia as a marker for unsuspected hemifacial microsomia. Arch Otolaryngol Head Neck Surg. 2007;133:997–1001.
3. Hartsfield JK. Review of the etiologic heterogeneity of the oculo-auriculo-vertebral spectrum (Hemifacial Microsomia). Orthod Craniofac Res. 2007;10: 121–8.
4. Mccarthy JG, Schreiber J, Karp N, Thorne CH, Grayson BH. Lengthening the human mandible by gradual distraction. Plast Reconstr Surg. 1992;89:1–08 9-10.
5. Han R, Tremper KK, Kheterpal S, O'Reilly M. Grading scale for mask ventilation. Anesthesiology. 2004;101:267.
6. Cormack RS, Lehane J. Difficult tracheal intubation in obstetrics. Anaesthesia. 1984;39:1105–11.
7. Mallampati SR, Gatt SP, Gugino LD, Desai SP, Waraksa B, Freiberger D, et al. A clinical sign to predict difficult tracheal intubation: a prospective study. Can Anaesth Soc J. 1985;32:429–34.
8. Schmitt HJ, Kirmse M, Radespiel-Troger M. Ratio of patient's height to thyromental distance improves prediction of difficult laryngoscopy. Anaesth Intensive Care. 2002;30:763–5.
9. Kondo I, Kobayashi H, Suga Y, Suzuki A, Kiyama S, Uezono S. Effect of availability of video laryngoscopy on the use of fiberoptic intubation in school-aged children with microtia. Paediatr Anaesth. 2017;27:1115–9.
10. Sun Y, Lu Y, Huang Y, Jiang H. Pediatric video laryngoscope versus direct laryngoscope: a meta-analysis of randomized controlled trials. Paediatr Anaesth. 2014;24:1056–65.
11. Schmidt AR, Weiss M, Engelhardt T. The paediatric airway: basic principles and current developments. Eur J Anaesthesiol. 2014;31:293–9.
12. Nargozian C, Ririe DG, Bennun RD, Mulliken JB. Hemifacial microsomia: anatomical prediction of difficult intubation. Paediatr Anaesth. 1999;9:393–8.
13. Saman M, Abramowitz JM, Buchbinder D. Mandibular osteotomies and distraction osteogenesis: evolution and current advances. JAMA Facial Plast Surg. 2013;15:167–73.
14. Zanaty O, El MS, Abo AD, Medra A. Improvement in the airway after mandibular distraction osteogenesis surgery in children with temporomandibular joint ankylosis and mandibular hypoplasia. Paediatr Anaesth. 2016;26:399–404.
15. Abramson ZR, Susarla SM, Lawler ME, Peacock ZS, Troulis MJ, Kaban LB. Effects of mandibular distraction osteogenesis on three-dimensional airway anatomy in children with congenital micrognathia. J Oral Maxillofac Surg. 2013;71:90–7.
16. Rachmiel A, Aizenbud D, Pillar G, Srouji S, Peled M. Bilateral mandibular distraction for patients with compromised airway analyzed by three-dimensional CT. Int J Oral Maxillofac Surg. 2005;34:9–18.

3

Comparison of vocal cord view between neutral and sniffing position during orotracheal intubation using fiberoptic bronchoscope

Sanghee Park[1], Hyung Gon Lee[1], Jeong Il Choi[1], Seongheon Lee[1], Eun-A Jang[1], Hong-Beom Bae[1], Jeeyun Rhee[1], Hyung Chae Yang[2] and Seongtae Jeong[1]* (iD)

Abstract

Background: In intubation using fiberoptic bronchoscope (FOB), partial or complete obstruction of upper airway makes the FOB insertion difficult. Thus, maneuvers to relieve such obstructions are recommended. There have been no studies to determine whether the sniffing or neutral position is superior for this purpose. Therefore, this study was performed to examine the effects of these two positions including vocal cord view.

Methods: Fifty-four patients scheduled to receive general anesthesia by orotracheal intubation were eligible for inclusion in the study with informed consent. After confirmation of proper head positioning depending on the group, the view of the vocal cord was acquired in each position. Images were reviewed using the percentage of glottic opening (POGO) score.

Results: A total of 106 images of vocal cords from 53 patients were obtained. The mean of difference of POGO score was 11.09, higher for the neutral position and standard deviation was 23.73 ($p = 0.002$). Neutral position increased POGO score in 31 patients and decreased POGO score in 13 patients compare to sniffing position ($p = 0.017$). There were no significant differences between the two head positions with regard to intubation time or degree of convenience during intubation.

Conclusions: Neutral position improved the view of glottic opening than sniffing position during oral fiberoptic intubation. However, there was no difference in the difficulty of tube insertion between the two positions.

Keywords: Airway management, Fiberoptic bronchoscope, Intubation, Patient positioning

Background

In intubation using fiberoptic bronchoscope (FOB), partial or complete obstruction of upper airway makes the FOB insertion difficult [1], and many methods to relieve the obstruction have been reported. As FOB has become a strategic tool for endotracheal intubation [2, 3], efficient positions for fiberoptic endotracheal intubation including patient head position, have been studied [4–8].

In the sedated state, the soft palate, tongue base, and epiglottis move posteriorly, thereby obstructing the airway patency [9, 10]. A number of positions including head tilt, jaw thrust, or lingual traction have been recommended for fiberoptic intubation to relieve the obstruction at these three points [4, 5, 11]. These positions move the oropharyngeal structures anteriorly with the mouth open and an empty oropharyngeal airspace, thus enabling advancement of the FOB. However, there have

* Correspondence: anesjst@jnu.ac.kr
[1]Department of Anesthesiology and Pain Medicine, Chonnam National University Medical School, Chonnam National University Hospital, 42 Jebong-ro, Dong-gu, Gwangju 61469, South Korea

been no studies to determine whether the sniffing or neutral position is superior for this purpose. Although the sniffing position has been recommended for laryngoscopic endotracheal intubation, its clinical benefit is controversial, and it is unclear whether this position is suitable for fiberoptic intubation [12–14].

In intubation using FOB, a previous endoscopic study indicated that the most common point where endotracheal tube advancement is blocked is the right arytenoid process [15]. Furthermore, the head position with neck flexion using a 7 cm high pillow aggravates the epiglottic lift and can induce the bumps between the endotracheal tube and the arytenoid process [16]. From these consequences, we deduced that the neck flexion would obstruct the advancement of endotracheal tube with limiting the view of FOB during orotracheal intubation. Therefore, we hypothesized the neutral position give better vocal cord view and ease of intubation than the sniffing position during fiberoptic orotracheal intubation.

Methods

This prospective randomized crossover trial was approved by the Institutional Review Board of Chonnam National University Hwasun Hospital (CNUHH-2016-120) and was registered in the ClinicalTrials.gov public registry (NCT02931019). The study was conducted at the Department of Anesthesiology of Chonnam National University Hwasun Hospital, Republic of Korea, between 13 October 2016 and 2 December 2016.

Patient selection and enrolment

Patients aged 19 to 70 years, with an American Society of Anesthesiologists classification of I–II, who were scheduled to receive general anesthesia for surgery of the thyroid, breast, stomach, colon, and uterus with orotracheal intubation, were eligible for the study. To minimize the effects of airway variation, a preoperative airway evaluation was conducted the day before surgery using the total airway score (TAS) including the Mallampati classification, thyromental distance, head and neck movement, body mass index, buck teeth, inter-incisor gap, and upper lip bite test [17]. Patients with a total airway score > 6 points or determined to be class III in the upper lip bite test were defined as being difficult to intubate and were thus excluded. Patients with a history of difficult intubation, cervical spine defect, previous head and neck surgery, or risk of pulmonary aspiration were also excluded. After the examination of 65 patients, 54 qualified for study participation and provided written informed consent.

Study design and data collection

The patients were divided into two groups according to the order of head position: S-N group, the sniffing (S) position followed by the neutral (N) position; and the N-S group, the neutral position followed by the sniffing position. The sequence of positions was randomized by a computer-generated list of random numbers. For the neutral position, patients were placed on the operating table in the supine position without a pillow, and for the sniffing position they were kept in the supine position with a 7 cm high pillow placed under the occiput. Upon arrival in the operating room, all patients were monitored with an electrocardiogram, pulse oximeter, non-invasive blood pressure unit (Aisys; GE Healthcare, Waukesha, WI, USA) and bispectral index score (BIS; Medtronic-Covidien, Dublin, Ireland). Patients were given 0.1 mg glycopyrrolate intravenously to suppress salivation, and anesthesia was induced with 2 mg kg^{-1} propofol followed first by remifentanil infusion of up to 3 ng mL^{-1} using a target-controlled infusion device (Orchestra Base Primea; Fresenius Kabi, Brezins, France), and then by 0.8 mg kg^{-1} rocuronium. Manual mask ventilation was provided until the patient's oxygen saturation reached 100% as determined by pulse oximetry. Neuromuscular monitoring was applied with train-of-four (TOF) monitoring (Aisys; GE Healthcare). At a TOF count of 0, an Ovassapian airway (Ovassapian Fiber Optic Intubating Airway; Teleflex, Wayne, PA, USA) was inserted to guide the scope insertion through the midline of the tongue base [18, 19]. Then a specific trained anesthesia nurse conducted the jaw thrust with mouth opening, grasping patient's both mandible angles and protruding the lower teeth until the FOB took a picture of tracheal inlet. All patients were intubated by experienced anesthesiologists using a FOB (MAF-TM Portable Bronchoscope; Olympus, Tokyo, Japan). Under the guidance of the Ovassapian airway, the FOB was inserted until just passing the tongue base and adjusted to get the best view of vocal cord with the epiglottis was acquired. At this point, the glottic opening formed by the epiglottis, vocal cord, and arytenoid cartilage was imaged (vocal cord view). Second images were taken after changing the position according to the patient group, and the FOB was passed into the trachea until it was located just above the carina. With the FOB position maintained, the Ovassapian airway was removed and the endotracheal tube (ETT) advanced smoothly into the trachea. If resistance was detected during passage into the airway, the ETT was withdrawn, rotated 90° anticlockwise, and re-inserted. The time from acquisition of the second image until completion of endotracheal intubation and the number of re-insertion trials were recorded. After proper placement of the ETT above the carina was confirmed by fiberoptic bronchoscopy view, the FOB was removed, and the patient was administered routine anesthetic care. Hypoxia, defined as oxygen saturation (SpO$_2$) < 93%, and the lowest SpO$_2$ value during the study were documented. The procedure was terminated if any adverse events occurred.

The epiglottic view of each position was assessed by the percentage of glottic opening (POGO) score to evaluate the practitioner's first vision of glottic opening during fiberoptic intubation [6, 20].

Sample size justification and statistical analyses

The POGO score was used to compare the visual range of tracheal inlet during fiberoptic intubation. The sample size calculation for the present study was based on changes in POGO score between two head positions (paired t-test). According to pilot study ($n = 12$), the difference of POGO scores showed normal distribution by Kolmogorov-Smirnov test, we obtained a mean of difference = 13.80, SD of difference = 37.86 (effect size = 0.3644069) for paired t-test. Thus, 48 patients yielded a power of 80% and a type I error of 0.05. Assuming a dropout rate, 54 patients were needed for the study. The patients were allocated to the S-N or N-S group using a randomization table. POGO scores were assigned by three other anesthesiologists who were blinded to the head position group. Numerical data, including the POGO score of vocal cord images, were analyzed using the paired *t*-test because it follows the normal distribution by the Kolmogorov-Smirnov test. Changes in the number of

patients in POGO score between positions were analyzed using McNemar test. Time to completion of intubation and the difficulty of tube insertion were analyzed using the Mann–Whitney U test. The relationship between difficulty of tube insertion and time to intubation was assessed by Pearson's correlation coefficient. Data are expressed as mean ± standard deviation or as numerical values. In all of the analyses, $P < 0.05$ was taken to indicate statistical significance.

Results

Sixty-five patients were initially enrolled in this study, and 11 were excluded. Detailed information on patients including those who were excluded is provided in Fig. 1. The characteristics of these patients are listed in Table 1. The lowest SpO_2 reading by pulse oximetry was 94%, recorded in one patient in the N-S group. No adverse events were observed in either group, nor were there significant differences in the hemodynamic parameters between the two groups during the study period.

As this study had a crossover design and images of each head position from 53 patients were taken, 106 images (53 images for sniffing position and 53 images

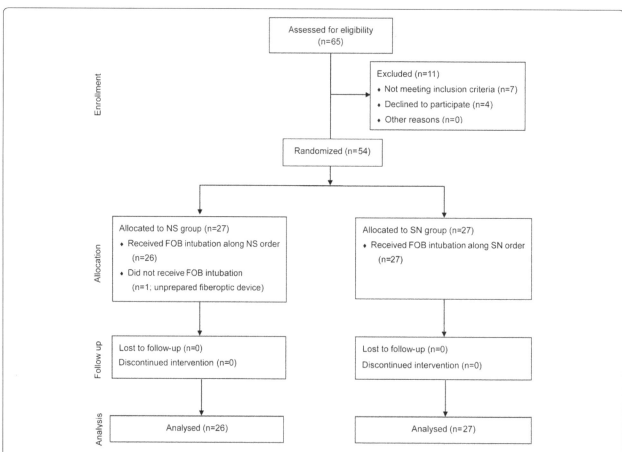

Fig. 1 CONSORT flowchart showing the flow of patients through the trial. Group NS: Neutral position followed by sniffing position, Group SN: Sniffing position followed by neutral position, FOB = fiberoptic bronchoscope

Table 1 Characteristics of the subjects and results of preoperative airway evaluation

Characteristic	Group NS	Group SN
Subjects (n = 53)	26	27
Age [yr: mean (range)]	53 (32–69)	52 (38–70)
Height [cm: mean (SD)]	161 (7.8)	159 (8.1)
Weight [kg: mean (SD)]	65 (8.9)	63 (13.1)
BMI [kg m^{-2}: mean (SD)]	25 (2.8)	25 (3.6)
Preoperative airway evaluation		
Mallampati class		
Class I	20	19
Class II	6	7
Class III-IV	0	1
ULBT		
Class I	21	23
Class II	5	3
Class III	0	1
Total airway score [mean (SD)]	1.15 (1.02)	1.22 (1.53)

Group NS Neutral position followed by sniffing position, *Group SN* Sniffing position followed by neutral position

for neutral position) of the vocal cord view were obtained. The mean of difference of POGO score was 11.09, higher for the neutral position and standard deviation was 23.73 ($p = 0.002$) (Fig. 2). Neutral position increased POGO score in 31 patients and decreased POGO score in 13 patients compare to sniffing position ($p = 0.017$) (Fig. 2). There were no significant differences in blockade during endotracheal tube insertion based on

the number of repositioning events or handling of the FOB (Table 2) [21] between the two groups ($p = 0.355$). The times from obtaining images to completion of intubation were 23.3 ± 6.5 s in the sniffing position and 23.4 ± 11.5 s in the neutral position ($p = 0.626$). POGO score and time to completion of intubation showed a correlation of - 0.118 ($p = 0.403$).

Discussion

In the present study, the POGO score indicating the non-obstructing area of glottic opening was significantly higher in the neutral position than in the sniffing position. This difference could be attributed to the anterior aspect of the vocal cord, which is covered by the epiglottis (Fig. 3). In the sniffing position, because the epiglottis is closer to the posterior pharyngeal wall [22] due to the stretched and collapsed retropharyngeal muscles at the neck flexion point, the area of vocal cord obscured by the epiglottis is wider than in the neutral position. In sedated patients, this tendency is stronger because of the reduced muscle tone of the retropharyngeal structure and soft palate [11, 23].

The sniffing position, achieved using a pillow, was recommended by Magill in 1936 as being better than the neutral position during endotracheal intubation using laryngoscopy [24]. The average head height needed to obtain an optimal laryngeal view was 55 mm (range: 31–71 mm) [25]. The anatomical basis of this recommendation is the three axes (oral, pharyngeal and laryngeal) alignment theory. Bannister and Macbeth suggested that the alignment of these three

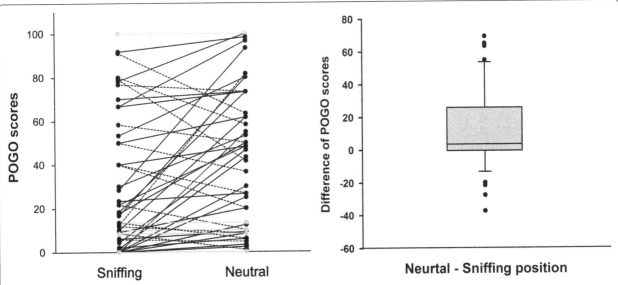

Fig. 2 Comparison of the POGO (percentage of glottic opening) scores. A Solid line (—): Neutral position increased POGO score compare to Sniffing position (n = 31); a dot line (--): decreased POGO score (n = 13); a grey line: no changes in POGO score (n = 9). The mean of difference of POGO score was 11.09, higher for the neutral position and standard deviation was 23.73 (p = 0.002). Neutral position significantly increased the number of patients with increased POGO score compare to sniffing position (p = 0.017)

Table 2 Grading for difficulty of tube insertion (DTI) and the result

Grade	Difficulty
0	No hold-up encountered
1	Hold-up on initial attempt, relieved by withdrawal and rotation of tube 90° anticlockwise.
2	Hold-up on initial attempt requiring more than one manipulation of the tube, alteration in head or neck position or external manipulation

Position	DTI Grading	Number of patients
Sniffing	0	22
	1	3
	2	1
Neutral	0	25
	1	1
	2	1

axes provides a better view of the vocal cords for endo-tracheal intubation using a laryngoscope [26].

However, the oral axes or line of view can be ignored during endotracheal intubation using FOB, because the view inside the oral cavity can be secured and the fiber-optic endoscope passed through the patient's mouth. Thus, only the angle between the pharyngeal and laryngeal axes is important during intubation using FOB. According to a previous MRI-based study, this angle is wider in the sniffing position as the pharyngeal axes lean posteriorly with atlanto-occipital extension [27], and poorer visualization of the vocal cord during fiberoptic endotracheal intubation is assumed.

As glottic view is one of determining factor for Fremantle score using videolaryngoscopic intubation which supplies the direct glottic view [28], the better glottic view can lead the successful intubation using FOB. In the previous studies about fiberoptic intubation, there was no consistent evaluating tool for assessment of glottis view [11, 16]. Therefore, to assess the visualization of vocal cord we used the POGO score which is invented to estimate the glottic inlet in conventional laryngoscopic

intubation. A validated scoring system of the percentage of glottic opening (POGO) score is used to investigate about a degree of glottic airway narrowing [29], and has high accuracy and inter-rater reliability during videolaryngoscopic intubation [30]. For applying the POGO score to the fiberoptic view which has wide angle view, we paid attention to maintain the consistency along the pictures using ovassapian airway. Also, to compensate the inconsistency of the location taking pictures between two head positions, we selected the images viewing the widest glottic opening for scoring the POGO.

In the present study, despite the apparent difference in vocal cord view between the two positions, there were no differences in the ease of intubation and the time for the endotracheal tube insertion. These observations suggested that two different positions do not affect time or ease of orotracheal intubation using FOB. Also, while visualization of the vocal cord affects the difficulty of laryngoscopic endotracheal intubation [31], the effects of vocal cord view on duration or ease of fiberoptic intubation are unclear. The time for tube insertion and the difficulty of tube insertion showed no relationship with better vocal cord view. These observations suggested that visualization of the vocal cord does not affect time or ease of orotracheal intubation using FOB.

The present study has several limitations. First, the intubation time was not measured during whole procedure but only measured from acquiring images to completion of tube insertion. There could be the difference in the time getting the best view of glottis opening between two head position. Measurement of whole intubation time may reveal the relationship between head position and intubation time. Second, we included patients with low TAS score for reducing the airway variation of subjects, excluding patients expected difficult intubation. In patients with difficult direct laryngoscopic intubation (Cormack & Lehane grade III), elevation of the head and neck beyond the sniffing position improved visualization of glottic structures [32]. In addition, sniffing position

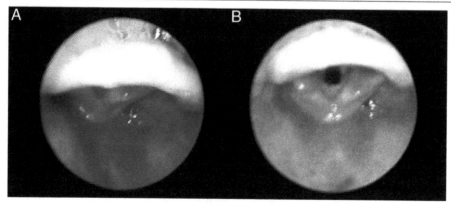

Fig. 3 Fiberoptic bronchoscopy views of vocal cord during (**a**) sniffing position and (**b**) neutral position

relieves obstruction of upper airway in patients with obstructive sleep apnea indicating difficult laryngoscopic intubation [33]. These results limit the application of this study's result to various clinical situations. To validate the superiority of different head positions during fiberoptic intubation, further studies are required with larger patient populations including various airway difficulty including measurement of the entire procedure time.

Conclusions
Neutral position improved the view of glottic opening than sniffing position during oral fiberoptic intubation. However, there was no difference in the difficulty of tube insertion between the two positions.

Abbreviations
BIS: Bispectral index score; ETT: Endotracheal tube; FOB: Fiberoptic bronchoscope; POGO: Percentage of glottic opening; SpO_2: Oxygen saturation; TAS: Total airway score; TOF: Train-of-four

Acknowledgements
None.

Authors' contributions
SJ, JIC designed the study. SJ and SP drafted manuscript. SP performed study and obtained data. EAJ, HBB and JR performed study and image analysis. SJ and SL performed statistical analysis. HGL and JR assisted literature search and data collection. JIC and HGL reviewed statistical analysis. HCY assisted study design and image analysis. All authors read and approved the final manuscript.

Author details
[1]Department of Anesthesiology and Pain Medicine, Chonnam National University Medical School, Chonnam National University Hospital, 42 Jebong-ro, Dong-gu, Gwangju 61469, South Korea. [2]Department of Otolaryngology-Head and Neck Surgery, Chonnam National University Medical School, Chonnam National University Hospital, Gwangju, South Korea.

References
1. Umutoglu T, Gedik AH, Bakan M, et al. The influence of airway supporting maneuvers on glottis view in pediatric fiberoptic bronchoscopy. Braz J Anesthesiol. 2015;65:313–8.
2. Murphy P. A fibre-optic endoscope used for nasal intubation. Anaesthesia. 1967;22:489–91.
3. Apfelbaum JL, Hagberg CA, Caplan RA, Blitt CD, Connis RT, Nickinovich DG, et al. American Society of Anesthesiologists Task Force on Management of the Difficult a. Practice guidelines for management of the difficult airway: an updated report by the American Society of Anesthesiologists Task Force on management of the difficult airway. Anesthesiology. 2013;118:251–70.
4. Iqbal R, Gardner-Thorpe C, Thompson J, Popat MT, Yentis SM, Pandit JJ. A comparison of an anterior jaw lift manoeuvre with the Berman airway for assisting fibreoptic orotracheal intubation. Anaesthesia. 2006;61:1048–52.
5. Durga VK, Millns JP, Smith JE. Manoeuvres used to clear the airway during fibreoptic intubation. Br J Anaesth. 2001;87:207–11.
6. Stacey M, Rassam S, Sivasankar R, Hall J, Latto I. A comparison of direct laryngoscopy and jaw thrust to aid fibreoptic intubation. Anaesthesia. 2005; 60:445–8.
7. Aoyama K, Takenaka I, Nagaoka E, Kadoya T. Jaw thrust maneuver for endotracheal intubation using a fiberoptic stylet. Anesth & Analg. 2000;90: 1457–8.
8. Han S, Oh A, Jung C, Park S, Kim J, Nahm F. The effect of the jaw-thrust manoeuvre on the ability to advance a tracheal tube over a bronchoscope during oral fibreoptic intubation. Anaesthesia. 2013;68:472–7.
9. Nandi P, Charlesworth C, Taylor S, Nunn J, Dore C. Effect of general anaesthesia on the pharynx. Br J Anaesth. 1991;66:157–62.
10. Sutthiprapaporn P, Tanimoto K, Ohtsuka M, Nagasaki T, Iida Y, Katsumata A. Positional changes of oropharyngeal structures due to gravity in the upright and supine positions. Dentomaxillofac Radiol. 2008;37:130–5.
11. Uzun L, Ugur MB, Altunkaya H, Ozer Y, Ozkocak I, Demirel CB. Effectiveness of the jaw-thrust maneuver in opening the airway: a flexible fiberoptic endoscopic study. ORL J Otorhinolaryngol Relat Spec. 2005;67:39–44.
12. Adnet F, Baillard C, Borron SW, Denantes C, Lefebvre L, Galinski M, et al. Randomized study comparing the "sniffing position" with simple head extension for Laryngoscopic view in elective surgery patients. Anesthesiology. 2001;95:836–41.
13. Akihisa Y, Hoshijima H, Maruyama K, Koyama Y, Andoh T. Effects of sniffing position for tracheal intubation: a meta-analysis of randomized controlled trials. Am J Emerg Med. 2015;33:1606–11.
14. Common Practice IS. Concepts in anesthesia: time for ReassessmentIs the sniffing position a "gold standard" for laryngoscopy? Anesthesiology. 2001; 95:825–7.
15. Johnson DM, From AM, Smith RB, From RP, Maktabi MA. Endoscopic study of mechanisms of failure of endotracheal tube advancement into the trachea during awake fiberoptic orotracheal intubation. Anesthesiology. 2005;102:910–4.
16. Cheng KI, Yun MK, Chang MC, Lee KW, Huang SC, Tang CS, et al. Fiberoptic bronchoscopic view change of laryngopharyngeal tissues by different airway supporting techniques: comparison of patients with and without open mouth limitation. J Clin Anesth. 2008;20:573–9.
17. Seo SH, Lee JG, Yu SB, Kim DS, Ryu SJ, Kim KH. Predictors of difficult intubation defined by the intubation difficulty scale (IDS): predictive value of 7 airway assessment factors. Korean J Anesthesiol. 2012;63:491–7.
18. Aoyama K, Seto A, Takenaka I. Simple modification of the Ovassapian Fiberoptic intubating airway. Anesthesiology. 1999;91:897–7.
19. Ravindran RS. Another advantage of marking Ovassapian Fiber-optic intubating airway. Anesthesiology. 2000;92:1843–3.
20. Ochroch EA, Hollander JE, Kush S, Shofer FS, Levitan RM. Assessment of laryngeal view: percentage of glottic opening score vs Cormack and Lehane grading. Can J Anaesth. 1999;46:987–90.
21. Greer JR, Smith SP, Strang T. A comparison of tracheal tube tip designs on the passage of an endotracheal tube during oral fiberoptic intubation. Anesthesiology. 2001;94:729–31.
22. Hagberg CA. Benumof's airway management. Elsevier Health Sciences. 2007.
23. Mathru M, Esch O, Lang J, Herbert ME, Chaljub G, Goodacre B, et al. Magnetic resonance imaging of the upper airway. Effects of propofol anesthesia and nasal continuous positive airway pressure in humans. Anesthesiology. 1996;84:273–9.
24. Magill IW. Endotracheal anesthesia. Am J Surg. 1936;34:450–5.
25. Horton WA, Fahy L, Charters P. Defining a standard intubating position using "angle finder". Br J Anaesth. 1989;62:6–12.
26. Bannister F, Macbeth R. Direct laryngoscopy and tracheal intubation. Lancet. 1944;244:651–4.
27. Adnet F, Borron SW, Dumas JL, Lapostolle F, Cupa M, Lapandry C. Study of the "sniffing position" by magnetic resonance imaging. Anesthesiology. 2001;94:83–6.
28. Swann AD, English JD, O'Loughlin EJ. The development and preliminary evaluation of a proposed new scoring system for videolaryngoscopy. Anaesth Intensive Care. 2012;40:697–701.
29. Meier S, Geiduschek J, Paganoni R, Fuehrmeyer F, Reber A. The effect of Chin lift, jaw thrust, and continuous positive airway pressure on the size of the Glottic opening and on stridor score in anesthetized, spontaneously breathing children. Anesth Analg. 2002;94:494–9.
30. O'Loughlin EJ, Swann AD, English JD, Ramadas R. Accuracy, intra- and inter-rater reliability of three scoring systems for the glottic view at videolaryngoscopy. Anaesthesia. 2017;72:835–9.
31. Adnet F, Borron SW, Racine SX, Clemessy J-L, Fournier J-L, Plaisance P, et al. The intubation difficulty scale (IDS): proposal and evaluation of a new score characterizing the complexity of endotracheal intubation. Anesthesiology. 1997;87:1290–7.
32. Schmitt HJ, Mang H. Head and neck elevation beyond the sniffing position improves laryngeal view in cases of difficult direct laryngoscopy. J Clin Anesth. 2002;14:335–8.
33. Isono S, Tanaka A, Ishikawa T, Tagaito Y, Nishino T. Sniffing position improves pharyngeal airway patency in anesthetized patients with obstructive sleep apnea. Anesthesiology. 2005;103:489–94.

4

A prospective, randomized comparison of the LMA-protector™ and i-gel™ in paralyzed, anesthetized patients

Jee-Eun Chang[1], Hyerim Kim[1], Jung-Man Lee[1], Seong-Won Min[1,2], Dongwook Won[1], Kwanghoon Jun[3] and Jin-Young Hwang[1,2]* (iD)

Abstract

Background: In the present study, we compare the LMA-Protector™ and the i-gel™ in terms of adequacy of the airway seal, insertion time, ease and accuracy of insertion, and the incidence of postoperative sore throat.

Methods: In 110 anesthetized and paralyzed adult patients, the i-gel™ ($n = 55$) or the LMA-Protector™ ($n = 55$) was inserted. The primary outcome was airway leak pressure. The secondary outcomes included the first-attempt success rate, insertion time, ease and accuracy of the device insertion, ease of gastric tube placement, blood staining on the device after removal, and incidence and severity of postoperative sore throat.

Results: The airway leak pressure was higher with the LMA-Protector™ than with the i-gel™ (31 [7] cmH$_2$O vs. 27 [6] cmH$_2$O, respectively; $P = 0.016$). Insertion time was longer with the LMA-Protector™ than with the i-gel™ (27 [16] sec vs. 19 [16] sec, respectively, $P < 0.001$), but ease of insertion and the first-attempt success rate were not different between the two groups. The LMA-Protector™ provided a worse fiberoptic view of the vocal cords and more difficult gastric tube insertion than the i-gel™ (both $P < 0.001$). Blood staining on the device was more frequent with the LMA-Protector™ than with the i-gel™ ($P = 0.033$). The incidence and severity of postoperative sore throat were not different between the two groups.

Conclusion: The LMA-Protector™ provided a better airway sealing effect than the i-gel™. However, it required a longer insertion time, provided a worse fiberoptic view of the vocal cords, and caused more mucosal injury compared to the i-gel™.

Keywords: I-gel, LMA-protector™, Airway sealing

Background

The supraglottic airway device is widely used for airway management in the anesthetic field, critical care, and emergency situations. It is also especially effective in difficult airway management. Since the introduction of the classic laryngeal mask airway (LMA), several innovative supraglottic airway devices have been developed which address such aspects as shape, quality, and function.

The i-gel™ (Intersurgical Ltd., Wokingham, UK) is made of a medical-grade thermoplastic elastomer and designed to anatomically fit the perilaryngeal structures with a non-inflatable gel-like cuff that provides easier insertion and avoids compression trauma [1]. Its advantages, including easier insertion, minimal compression trauma, and sufficient airway sealing pressure have been well identified in the clinical practice [2–5]. The LMA-Protector™ (Teleflex Medical, Co. Westmeath, Ireland) is a recently developed supraglottic airway device made of medical-grade silicone which makes it more flexible and less traumatic than previous LMA devices made of polyvinylchloride. It has a fixed, curved structure for easier insertion with an inflatable

* Correspondence: mistyblue15@naver.com
[1]Department of Anesthesiology and Pain Medicine, SMG-SNU Boramae Medical Center, Boramae-ro, Dongjak-gu, Seoul 156-707, Republic of Korea
[2]College of Medicine, Seoul National University, Seoul, Republic of Korea

airway cuff. It distinctively has two drain channels which emerge proximally as separate ports and enter a chamber behind the cuff bowl. This chamber narrows distally into the orifice located at the end of the cuff which communicates distally with the upper esophageal sphincter. Additionally, the LMA-Protector™ is available with a pilot balloon or the integrated Cuff Pilot™ that provides easier adjustment of the intracuff pressure (Fig. 1) [6].

A preliminary assessment of the LMA-Protector™ showed that it is easy to insert and provides a reliable and adequate seal [7], and a recent primary evaluation of the LMA-Protector™ reported that the LMA-Protector™ provides a high pharyngeal seal [8]. However, its performance, particularly airway sealing effect, has not been compared with other well-identified supraglottic airway devices such as the i-gel™. The i-gel™ has been widely used in the clinical practice and has been reported to show a comparable performances including airway sealing effect compared to previous LMA devices [5, 9, 10]. We hypothesized that the LMA-Protector™ would provide an improved airway seal than the i-gel™, and compared the clinical performance of the LMA-Protector™ and the i-gel™ in terms of the adequacy of airway seal, insertion time, ease and accuracy of insertion, and the incidence of postoperative sore throat in paralyzed and anesthetized patients.

Methods

This study was approved by the Institutional Review Board of our hospital (20,170,228/26–2017-33/032), and registered at ClinicalTrials.gov (NCT03078517). After obtaining written informed consents, patients scheduled for elective surgery under general anesthesia were recruited to the study. The exclusion criteria were the presence of an upper airway anatomic variation or pathology, aspiration tendency (full stomach, history of stomach surgery, gastroesophageal reflux, hiatal hernia), a body mass index greater than $30 \, kg/m^2$, a known or predicted difficult airway,

surgery requiring lateral or prone position, head and neck surgery, or requirements for postoperative ventilator care.

Patients were randomly allocated to the i-gel™ or LMA-Protector™ group, using a computer-generated program (Random Allocation Software, ver. 1.0; Isfahan University of Medical Sciences, Isfahan, Iran). General anesthesia was induced with intravenous propofol 1.5–2 mg/kg, fentanyl 1–2 µg/kg and rocuronium 0.6 mg/kg. After 100 s of mask ventilation with sevoflurane in 100% oxygen, the i-gel™ or LMA-Protector™ was inserted by two board-certified staff anesthesiologists according to the manufacturer's instruction. They inserted them alternately in each group to achieve a similar distribution for using them. The lubricated i-gel™ was inserted into the mouth and introduced along the hard palate with a continuous and gentle push in the sniffing position until resistance was felt in the hypopharynx. The LMA-Protector™ was lubricated on the posterior surface of the mask with the cuff delated. In the sniffing position, it was introduced pressing against the hard and soft palate with a circular motion until resistance was felt in the hypopharynx. The anesthesiologists had performed more than 30 insertions with the LMA-Protector™ and more than 100 insertions with the i-gel™. The size selection was made according to the manufacturer's recommendation: for the i-gel™, a size three for patients less than 50 kg, a size four for those between 50 and 90 kg, and a size five for those over 90 kg; for the LMA Protector™, a size three for patients less than 50 kg, a size four for those between 50 and 70 kg, and a size five for those over 70 kg [1, 6].

During insertion of the device, the following manipulations were allowed: jaw thrust, adjusting insertion depth, or head extension and flexion beyond the sniffing position. If required, any maneuvers among the three were chosen at the discretion of anesthesiologists. Three attempts were allowed, and each attempt proceeded for 60 s. If the insertion was not performed within 60 s, the next attempt was

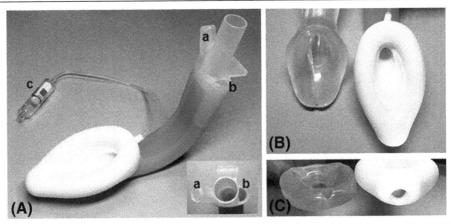

Fig. 1 (**a**) LMA-Protector™. **a**, male suction port; **b**, female drainage port; **c**, integrated Cuff Pilot™ (**b**) Cuff of the i-gel™ and LMA-Protector™ (**c**) Distal orifice of gastric channel of the i-gel™ and LMA-Protector™. Size 4 LMA-Protector™ and i-gel™ were used for this photograph

made after manual ventilation. When the placement failed after three attempts, the insertion was recorded as a failure, and tracheal intubation was performed using a direct laryngoscope. The correct insertion was assessed by proper chest expansion, the presence of a square waveform on the capnogram, absence of an audible leak, and lack of gastric insufflations, as determined by epigastric auscultation. Insertion time was defined as the time from picking up the i-gel™ or LMA-Protector™ to observing the end-tidal CO_2 waveform, and was calculated by adding the time taken for each attempt. Ease of insertion was evaluated according to the required maneuvers (jaw thrust, adjusting insertion depth, or head extension and flexion) during insertion as follows: easy for no maneuver, fair for one type of maneuver, difficult for more than one type of maneuver. The intracuff pressure of the LMA-Protector™ was set at 60 cmH$_2$O, and monitored and adjusted every 30 min. The anatomic position of the devices was evaluated using a fiberoptic bronchoscope and graded on a scale of one to four as follows: four, only the vocal cords seen; three, vocal cords and posterior part of the epiglottis seen; two, vocal cords and anterior part of the epiglottis seen; one, vocal cords not seen, but adequate ventilation [11]. Airway leak pressure was determined by closing the expiratory valve of the circle system at a fresh gas flow of three L min^{-1} and observing the airway pressure at equilibrium by auscultating the leak sound over the thyroid cartilage using a stethoscope. Airway pressure was allowed up to 40 cm H$_2$O. A lubricated gastric tube was inserted through the gastric channel (size 12 Fr for i-gel™, and size 14 Fr for the LMA-Protector™). The correct placement of the gastric tube was confirmed through the injected air by auscultation of the epigastrium and aspiration of gastric content. Ease of gastric tube placement was graded as follows: one, first attempt; two, second attempt; three, impossible. Investigators who inserted the supraglottic airway device, assessed the airway leak pressure and the anatomic position of the device, and inserted the gastric tube and the observers who recorded data were not blinded to the group assignment. At the end of surgery, residual neuromuscular block was reversed by pyridostigmine and glycopyrrolate. After confirming full recovery of the spontaneous ventilation by the presence of regular and adequate trace of end-tidal CO_2 waveform and proper chest rise without assistance, the supraglottic airway devices were removed, and the presence of blood on the device was recorded by anesthesiologists unblinded to the group assignment. The sore throat was evaluated at 1 and 24 h after surgery. A 0- to 100-mm numerical rating scale was used to evaluate the severity of sore throat (0, no pain; 100, worst pain imaginable) by investigators unaware of the group allocation. Postoperative analgesic medications was recorded for the first 24 h after surgery.

The primary outcome was the airway leak pressure. The secondary outcomes included the success rate at the first attempt, insertion time, ease and accuracy of supraglottic airway device insertion, ease of gastric tube placement, the presence of blood on the device, and incidence and severity of postoperative sore throat at 1 and 24 h after surgery.

A preliminary study was performed in 30 patients (15 per each group), and the airway leak pressure was 27.0 (6.4) cmH$_2$O with the i-gel™ and 30.8 (6.6) cmH$_2$O the LMA-Protector™. Based on the results of a preliminary study, a sample size calculation was performed assuming as a clinically significant difference in the airway leak pressure of 3.8 cmH$_2$O between the two devices, and 50 patients per group were required at a significance level of 95% and with a power of 80%. Considering the possible dropouts, 55 patients per group were enrolled.

SPSS version 20 for Windows (IBM, Armonk, NY, USA) was used for the statistical analyses. Normality of the data was tested using the Shapiro-Wilk test. Data are expressed as mean (SD) or patient numbers (%). Student's t-test or Mann-Whitney U test was used to compare the airway leak pressure, insertion time, and the severity of postoperative sore throat. The number of insertion attempts, ease of airway device, anatomic position of the device, ease of gastric tube placement, presence of blood on the device, and the occurrence of postoperative sore throat were compared using the chi-square test or Fisher's exact test. A P-value < 0.05 was considered statistically significant.

Results

A total of 138 patients were recruited from May 2017 to January 2018. Twenty patients did not fulfil the inclusion criteria, and eight patients declined to participate. One hundred and ten patients were enrolled in the study, and included in the analysis (Fig. 2). Patient characteristics, type of surgery, postoperative analgesic medications, and duration of surgery and anesthesia are presented in Table 1.

Data related to the device insertion are presented in Table 2. The airway leak pressure was significantly higher with the LMA-Protector™ than with the i-gel™ (31 [7] cmH$_2$O vs. 27 [6] cmH$_2$O, respectively; $P = 0.016$) Insertion time was significantly longer with the LMA-Protector™ than with the i-gel™ (27 [16] sec vs. 19 [16] sec, respectively, $P < 0.001$), but ease of insertion and the success rate on the first attempt were not different between the two groups. During the fiberoptic examination of the position of the devices, the vocal cords were totally and exclusively visualized more frequently through the i-gel™ than through the LMA-Protector™ (80% vs. 16%, respectively; $P < 0.001$). Gastric tube placement was more difficult through the LMA-Protector™ than through the i-gel™ ($P < 0.001$), and it failed in one patient through the i-gel™ and nine patients through the LMA-Protector™. Blood staining after removal of the devices was more often observed in the LMA-Protector™

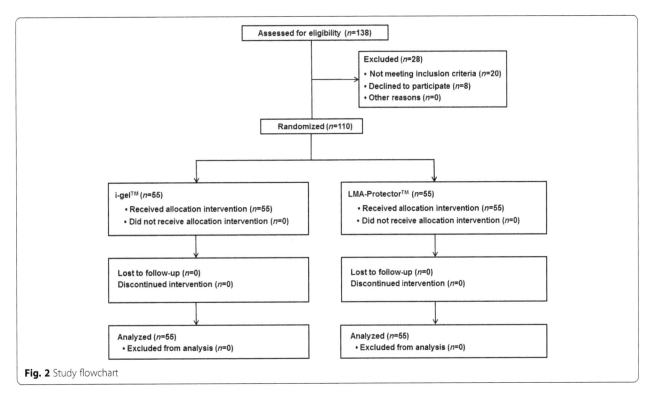

Fig. 2 Study flowchart

group than in the i-gel™ group (24% vs. 7%, respectively; $P = 0.033$).

The incidence and severity of postoperative sore throat at 1 and 24 h were not different between the two groups (Table 3).

Table 1 Patient characteristics and surgery-related data

	i-gel™ (n = 55)	LMA-Protector™ (n = 55)
Age (years)	59 (14)	57 (18)
Gender (M/F)	28/27	27/28
Weight (kg)	65 (9)	64 (11)
Height (cm)	163 (7)	163 (8)
Postoperative analgesia		
PCA with fentanyl	32	33
Ketorolac tromethamine	7	6
Acetaminophen	4	4
Tramadol	5	5
Demorol	3	4
None	4	3
Type of surgery		
Orthopedic surgery	25	28
Urologic surgery	20	20
General surgery	10	7
Duration of surgery (min)	59 (31)	58 (38)
Duration of anesthesia (min)	90 (32)	91 (41)

Values are means (SD) or number of patients. PCA, patient-controlled analgesia

Discussion

This study showed that the LMA-Protector™ provides a better airway sealing effect than the i-gel™, however, the LMA-Protector™ required a longer insertion time, provided a worse fiberoptic view of the vocal cords, and caused more mucosal injury.

In the present study, the mean airway leak pressure was higher with the LMA-Protector™ (31 cmH₂O) than with the i-gel™ (27 cmH₂O), consistent with the results of the previous studies showing values of 23–29 cmH₂O for the i-gel™ [5, 9, 10, 12]. The oropharyngeal airway seal, quantified by the airway leak pressure, is essential for the prevention of aspiration and ventilator efficiency. Higher airway leak pressure results from the closer contact between the cuff and the adjacent soft tissues. The LMA-Protector™ cuff, made of medical-grade silicone, may provide a more individualized fit in the pharynx and hypopharynx. According to a preliminary evaluation, the median pharyngeal seal pressure of the LMA-Protector™ was 34 cmH₂O [8]. In another preliminary assessment in non-paralyzed female patients with the LMA-Protector™ size three [7], median oropharyngeal leak pressure was 25.2 cmH₂O. In the present study, we used the different sized devices (size three, four or five) according to the manufacturer's recommendation based on the patient's weight in paralyzed males and females. Several factors such as the use of neuromuscular blockade and the size of the device, may have affected the airway leak pressure.

In the present study, the mean airway leak pressure was slightly higher with the LMA-Protector™ than with

Table 2 Factors related to the device insertion

	i-gel™ (n = 55)	LMA-Protector™ (n = 55)	P-value
Number of insertion attempts			
one	51 (93)	50 (91)	1.000
two	4 (7)	5 (9)	
three	0 (0)	0 (0)	
Insertion time (sec)	19 (16)	27 (16)	< 0.001
Airway leak pressure (cmH$_2$O)	27 (6)	31 (7)	0.016
Ease of insertion			
Easy	45 (82)	37 (67)	0.125
Fair	10 (18)	18 (33)	
Difficult	0 (0)	0 (0)	
Fibreoptic examination			
Only vocal cords	44 (80)	9 (16)	< 0.001
Vocal cords and posterior part of the epiglottis	8 (15)	28 (51)	
Vocal cords and anterior part of the epiglottis	3 (5)	11 (20)	
Vocal cords not seen, but adequate ventilation	0 (0)	7 (13)	
Ease of gastric tube insertion			
First attempt	51 (93)	27 (49)	< 0.001
Second attempt	3 (5)	19 (35)	
Impossible	1 (2)	9 (16)	
Blood staining on the device	4 (7)	13 (24)	0.033

Values are means (SD) or number of patients (%)

the i-gel™, which might be clinically insignificant. However, this result should not be ignored because it may also suggest that the LMA-Protector™ can be a choice in some clinical situations where a higher airway leak pressure is required such as laparoscopic surgery, although it was not evaluated in this study.

The success rate of the device insertion at the first attempt (91% vs. 93%, LMA-Protector™ vs. i-gel™, respectively), and ease of insertion were not different between the two devices, but the insertion time was longer with the LMA-Protector™ than with the i-gel™. The i-gel™ has a non-inflatable cuff, whereas the LMA-Protector™ has a longer and larger inflatable cuff, therefore, it might take

Table 3 Incidence and severity of postoperative sore throat

	i-gel™ (n = 55)	LMA-Protector™ (n = 55)	P – value
Incidence			
1 h after surgery	11 (20)	16 (29)	0.376
24 h after surgery	8 (15)	9 (16)	1.000
Severity			
1 h after surgery	4 (11)	9 (17)	0.168
24 h after surgery	3 (7)	3 (8)	0.794

Values are means (SD) or number of patients (%). Severity of postoperative sore throat was assessed using a 0- to 100-mm numerical rating scale (0, no pain; 100, worst pain imaginable)

more time to introduce the larger cuff into the oropharyngeal space and inflate it. Moreover, anesthesiologists had more familiarity with the i-gel™ than the LMA-Protector™, which may influence insertion time.

The i-gel™ and LMA-Protector™ can be used as an intubation conduit, and proper alignment of the ventilation pathway with the vocal cords is crucial for successful tracheal intubation. In the present study, ventilation was adequate in all patients, but the i-gel™ had a better fiberoptic view of the glottis with less epiglottic down-folding than the LMA-Protector™. This finding was consistent with previous studies in which the i-gel™ provided an acceptable fiberoptic view of the vocal cords in more than 80% of subjects [5, 10]. The i-gel™ has an epiglottic rest preventing the epiglottis from down-folding or obstructing the distal opening the airway [1], whereas the LMA-Protector™ has no component to prevent epiglottic down-folding, such as the epiglottic elevating bar in the LMA-Fastrach™ [13, 14].

The i-gel™ has one gastric channel, similar to other pre-existing supraglottic airway devices. The newly developed LMA-Protector™ distinctively contains two gastric channels, a suction port and a drainage port, which emerge proximally as separate ports, entered a chamber located behind the cuff bowl, and communicates distally with the upper esophageal sphincter (Fig. 1). The gastric fluid can be removed by attaching suction to the suction port or by inserting a gastric tube through the drainage port to the stomach. The internal volume of the drainage pathway in the LMA-Protector™ (31 mL for size three; 41 mL for size four; 42 mL for size five) [13] is much larger than that of the i-gel™. Thus, the LMA-Protector™ may be more efficient at reducing the risk of pulmonary aspiration of gastric contents. Nevertheless, in the present study, the gastric tube insertion was more difficult through the LMA-Protector™ than through the i-gel™ despite of adequate ventilation in all patients. We failed to insert the gastric tube in nine patients through the LMA-Protector™ and one patient through the i-gel™. This finding might be associated with the size of the gastric tube used with the LMA-Protector™. According to the instructions for use of each device, the recommended maximum size of the gastric tube was 12 or 14 Fr for the i-gel™ (12 Fr for sizes three and four; 14 Fr for size five) and 16 or 18 Fr for the LMA-Protector™ (16 Fr for size three; 18 Fr for sizes four and five) [1, 6]. In the present study, we used the gastric tube size 12 Fr for the i-gel™ and size 14 Fr for the LMA-Protector™. The selection of the 14 Fr gastric tube for the LMA-Protector™ was based on a preliminary study using the LMA-Protector™ size three in female patients in which the 14 Fr gastric tube was successfully inserted in 24 of 25 patients [7]. In this study, we inserted the 14 Fr gastric tube through the size three, four or five LMA-Protector™, and considered that it was difficult to introduce the relatively thin and flexible gastric tube within the large drainage pathway. Thus, the use of a larger sized gastric tube might facilitate the passage through the gastric channel of the LMA-Protector™ although it was not evaluated in this study. Moreover, the LMA-Protector™ has a large gastric pathway, which may provide a potential advantage at risk of pulmonary aspiration. Thus, a further study is required regarding the protective effect of the LMA-Protector™ against pulmonary aspiration.

In the present study, blood staining indicative of mucosal injury was more frequent with the LMA-Protector™ (24%) than with the i-gel™ (7%). In some previous studies, blood staining was observed in 0–13% of patients with the i-gel™ [9, 15–17]. The i-gel™ has a non-inflatable cuff made of a soft, gel-like medical-grade thermoplastic elastomer, potentially reducing the oropharyngeal tissue injury [18]. Although the LMA-Protector™ is made of flexible medical-grade silicone, it has a strongly tapered leading tip and a longer and larger inflatable cuff compared to the i-gel™, which may cause more mucosal injury. The incidence and severity of postoperative sore throat, however, were not different between the two devices.

This study had several limitations. First, the investigators who inserted the supraglottic airway device were not blinded to the group assignment due to the nature of the study. They followed the standardized and detailed study protocol. The investigators that evaluated postoperative sore throat, and all patients were blinded to the group allocation. Yet, there is still the potential for bias. Second, the investigators who inserted the supraglottic airway device had more experience with the i-gel™ (more than 100 insertions) than with the LMA-Protector™ (more than 30 insertions). They did have experience with more than 50 insertions of the LMA-Supreme™ which has a similar insertion method to the LMA-Protector™. However, a conscious (or unconscious) bias against the newer device, LMA-Protector™, might affect the results. Furthermore, the difference in experience with the two devices, especially less experience with the newer device, may be a possible source of bias. Third, this study was performed in anesthetized and paralyzed patients with normal airways. Thus, our results cannot be generalized to non-paralyzed patients, patients during spontaneous ventilation, and patients with difficult airways. Fourth, this study was conducted in patients with a mean body mass index of 24 kg/m², not in obese patients, and our results may not be applicable to obese patients.

Conclusions

LMA-Protector™ provided a higher airway sealing effect, but provided a worse fiberoptic view of the vocal cords, and caused more mucosal injury compared to the i-gel™. The gastric tube placement was more difficult with the LMA-Protector™ than with the i-gel™, however this may be related to the gastric tube size used in our study. A larger sized gastric tube, within the range of recommended sizes, might better facilitate the passage through the gastric channel of the LMA-Protector™. Moreover, the LMA-Protector™ has a distinctively large gastric pathway, and a further study is required regarding the protective effect of the LMA-Protector™ against pulmonary aspiration.

Abbreviations
LMA: laryngeal mask airway; PCA: patient-controlled analgesia

Acknowledgements
The authors would like to thank Sohee Oh, PhD of the Department of Biostatistics in Seoul Metropolitan Government Seoul National University Boramae Medical Center for statistical advice.

Authors' contributions
JEC designed the study, conducted the study, analyzed the data, and wrote and revised the manuscript. HK designed the study, conducted the study, analyzed the data, and helped revise the manuscript. JML designed the study, conducted the study, analyzed the data, and wrote the manuscript. SWM designed the study, conducted the study, analyzed the data, and wrote and revised the manuscript. DW designed the study, conducted the study, analyzed the data, and wrote the manuscript. KJ conducted the study, analyzed the data, and helped write the manuscript. JYH designed the study, conducted the study, analyzed the data, and wrote and revised the manuscript. All authors read and approved the final manuscript.

Author details
[1]Department of Anesthesiology and Pain Medicine, SMG-SNU Boramae
Medical Center, Boramae-ro, Dongjak-gu, Seoul 156-707, Republic of Korea.
[2]College of Medicine, Seoul National University, Seoul, Republic of Korea.
[3]Department of Anesthesiology and Pain Medicine, Seoul National University
Hospital, Seoul, Republic of Korea.

References
1. i-gel User Guide. Wokingham. UK: Intersurgical ltd; 2009.
2. Bamgbade OA, Macnab WR, Khalaf WM. Evaluation of the i-gel airway in
    300 patients. Eur J Anaesthesiol. 2008;25:865–6.
3. Gatward JJ, Cook TM, Seller C, Handel J, Simpson T, Vanek V, et al.
    Evaluation of the size 4 i-gel airway in one hundred non-paralysed patients.
    Anaesthesia. 2008;63:1124–30.
4. Richez B, Saltel L, Banchereau F, Torrielli R, Cros AM. A new single use
    supraglottic airway device with a noninflatable cuff and an esophageal
    vent: an observational study of the i-gel. Anesth Analg. 2008;106:1137–9.
5. Francksen H, Renner J, Hanss R, Scholz J, Doerges V, Bein B. A comparison
    of the i-gel with the LMA-unique in non-paralysed anaesthetised adult
    patients. Anaesthesia. 2009;64:1118–24.
6. LMA-Protector Instructions for use, Athlone, Ireland, Teleflex Medical, 2015.
7. Sng BL, Ithnin FB, Mathur D, Lew E, Han NR, Sia AT. A preliminary
    assessment of the LMA protector in non-paralysed patients. BMC
    Anesthesiol. 2017;17:26.
8. Eckardt F, Engel J, Mann ST, Muller M, Zajonz T, Koerner CM, et al. LMA
    protector airway: first experience with a new second generation laryngeal
    mask. Minerva Anestesiol. 2019;85:45–52.
9. Eschertzhuber S, Brimacombe J, Kaufmann M, Keller C, Tiefenthaler W.
    Directly measured mucosal pressures produced by the i-gel and laryngeal
    mask airway supreme in paralysed anaesthetised patients. Anaesthesia.
    2012;67:407–10.
10. Joly N, Poulin LP, Tanoubi I, Drolet P, Donati F, St-Pierre P. Randomized
    prospective trial comparing two supraglottic airway devices: i-gel and LMA-
    supreme in paralyzed patients. Can J Anaesth. 2014;61:794–800.
11. Brimacombe J, Berry A. A proposed fiber-optic scoring system to standardize
    the assessment of laryngeal mask airway position. Anesth Analg. 1993;76:457.
12. Uppal V, Gangaiah S, Fletcher G, Kinsella J. Randomized crossover
    comparison between the i-gel and the LMA-unique in anaesthetized,
    paralysed adults. Br J Anaesth. 2009;103:882–5.
13. Van Zundert AA, Skinner MW, Van Zundert TC, Luney SR, Pandit JJ. Value of
    knowing physical characteristics of the airway device before using it. Br J
    Anaesth. 2016;117:12–6.
14. Gerstein NS, Braude DA, Hung O, Sanders JC, Murphy MF. The Fastrach
    intubating laryngeal mask airway: an overview and update. Can J Anaesth.
    2010;57:588–601.
15. Shin WJ, Cheong YS, Yang HS, Nishiyama T. The supraglottic airway I-gel in
    comparison with ProSeal laryngeal mask airway and classic laryngeal mask
    airway in anaesthetized patients. Eur J Anaesthesiol. 2010;27:598–601.
16. Teoh WH, Lee KM, Suhitharan T, Yahaya Z, Teo MM, Sia AT. Comparison of
    the LMA supreme vs the i-gel in paralysed patients undergoing
    gynaecological laparoscopic surgery with controlled ventilation.
    Anaesthesia. 2010;65:1173–9.
17. Kim HC, Yoo DH, Kim HJ, Jeon YT, Hwang JW, Park HP. A prospective
    randomised comparison of two insertion methods for i-gel placement in
    anaesthetised paralysed patients: standard vs. rotational technique.
    Anaesthesia. 2014;69:729–34.
18. Levitan RM, Kinkle WC. Initial anatomic investigations of the I-gel airway: a
    novel supraglottic airway without inflatable cuff. Anaesthesia. 2005;60:1022–6.

5

Intubation of non-difficult airways using video laryngoscope versus direct laryngoscope

De-Xing Liu, Ying Ye, Yu-Hang Zhu, Jing Li, Hong-Ying He, Liang Dong and Zhao-Qiong Zhu[*]

Abstract

Background: The video laryngoscope is recommended for intubating difficult airways. The present study aimed to determine whether the video laryngoscope can further improve intubation success rates compared with the direct laryngoscope in patients with non-difficult airways.

Methods: In total, 360 patients scheduled for elective abdominal surgeries were randomly assigned to undergo intubation using either a video laryngoscope ($n = 179$) or a direct laryngoscope ($n = 181$). The following parameters were measured: mouth opening; thyromental distance; sternomental distance; shape angle of the tracheal catheter; and glottic exposure grade.

Results: The percentage of patients with level I-II of total glottic exposure in the video laryngoscope group was 100% versus 63.5% in the direct laryngoscope group ($P < 0.001$). The one-attempt success rate of intubation was 96.1% using a video laryngoscope versus 90.1% using a direct laryngoscope ($P = 0.024$). The intubation success rate using a video laryngoscope was 100% versus 94.5% using a direct laryngoscope ($P = 0.004$). Immediate oropharyngeal injury occurred in 5.1% of patients intubated using a direct laryngoscope versus 1.1% using a video laryngoscope ($P = 0.033$). On postoperative day 1, obvious hoarseness was exhibited by 7.9% of patients intubated using a direct laryngoscope versus 2.8% using a video laryngoscope ($P = 0.035$). The grade of glottic exposure and catheter shape angle were independent risk factors for tracheal intubation failure. Thyromental distance, shape angle, glottic exposure time, and surgical position were independent risk factors for postoperative complications. Thyromental distance and glottic exposure time were independent risk factors for complications lasting > 2 days.

Conclusions: Intubation using a video laryngoscope yielded significantly higher intubation success rates and significantly fewer postoperative complications than direct laryngoscopy in patients with non-difficult airways.

Keywords: Intubation, Anesthesia, Glottic exposure, Abdominal surgery

* Correspondence: ganzhuzhaoqiong@hotmail.com
Department of Anesthesiology, Affiliated Hospital of Zunyi Medical College, No. 149 Dalian Road, Zunyi 563000, China

Background

The success rate of tracheal intubation in cases of difficult airways has increased significantly with the use of video laryngoscopes and improvements in the degree of glottic exposure [1–3]. The 2013 Guidelines from the American Association of Anesthesiologists for Difficult Airway Treatment recommended the video laryngoscope as the first choice after the failure of direct laryngoscope intubation [4]. Due to the unique lens design of most video laryngoscopes, in which the distal end is tilted upward and the angle with the horizontal plane is significantly larger than that of the direct laryngoscope, neck extension is not necessary after mastering the intubation skills. Moreover, during intubation, throat structure is always within the operator's field of view, and cricoid pressure and external laryngopharyngeal operations are also diminished to reduce the incidence of throat injury [5, 6].

The video laryngoscope can reduce the complications of tracheal intubation associated with difficult airways; therefore, an analysis of its potential for completely replacing direct laryngoscopy is warranted. The present study aimed to compare the video laryngoscope with the direct laryngoscope for tracheal intubation in patients with non-difficult airways scheduled for elective abdominal surgeries.

Methods

Patients

The present study was approved by the Ethics Committee of the Affiliated Hospital of Zunyi Medical College (No. 2015062901). All patients were recruited from the Affiliated Hospital of Zunyi Medical College (Guizhou province, China) between April and December 2017. Before study enrollment, all participants provided informed written consent for participation. The trial was retrospectively registered at the China Clinical Trial Registration Center (www.chictr.org.cn, ChiCTR-IOR-16009023; Principal investigator, Liu Dexing; date of registration, August 14, 2016) before patient enrollment, and is not ongoing. Our study adheres to the CONSORT guidelines.

The inclusion criteria were: [1] age ≥ 18 years; [2] scheduled for elective abdominal surgery and; [3] required tracheal intubation under general anesthesia. Patients with a history of a neck injury, those with a difficult airway, those who had participated in other clinical trials within the previous 3 months or who had other contraindications to intubation, were excluded. Patients with any of the following conditions were predicted to have a difficult airway: [1] thyromental distance < 6 cm; [2] mouth opening < 3 cm; [3] cervical ankylosis; [4] a class IV Mallampati score. The patient inclusion process is illustrated in Fig. 1.

Anesthesia protocol

After the patient entered the operating room, the thyromental distance and sternomental distance were recorded. Intravenous access was established and monitors were connected. Patients were monitored for electrocardiogram, non-invasive blood pressure, oxygen saturation, heart rate, and end-tidal carbon dioxide ($PEtCO_2$). A reinforced endotracheal tube with an inner diameter of 7.0 mm was used for females, while a reinforced endotracheal tube with an inner diameter of 7.5 mm was used for males. Midazolam 2 mg, sufentanil 0.4 μg/kg, etomidate 0.3 mg/kg, and rocuronium 0.8 mg/kg were administrated intravenously. Tracheal intubation was performed 90 s after rocuronium injection. Mechanical ventilation was initiated after completion of intubation.

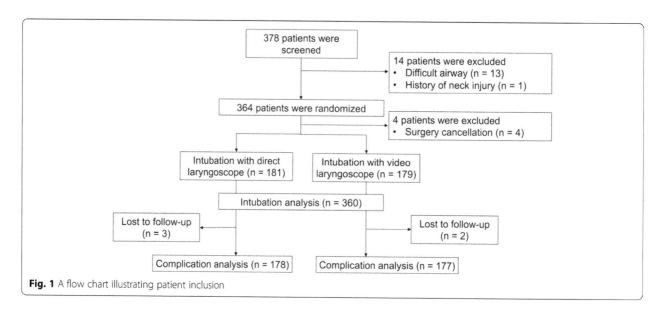

Fig. 1 A flow chart illustrating patient inclusion

The parameter settings included a tidal volume of 10 ml/kg and a respiratory rate of 12 breaths/min; respiratory parameters were adjusted according to PEtCO$_2$ during the operation. Propofol and remifentanil were injected by the intravenous compound pump, with the use of sevoflurane to maintain anesthesia.

For intubation using a direct laryngoscope, the mirror handle was held in the left hand while the right hand was used to open the mouth. With the neck in the extended position, the laryngoscope lens was placed at the root of the epiglottis to expose the glottis. The exposure classification (Wilson-CL classification) was recorded. The tracheal tube, of which the shape angle was recorded, was then placed. If the number of consecutive intubation failures exceeded 2, a change to an alternative intubation method was performed or was attempted by another qualified intubation personnel. Glottic exposure grade, glottic exposure time, and total time of tracheal intubation were recorded.

For intubation using a video laryngoscope (Fig. 2; TOSIGHT, Shanghai Jingshen Electronic Technology, China), the patient's neck was not extended, and the remaining maneuvers were the same as those used for the direct laryngoscope.

In the direct laryngoscope group, a video laryngoscope was used upon two consecutive intubation failures with the direct laryngoscope. If the video laryngoscope also failed, intubation with an additional fiber bronchoscope is considered. In the video laryngoscope group, an additional fiber bronchoscope is used upon two consecutive intubation failures.

Before induction, the endotracheal tube was modified to be linearly shaped 1 cm after the cuff. The shape was adjusted by the operators according to their experience and the researchers did not interfere during such adjustments. The angle was traced on sterile non-woven fabric and measured.

Patient evaluation

The basic information included: age; sex; weight; height, risk factors for difficult mask ventilation; American Society of Anesthesiologists (ASA) score, modified Mallampati grade; type of surgery; surgical position; and duration of surgical anesthesia. The primary outcomes included intubation success rate, intubation complications, intubation time, immediate intubation injury, and postoperative 7-days complications after, of which the definitions are presented in Table 1. The secondary outcomes included: anatomical parameters (mouth opening, thyromental distance, and sternomental distance); shape angle of the tracheal catheter; and glottic exposure according to the Wilson-C-L grading.

Statistical analyses

The sample size calculation was based on the results of a pre-experiment. This pre-experiment performed to include the maximum sample size comprised the following tests: a superiority test of the success rate of intubation in one of the two groups, the non-inferiority test of glottic exposure time in both groups, and the non-inferiority test of the total intubation time in the two groups. Finally, a superiority test for the success rate of intubation in one of the two groups was performed as the

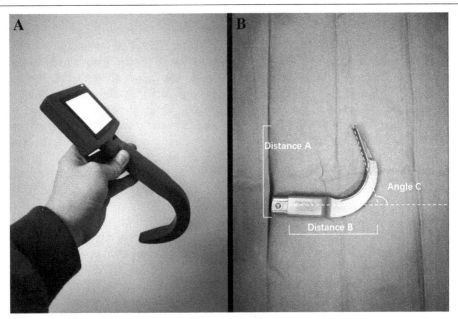

Fig. 2 A picture of the video laryngoscope. **a** The video laryngoscope. **b** The parameters. Distance A, 11.5 cm. Distance B, 11.5 cm. Angle C, 120°

Table 1 Main observational indicators and their definitions

Main observational indicator	Definition
Immediate intubation injury	Immediate mouth, pharynx and larynx injury, or incisor injury after intubation
Postoperative intubation complications	Postoperative intubation complications in patients including neck pain, pharyngeal pain, dysphagia, hoarseness, dysphonia, and dislocation of the cricoarytenoid joint.
Grade of voice hoarseness	
Mild	Conscious hoarseness
Moderate	Obvious hoarseness can be heard
Severe	Dysphonia
Glottic exposure time	Time between the cessation of oxygen supply until the glottis is exposed, and determines when it is possible to intubate
Total duration of tracheal intubation	Time between the cessation of oxygen supply until the waveform is confirmed with end tidal carbon dioxide monitoring

calculation basis for sample size. It was assumed that the test delta (Δ) was 0.05, the loss to follow-up rate and drop-out rate was 20%, and the statistical power was 95%, with a significance level of $\alpha = 0.05$. A total of 364 subjects were required; 182 subjects in each group participated in randomization. According to the work experience of the intubating anesthetist, the patients in each group were again randomly allocated into groups with a senior anesthetist or a junior anesthetist, with 91 cases in each group. More specifically, they were randomly divided into the following groups: video laryngoscope by a senior anesthetist; video laryngoscope by a junior anesthetist; direct laryngoscope by a senior anesthetist; and direct laryngoscope by a junior anesthetist.

Randomized comparisons were performed in this study. Before the patients were formally included in the trial, random numbers were generated by an individual other than the operator, and an opaque random envelope was prepared. After the patients were formally included and the statistics of their baseline data collated, the researchers, who did not participate in the operation, randomly grouped the patients according to the random number within the envelope. After the completion of surgery, the researchers submitted the case questionnaire with only the random numbers but hid the random groups from the follow-up staff who performed the follow-up investigation.

Continuous data are presented as mean and standard deviation and were compared using the Student's t-test. Categorical data are presented as frequencies or percentages and were compared using the Chi-squared test. Logistic regression analysis was used to analyze risk factors for tracheal intubation failure and postoperative

complications. All statistical analyses were performed using the SPSS version 21.0 (IBM Corporation, Armonk, NY, USA); $p < 0.05$ was statistically significant.

Results

Among the 364 patients, 4 were excluded due to surgery cancellations. Therefore, a total of 360 patients were included in the study: 181 in the direct laryngoscope group and 179 in the video laryngoscope group. Of these patients, 290 were female and 70 were male. There were no statistical differences in patient sex, age, height, weight, body mass index, ASA grade, anatomical parameters such as mouth opening, and surgical information between the direct laryngoscope and video laryngoscope groups ($p > 0.05$) (Table 2).

The tracheal intubation operators included the following individuals. "Dr. A" was a senior anesthetist assigned to the video laryngoscope group and had 12 years' clinical work experience. He had cumulatively completed or guided complete tracheal intubation in > 6000 cases and had provided video laryngoscope intubation training in > 30 cases before patients were included. "Dr. B" was a junior anesthetist assigned to the video laryngoscope group and had 5 years' clinical work experience. He had cumulatively completed or guided complete tracheal intubation in > 1500 cases and had provided video laryngoscope intubation training in > 30 cases before patients were included "Dr. C" was a senior anesthetist assigned to the direct laryngoscope group and had 11 years' clinical work experience. He had cumulatively completed or guided complete tracheal intubation in > 5000 cases. Finally, "Dr. D" was a junior anesthetist assigned to the direct laryngoscope group and had 5 years' clinical work experience. He had cumulatively completed or guided complete tracheal intubation in > 1800 cases.

The percentage of patients with levels I-II of total glottic exposure in the video laryngoscope group was 100%, which was higher than that in the direct laryngoscope group (63.5%). Glottic exposure times in the video laryngoscope group were all shorter than those in the direct laryngoscope group. The total intubation time of the video laryngoscope group was also shorter than that of the direct laryngoscope group. In the direct laryngoscope group, the total intubation time of the senior anesthetists was shorter than that of the junior anesthetists (Table 3).

In total, 172 (96.1%) patients in the video laryngoscope group were successfully intubated in one attempt, which was higher than that in the direct laryngoscope group (163 cases [90.1%]). The success rate in the senior group (97.7%) was higher than that in the junior group (94.5%). In the comparison of overall intubation success rate, all 179 patients (100%) in the video laryngoscope group were successfully intubated, which was higher than the

Table 2 Patient characteristics

	Direct laryngoscope (n = 181)	Video laryngoscope (n = 179)	P
Patient characteristic			
Male/female	31 (17.1)/150 (82.9)	39 (21.8)/140 (78.2)	0.264
Age (y)	41.7 ± 10.2	40.7 ± 10.9	0.313
Height (cm)	159.7 ± 6.6	159.8 ± 7.5	0.731
Weight (kg)	61.0 ± 10.6	59.7 ± 10.7	0.309
Body mass index (kg/m^2)	23.9 ± 3.5	23.3 ± 3.3	0.158
ASA classification			
I	87 (48.1)	87 (48.6)	0.919
II	94 (51.9)	92 (51.4)	0.919
DMV risk factors	100 (55.2)/81 (44.8)	94 (52.5)/85 (47.5)	0.603
Mallampati			
1	40 (22.1)	49 (27.4)	0.246
2	128 (70.7)	117 (65.4)	0.276
3	13 (7.2)	13 (7.3)	0.977
Anatomical parameters			
Mouth opening (cm)	4.0 ± 0.6	4.0 ± 0.5	0.707
Thyromental distance (cm)	8.6 ± 1.3	8.5 ± 1.1	0.342
Sternomental distance (cm)	15.1 ± 2.0	15.0 ± 1.9	0.717
Type of surgery			
Gynecology	76 (42.0)	72 (40.2)	0.734
Hepatobiliary	100 (55.2)	100 (55.9)	0.906
Urology	2 (1.1)	1 (0.6)	1
Gastrointestinal	3 (1.7)	6 (3.4)	0.489
Surgical position			
Low head and high foot	71 (39.2)	66 (36.9)	0.645
High head and low foot	101 (55.8)	102 (57.0)	0.821
Supine position	9 (5.0)	10 (5.6)	0.794
Side position	0	1 (0.6)	0.497
Surgical site			
Upper abdomen	100 (55.2)	100 (55.9)	0.906
Midsection	2 (1.1)	1 (0.6)	1
Lower abdomen	79 (43.6)	78 (43.6)	0.989
Operation time (min)	80.5 ± 53.3	88.4 ± 73.1	0.724

171 patients (94.5%) in the direct laryngoscope group. In the analysis of intubation failure, 7 (3.9%) patients in the direct laryngoscope group were switched to the video laryngoscope; however, there was no tool replacement in the video laryngoscope group; the difference between the two groups was statistically significant (Table 4).

Overall, 5 cases were lost to follow-up after the operation, and a total of 355 cases were included in the complication analysis: 5.1% of patients (9 cases) in the direct laryngoscope group experienced immediate oropharyngeal injury after intubation, which was higher than the 1.1% of patients (2 cases) in observed in the video laryngoscope group (p = 0.033). After intubation using the video laryngoscope, the incidence of postoperative

pharyngeal pain in the junior anesthetist group was 7.7% (7 cases). This was lower than the 19.8% (17 cases) of cases assigned to the senior anesthetists in the same group and was also lower than the 22% (20 cases) of cases assigned to the junior anesthetists in the direct laryngoscope group. When comparing hoarseness on the first day after the surgery, 7.9% of patients (n = 14) in the direct laryngoscope group exhibited obvious hoarseness. This was higher than the 2.8% of patients (5 cases) seen in the video laryngoscope group. Ten cases (11.0%) with hoarseness were observed in the junior anesthetist group using the direct laryngoscope and this was higher than the 2 cases (2.2%) observed in the junior group using the video laryngoscope. There was no statistical

Table 3 Comparison of glottic exposure grading, glottic exposure time, and total intubation time in each group (%, s)

	n	Glottic exposure		Intubation	
		Glottic exposure [1, 2]	Glottic exposure (≥3)	Glottic exposure time (s)	Total intubation time (s)
Direct laryngoscope	181	115 (63.5)	66 (36.5)	15.7 (10.3,22.6)	49.9 (40.6,64.0)
Junior	91	57 (62.6)	34 (37.4)	16.4 (11.1,22.7)	55.2 (44.6,71.6)
Senior	90	58 (64.4)	32 (35.6)	14.3 (10.0,21.9)	44.8 (37.7,58.2)[d]
Video laryngoscope	179	179 (100)[a]	0[a]	9.5 (7.7,12.0)[a]	46.6 (41.6,53.5)[a]
Junior	91	91 (100)[b]	0[b]	9.1 (7.8,13.1)[b]	45.5 (40.1,53.2)[b]
Senior	88	88 (100)[c]	0[c]	9.7 (7.7,11.1)[c]	47.5 (42.5,53.9)

a: compared with group direct laryngoscopy, P < 0.05
b: compared with group direct laryngoscopy (junior), P < 0.05
c: compared with group direct laryngoscopy (senior), P < 0.05
d: compared with group direct laryngoscopy (junior), P < 0.05

difference between the two groups with regards to severe hoarseness or dislocation of the cricoarytenoid joint (Table 5).

Logistic regression was used to analyze independent risk factors for tracheal intubation failure. Analysis revealed that the grade of glottic exposure and catheter shape angle were independent risk factors for the failure of tracheal intubation; however, laryngoscopy classification was not an independent risk factor for intubation failure. Logistic regression revealed that thyromental distance, shape angle, glottic exposure time, and surgical position were the independent risk factors for postoperative complications, although laryngoscope classification was not an independent risk factor. Logistic regression demonstrated that thyromental distance and glottic exposure time were independent risk factors for tracheal intubation complications lasting > 2 days. Laryngoscopy classification was not an independent risk factor (Table 6).

Discussion

The results of the present study demonstrated no significant differences between the senior and junior anesthetists in either group. This indicated that the glottic exposure rate was the same for the same intubation devices and it was not affected by the level of experience. The amount of muscle relaxant and onset time is

directly related to glottic exposure during tracheal intubation. The induction and administration of muscle relaxants in this study and the wait time after drug administration were consistent with the pharmacokinetics and previous studies in both groups (rocuronium 0.8 mg/kg; tracheal intubation performed after 90 s of rocuronium injection) [7, 8]. However, the percentage of patients with Wilson-Cormack-Lehane classification levels I-II of glottic exposure in the video laryngoscope group was 100%, which was higher than that in the direct laryngoscope group (63.5%). Even the percentage of patients with Wilson-Cormack-Lehane classification I-II by the junior anesthetist in the video laryngoscope group (100%) was also higher than that by the senior anesthetist in the direct laryngoscope group (64.4%), indicating that the video laryngoscope could effectively improve glottic exposure in the tracheal intubation of patients undergoing elective surgery. The above results were similar to those reported in the literature addressing video laryngoscope use for difficult airways and video laryngoscope use by novice operators [9–11]. The results demonstrated that the visual equipment also had the advantage of providing good glottic exposure in patients undergoing elective surgery.

Similar to the success rate of 93.6% for one-time intubation with video laryngoscope reported in a study by Ibinson et al. [12], our results demonstrated that the in-

Table 4 Comparison of tracheal intubation in each group (n, %)

	n	1 attempt	2 attempts	Overall success rate	Intubation failure within two times	
					Change anesthetist	Change equipment
Direct laryngoscope	181	163 (90.1)	8 (4.4)	171 (94.5)	3 (1.7)	7 (3.9)
Junior	91	82 (90.1)	4 (4.4)	86 (94.5)	2 (2.2)	3 (3.3)
Senior	90	81 (90.0)	4 (4.4)	85 (94.4)	1 (1.1)	4 (4.4)
Video laryngoscope	179	172 (96.1)[a]	7 (3.9)	179 (100)[a]	0	0[a]
Junior	91	86 (94.5)	5 (5.5)	91 (100)	0	0
Senior	88	86 (97.7)[c]	2 (2.3)	88 (100)	0	0

a: compared with group direct laryngoscopy, P < 0.05
c: compared with group direct laryngoscopy (senior), P < 0.05

Table 5 Comparison of complications on the first day after operation in each group (n, %)

| | n | Oropharyngeal injury | Neck pain | Pharyngeal pain | Dysphagia | Hoarseness | | | Dysphonia | Dislocation of the cricoarytenoid joint |
						Mild	Moderate	Severe		
Direct laryngoscope	178	9 (5.1)	5 (2.8)	35 (19.7)	2 (1.1)	44 (24.7)	14 (7.9)	0	2 (1.1)	0
Junior	91	5 (5.5)	1 (1.1)	20 (22.0)	1 (1.1)	23 (25.3)	10 (11.0)	0	0	0
Senior	87	4 (4.4)	4 (4.6)	15 (17.2)	1 (1.1)	21 (24.1)	4 (4.6)	0	2 (2.3)	0
Video laryngoscope	177	2 (1.1)[a]	2 (1.1)	24 (13.6)	1 (0.6)	37 (20.9)	5 (2.8)[a]	1 (0.6)	0	0
Junior	91	2 (2.2)	0	7 (7.7)[be]	0	21 (23.1)	2 (2.2)[b]	1 (1.1)	0	0
Senior	86	0	2 (2.3)	17 (19.8)	1 (1.2)	16 (18.6)	3 (3.5)	0	0	0

a: compared with group direct laryngoscopy, $P < 0.05$
b: compared with group direct laryngoscopy (junior), $P < 0.05$
e: compared with group glidescope (junior), $P < 0.05$

tubation success rate for one-time intubation in the video laryngoscope group (96.1%) was higher than that in the direct laryngoscope group with the senior anesthetist (90.1%). The total intubation success rate in the two trials of the video laryngoscope group was 100%, which was higher than that of the direct laryngoscope group (94.5%). When using the direct laryngoscope, after intubation was blocked, the intubation operator had to switch to a video laryngoscope to complete tracheal intubation in 7 cases. However, re-intubation could have been avoided if the video laryngoscope was used in the first attempt. Earlier studies reported that, despite the significant advantage of glottic exposure using the video laryngoscope, the limitation was that, even if the operator clearly observed the glottis, difficulties may occur when placing the endotracheal tubes [5]; however,

appropriate limits on glottic exposure grading when using a direct laryngoscope may be better for tracheal intubation [13]. The reason was that the opening of the oral cavity was reduced during intubation using the video laryngoscope and the operable space of the oropharynx was also narrowed while the angle adjustment of the catheter in the oropharyngeal cavity became more difficult. Some investigators have used special equipment, such as a fibrobronchoscope or Infrared Red Intubation System (IRRIS) equipment, to assist in video laryngoscope intubation, which achieved more ideal outcomes [14, 15]. However, the use of such equipment would result in an increase in complexity and cost of conventional intubation, which is not conducive to regular large-scale application. Systemic evaluations performed by Lewis et al. recognized the value of visual

Table 6 Risk factors for ≥2 intubation failures, and postoperative intubation complications and complications lasting > 2 days

| | Intubation failure within two times | | | Postoperative intubation complications | | | Complications lasting longer than two days | | |
| | Univariate | Multivariate | OR (95% CI) | Univariate | Multivariate | OR (95% CI) | Univariate | Multivariate | OR (95% CI) |
	P	P		P	P		P	P	
Types of laryngoscope	0.004	0.995	/				0.018	0.651	/
Glottic exposure grading	< 0.001	0.042	4.38 (1.06 to 18.1)				0.017	0.904	/
Angle of tracheal catheter	0.029	0.011	6.28 (1.53 to 25.84)	< 0.001	0.004	2.72 (1.38 to 5.38)			
Glottic exposure time				0.013	0.007	2.00 (1.21 to 3.31)	< 0.001	0.043	3.69 (1.04 to 13.11)
Thyromental distance				< 0.001	0.001	2.36 (1.40 to 3.99)	0.009	0.017	2.983 (1.22 to 7.32)
Surgical position				0.002	0.015	1.92 (1.14 to 3.24)			
Anesthesia time				0.006	0.587	/			
The time with catheter				0.001	0.209	/			
Total intubation time							0.002	0.451	/

intubation devices in improving the success rate of intubation of difficult airways. However, they did not thoroughly analyze the differences in intubation success rates and the differences in postoperative complications of the different intubation devices for tracheal intubation in patients with non-difficult airways [16]. To explore reasons for this, a large number of studies have instead focused on the following: 1) the comparison of different types of laryngoscopes in the treatment of airway conditions in selected settings such as in an emergency, in obese patients, during cardiopulmonary resuscitation, during double-lumen intubation, among others [17–20]; 2) the salvage value of the video laryngoscope after the first intubation failure [21]; or 3) the difference in dealing with difficult airways between selected special methods and the video laryngoscope [22].

In our study, 6 cases of oropharyngeal hemorrhage, 2 cases of lip injury, and 1 case of incisor injury occurred after intubation in the direct laryngoscope group. However, only 2 cases of lip injury occurred in the video laryngoscope group. With respect to complications on postoperative day 1, obvious sound change could be heard in 14 patients in the direct laryngoscope group but could be heard in only 5 patients (2.8%) in the video laryngoscope group. From an anatomical perspective, with the head in a natural position, the respiratory tract forms four axes that form angles with one another. When the head is tilted back, the pharynx axis, the laryngeal axis, and the tracheal axis become aligned, which is advantageous for opening the glottis directly. However, the increased tissue tension of the throat caused by lifting the mandible using the direct laryngoscope leads to throat damage by the intubation device and catheter. Many previous studies have demonstrated that the video laryngoscope exerts a lower lifting force on the mandible than a direct laryngoscope in both normal and difficult airways [23–25]. Thus, when the endotracheal tube is inserted effectively, it decreases tension in throat tissue and reduces the damage caused by tracheal intubation. Because the sample size calculation criteria in this study were based on the success rate of tracheal intubation as a standard, there was no significant difference in the incidence of serious complications. However, we believe that if the program expanded the sample size, it is highly likely that differences would emerge in the incidence of serious complications.

All 360 cases were included in the regression analysis, and glottic exposure classification and catheter shape angle were independent risk factors for ≥2 failures. Receiver operating characteristic curve analysis was performed on the measured values of the shape angle, with intubation failure as the state variable. The stratified analysis was performed using the largest Youden index corresponding to the shape angle (86.5°) as the critical

point, of which the difference was statistically significant, prompting further binary logistic regression analysis. However, the type of laryngoscope itself was not a decisive factor in intubation failure. We believe that, regardless of whether a video laryngoscope, direct laryngoscope, or another type of visual intubation device is used, the success rate of intubation of non-difficult patients undergoing elective surgery can be increased as long as the level of glottic exposure can be improved. An excessively curved catheter may result in its inability to be adjusted within the mouth to face the glottis. In this case, the catheter must be removed for reshaping.

Similarly, laryngoscope types were not risk factors for postoperative complications and complications that lasted for ≥2 days. However, prolonged time of glottic exposure was an independent risk factor for postoperative complications and complications lasting > 2 days. In operations requiring tracheal intubation, the operator adjusts the position of the laryngoscope in the event of difficulty when the glottis is exposed. Similar to previous conclusions, we found that the longer the process, the greater the risk that the laryngoscope lens can damage the throat tissue. Therefore, any intubation device that can effectively shorten glottic exposure time can effectively mitigate the postoperative complications of intubation.

At the time of design, we randomly assigned the anesthetists' seniority, hoping to analyze whether anesthetists with more extensive clinical experience demonstrated better intubation ability than junior anesthetists. Unexpectedly, however, there was no significant difference in the use of special equipment such as video laryngoscope, by senior or junior anesthetists to perform intubation of non-difficult patients. The one-time intubation success rates of the junior anesthetists were higher than that of senior anesthetists (97.7% versus 94.5%). This result revealed that the method of operation of the video laryngoscope was very different from that of traditional tracheal intubation. Without receiving extensive training, however, most physicians may still use methods for the direct laryngoscope when initially operating a video laryngoscope. With the availability of such equipment, senior anesthetists and junior anesthetists were essentially at the same starting point. Ambrosio et al. studied first-year resident physicians using the video laryngoscope to approach difficult airways. They found that after learning methods involving both the video laryngoscope and direct laryngoscope, the anesthetists were significantly better at using the video laryngoscope than the direct laryngoscope [26]. Moreover, there were similar conclusions in the comparison of the two types of laryngoscopes among intern anesthetists [27]. However, the results of the present study may have been affected by the volume of intubations performed, in that the junior anesthetists had more opportunities for clinical intubations in the country where the study was performed. Although their experiences were still not as extensive as the senior anesthetists, the junior anesthetists experienced a high frequency of clinical intubations. Therefore, this result may not apply in other countries or regions with low frequencies. However, it is worth noting that there is a direct correlation between the proficiency of an intubation device and its effect in use [28]. In a national survey conducted in the United Kingdom, 91% of anesthesiology departments and 50% of intensive care units were equipped with video laryngoscopes in public hospitals; nevertheless, they were not prevalent in emergency or pediatric departments, or private hospitals [29]. The promotion of visual intubation equipment should not be limited to operating rooms.

Our study had limitations. First, a regression equation was not calculated for the risk factors for video laryngoscope intubation to improve the efficiency of video laryngoscope intubation. Because the sample involved in this study were regional cases, anatomical data may not be applicable due to differences in ethnicity. Second, only abdominal surgeries were included in the study, which did not involve surgeries that may affect the airway, such as neck surgery and neurosurgery. Therefore, the results of this investigation may still require many follow-up studies to continue the validation analysis.

Conclusions
Intubation using the video laryngoscope significantly improved the success rate of intubation and significantly lowered postoperative complications associated with intubation compared with direct laryngoscope in patients with non-difficult airways. The use of video laryngoscope is worth considering for intubation of non-difficult airways due to its ease of use and satisfactory safety profile.

Abbreviations
ASA: American Society of Anesthesiologists; IRRIS: Infrared Red Intubation System; PEtCO$_2$: End-tidal carbon dioxide

Acknowledgements
The authors would like to thank Qiu-Ying Zhang, Peng-Cheng Zhao, Yuan-Ping Zhong, and Chao Zhang of the Department of Anesthesiology, Affiliated Hospital of Zunyi Medical College for their assistance in patient's enrollment and therapy.

Authors' contributions
LDX designed the work and drafted the manuscript. YY, ZYH, and LJ conducted the study and contributed to the interpretation of data. HHY and DL performed the follow-up and the acquisition of data. ZZQ designed the study and randomization. They have agreed both to be personally accountable for the author's own contributions and to ensure that questions related to the accuracy or integrity of any part of the work. All authors have read this paper and have approved this submitted version.

References
1. Tabari M, Soltani G, Zirak N, Alipour M, Khazaeni K. Comparison of effectiveness of betamethasone gel applied to the tracheal tube and IV dexamethasone on postoperative sore throat: a randomized controlled trial. Iran J Otorhinolaryngol. 2013;25(73):215–20.
2. Cooper RM, Pacey JA, Bishop MJ, McCluskey SA. Early clinical experience with a new videolaryngoscope (GlideScope) in 728 patients. Can J Anaesth. 2005;52(2):191–8.
3. Hirabayashi Y, Hakozaki T, Fujisawa K, Yamada M, Suzuki H, Satoh M, et al. GlideScope videolaryngoscope: a clinical assessment of its performance in 200 consecutive patientsMasui. 2007;56(9):1059–64.
4. Apfelbaum JL, Silverstein JH, Chung FF, Connis RT, Fillmore RB, Hunt SE, et al. Practice guidelines for postanesthetic care: an updated report by the American Society of Anesthesiologists Task Force on Postanesthetic care. Anesthesiology. 2013;118(2):291–307.
5. Serocki G, Bein B, Scholz J, Dorges V. Management of the predicted difficult airway: a comparison of conventional blade laryngoscopy with video-assisted blade laryngoscopy and the GlideScope. Eur J Anaesthesiol. 2010; 27(1):24–30.
6. Jungbauer A, Schumann M, Brunkhorst V, Borgers A, Groeben H. Expected difficult tracheal intubation: a prospective comparison of direct laryngoscopy and video laryngoscopy in 200 patients. Br J Anaesth. 2009; 102(4):546–50.
7. Dong J, Gao L, Lu W, Xu Z, Zheng J. Pharmacological interventions for acceleration of the onset time of rocuronium: a meta-analysis. PLoS One. 2014;9(12):e114231.
8. Lee S, Ro YJ, Koh WU, Nishiyama T, Yang HS. The neuromuscular effects of rocuronium under sevoflurane-remifentanil or propofol-remifentanil anesthesia: a randomized clinical comparative study in an Asian population. BMC Anesthesiol. 2016;16(1):65.
9. Mahran EA, Hassan ME. Comparative randomised study of GlideScope((R)) video laryngoscope versus flexible fibre-optic bronchoscope for awake nasal intubation of oropharyngeal cancer patients with anticipated difficult intubation. Indian J Anaesth. 2016;60(12):936–8.
10. Abdellatif AA, Ali MA. GlideScope videolaryngoscope versus flexible fiberoptic bronchoscope for awake intubation of morbidly obese patient with predicted difficult intubation. Middle East J Anaesthesiol. 2014;22(4):385–92.
11. Wang PK, Huang CC, Lee Y, Chen TY, Lai HY. Comparison of 3 video laryngoscopes with the Macintosh in a manikin with easy and difficult simulated airways. Am J Emerg Med. 2013;31(2):330–8.
12. Ibinson JW, Ezaru CS, Cormican DS, Mangione MP. GlideScope use improves intubation success rates: an observational study using propensity score matching. BMC Anesthesiol. 2014;14:101.
13. Gu Y, Robert J, Kovacs G, Milne AD, Morris I, Hung O, et al. A deliberately restricted laryngeal view with the GlideScope(R) video laryngoscope is associated with faster and easier tracheal intubation when compared with a full glottic view: a randomized clinical trial. Can J Anaesth. 2016;63(8):928–37.
14. Liu WF, He HP, Xie WX, Weng PQ, Li SY. Effects of different nasotracheal intubations in obstructive sleep apnea hypopnea syndrome patients with uvulopalatopharyngoplasty. Zhonghua Yi Xue Za Zhi. 2012;92(43):3067–71.
15. Biro P, Fried E, Schlaepfer M, Kristensen MS. A new retrograde transillumination technique for videolaryngoscopic tracheal intubation. Anaesthesia. 2018;73(4):474–9.
16. Lewis SR, Butler AR, Parker J, Cook TM, Smith AF. Videolaryngoscopy versus direct laryngoscopy for adult patients requiring tracheal intubation. Cochrane Database Syst Rev. 2016;11:Cd011136.
17. Sakles JC, Douglas MJK, Hypes CD, Patanwala AE, Mosier JM. Management of Patients with predicted difficult Airways in an Academic Emergency Department. J Emerg Med. 2017;53(2):163–71.
18. Yumul R, Elvir-Lazo OL, White PF, Sloninsky A, Kaplan M, Kariger R, et al. Comparison of three video laryngoscopy devices to direct laryngoscopy for intubating obese patients: a randomized controlled trial. J Clin Anesth. 2016;31:71–7.
19. Kim JW, Park SO, Lee KR, Hong DY, Baek KJ, Lee YH, et al. Video laryngoscopy vs. direct laryngoscopy: which should be chosen for endotracheal intubation during cardiopulmonary resuscitation? A prospective randomized controlled study of experienced intubators. Resuscitation. 2016;105:196–202.
20. Belze O, Lepage E, Bazin Y, Kerourin P, Fusciardi J, Remerand F, et al. Glidescope versus Airtraq DL for double-lumen tracheal tube insertion in patients with a predicted or known difficult airway: a randomised study. Eur J Anaesthesiol. 2017;34(7):456–63.

21. Aziz MF, Brambrink AM, Healy DW, Willett AW, Shanks A, Tremper T, et al. Success of intubation rescue techniques after failed direct laryngoscopy in adults: a retrospective comparative analysis from the multicenter perioperative outcomes group. Anesthesiology. 2016;125(4):656–66.

22. Aziz MF, Abrons RO, Cattano D, Bayman EO, Swanson DE, Hagberg CA, et al. First-attempt intubation success of video laryngoscopy in patients with anticipated difficult direct laryngoscopy: a multicenter randomized controlled trial comparing the C-MAC D-blade versus the GlideScope in a mixed provider and diverse patient population. Anesth Analg. 2016;122(3):740–50.

23. Carassiti M, Biselli V, Cecchini S, Zanzonico R, Schena E, Silvestri S, et al. Force and pressure distribution using Macintosh and GlideScope laryngoscopes in normal airway: an in vivo study. Minerva Anestesiol. 2013;79(5):515–24.

24. Fiadjoe JE, Stricker P. Force and pressure distribution using Macintosh and GlideScope laryngoscopes. Br J Anaesth. 2012;108(4):698 author reply.

25. Carassiti M, Zanzonico R, Cecchini S, Silvestri S, Cataldo R, Agro FE. Force and pressure distribution using Macintosh and GlideScope laryngoscopes in normal and difficult airways: a manikin study. Br J Anaesth. 2012;108(1):146–51.

26. Ambrosio A, Pfannenstiel T, Bach K, Cornelissen C, Gaconnet C, Brigger MT. Difficult airway management for novice physicians: a randomized trial comparing direct and video-assisted laryngoscopy. Otolaryngol Head Neck Surg. 2014;150(5):775–8.

27. Aqil M, Khan MU, Hussain A, Khokhar RS, Mansoor S, Alzahrani T. Routine use of Glidescope and Macintosh laryngoscope by trainee anesthetists. J Coll Physicians Surg Pak. 2016;26(4):245–9.

28. Russell KA, Brook CD, Platt MP, Grillone GA, Aliphas A, Noordzij JP. The benefits and limitations of targeted training in flexible Transnasal laryngoscopy diagnosis. JAMA Otolaryngol Head Neck Surg. 2017;143(7):707–11.

29. Cook TM, Kelly FE. A national survey of videolaryngoscopy in the United Kingdom. Br J Anaesth. 2017;118(4):593–600.

6

Modified-ramped position: A new position for intubation of obese females

Ahmed Hasanin[1]*[ID], Hager Tarek[1], Maha M. A. Mostafa[1], Amany Arafa[1], Ahmed G. Safina[2], Mona H. Elsherbiny[1], Osama Hosny[1], Ahmed A. Gado[1], Tarek Almenesey[3], Ghada Adel Hamden[1], Mohamed Mahmoud[1] and Sarah Amin[1]

Abstract

Background: Endotracheal intubation requires optimum position of the head and neck. In obese females, the usual ramped position might not provide adequate intubating conditions. We hypothesized that a new position, termed modified-ramped position, during induction of anesthesia would facilitate endotracheal intubation through bringing the breasts away from the laryngoscope and would also improve the laryngeal visualization.

Methods: Sixty obese female patients scheduled for general anesthesia were randomly assigned into either ramped or modified-ramped position during induction of anesthesia. In the ramped position ($n = 30$), the patient head and shoulders were elevated to achieve alignment of the sternal notch and the external auditory meatus; while in the modified-ramped position ($n = 30$), the patient shoulders were elevated using a special pillow, and the head was extended to the most possible range. Our primary outcome was the incidence of failed laryngoscopic insertion in the oral cavity (the need for patient repositioning). Other outcomes included time till vocal cord visualization, time till successful endotracheal intubation, difficulty of the mask ventilation, and Cormack-Lehane grade for laryngeal view.

Results: Fourteen patients (47%) in ramped group required repositioning to facilitate introduction of the laryngoscope in the oral cavity in comparison to one patient (3%) in the modified-ramped position ($p < 0.001$). Modified-ramped position showed lower incidence of difficult mask ventilation, shorter time for glottic visualization, and shorter time for endotracheal tube insertion compared to the ramped position. The Cormack-Lehane grade was better in the modified-ramped position.

Conclusion: Modified-ramped position provided better intubating conditions, improved the laryngeal view, and eliminated the need for repositioning of obese female patients during insertion of the laryngoscope compared to ramped position.

Keywords: Obese, Female, Laryngoscopy, Ramped position, Modified-ramped position

* Correspondence: ahmedmohamedhasanin@gmail.com
[1]Department of anesthesia and critical care medicine, Cairo university, Giza, Egypt

Background

Adequate conditions for endotracheal intubation require appropriate positioning of head and neck. The most appropriate position for laryngeal visualization, termed "sniffing position" [1], requires flexion of the neck by 35° (achieved by head elevation), and extension of the head by 15° [2] to have the sternum at the same level of the external auditory meatus [3, 4]. Sniffing position maintains the alignment of the three axes, namely the oral, the pharyngeal, and the laryngeal axes, to reach the optimal laryngeal visualization [1]. In patients with obesity, the ramped position was suggested to achieve better intubating conditions [3, 5]. However, the data for the optimum position for intubating patients with obesity are conflicting [3, 5, 6]. Semler et al. pointed out that putting patients in the ramped position increased the numbers of intubation trials through wide-ranging of body mass indices [6]. Thus, it had been suggested that more research and modifications are warranted to reach the proper intubating position [7, 8].

In obese females, laryngoscopy is usually impeded by patients' breasts; therefore, the intubation process could be prolonged leading to serious hypoxia [9]. We hypothesized that using a special pillow (Fig. 1) to achieve a modified-ramped position, through slight neck extension than that offered in the ramped position, and more head extension, would improve the intubating conditions in obese females. We hypothesized that this slight head, and neck extension at the beginning of the laryngoscopy would bring the breasts away from the laryngoscope and would also improve the laryngeal visualization. The aim of this pilot study was to investigate the feasibility of using the modified-ramped position for laryngoscopy in obese females compared to the traditional ramped position.

Methods

This randomized controlled study was conducted in Cairo University Hospital after institutional board review

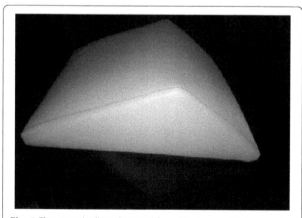

Fig. 1 The special pillow designed for achieving modified ramped position (Hasanin Pillow)

approval (N-107-2018) from September 2018 till February 2019. The study was registered before recruitment of the first participant at clinicaltrials.gov registry system on 21 August 2018 (NCT03640442). Written informed consents were obtained from all participants before enrollment. Randomization was achieved using computer-generated sequence. Concealment was achieved using opaque, closed envelopes by a research assistant who had no further involvement in the study.

The study included: obese female patients (body mass index above 35 kg/m^2), aged above 18 years, with American Society of Anesthesiologists class II or III, scheduled for any operation under general anesthesia with endotracheal intubation. Patients with facial or neck scars, edentulous patients, patients with unstable cervical spine, patients with limited neck extension and patients with airway masses were excluded. Five patients were excluded for the following reasons: edentulous (1 patient), limited neck extension (2 patients), refusal to participate (2 patients).

On arrival to the operating room, airway assessment for the patients was performed (Mallampati score, thyromental distance, mouth opening, and neck extension). Patients received the routine preoperative medications (metoclopramide 10 mg intravenous and ranitidine 50 mg intravenous). Routine monitors, including electrocardiogram, non-invasive blood pressure monitor, and pulse oximetry were applied before induction of anesthesia. End-tidal capnography was applied after endotracheal intubation. Before induction of anesthesia, patients were randomized to be initially settled into either ramped group ($n = 30$) or modified ramped group ($n = 30$).

Details of each position

Ramped position: This position was achieved by elevation of the shoulders and the head till achieving alignment of the sternal notch and the external auditory meatus (as shown in Fig. 2).

Modified ramped position: This position was achieved using a special pillow (Hasanin Pillow). The pillow's height and length were 15 cm and 60 cm (Fig. 3). The shoulders were elevated, and the head was extended to the most possible range to bring the breasts away from the laryngoscope.

Anesthesia was induced using propofol (2 mg/kg), atracurium (0.5 mg/kg), and fentanyl (2 mcg/kg). Ventilation was maintained using face mask for 3–4 min, then, the endotracheal tube (size 7–7.5 mm) was inserted by the same anesthesiologist (HT) using Macintosh blade (size 3). The laryngoscopic view was graded according to the Cormack-Lehane scale [10] without cricoid pressure.

If the laryngeal visualization was not sufficient in the modified-ramped position group, the head was manually elevated to achieve the ramped position. The position of endotracheal tube was confirmed using the capnography.

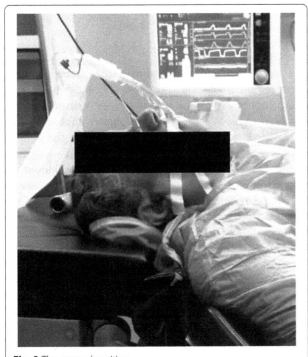

Fig. 2 The ramped position

The special pillow was removed after confirming successful intubation.

Primary outcome
Incidence of difficult laryngoscopy defined as "failure to insert the laryngoscope in the oral cavity due to large breasts with the need to reposition the patient to insert

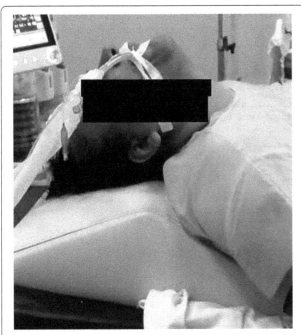

Fig. 3 The modified ramped position

the laryngoscope". The term "reposition" means: the need to make further elevation of the patient shoulders by the assistant in order to extend the patient neck and to move the breasts away from the handle of the laryngoscope.

Secondary outcomes
Time till complete visualization of the vocal cords: defined as the time from starting to handle the laryngoscope till visualization of the vocal cords.

Time of endotracheal intubation: time from starting to handle the laryngoscope till confirmation of the endotracheal tube position by capnography.

Cormack-Lehane [10] grade of vocal cord view (with and without cricoid pressure) as follows:
- Grade I: full visualization of the vocal cords.
- Grade II (a): partial visualization of the vocal cords.
- Grade II (b): only the posterior part of the vocal cords or the arytenoid cartilages are visualized.
- Grade III: only epiglottis is visualized.
- Grade IV: epiglottis is not visualized.

Incidence of relatively difficult mask ventilation: defined as the need of high force and/or oral airway insertion for maintenance of adequate mask ventilation.

Number of trials for endotracheal tube insertion.

Incidence of hypoxemia (defined as oxygen saturation less than 90%) during the period starting from induction of anesthesia till insertion of the endotracheal tube.

Oxygen saturation every 30 s starting from induction of anesthesia till confirmation of the position of endotracheal tube.

End-tidal CO_2 reading just after insertion of the endotracheal tube.

Incidence of airway trauma (teeth, lips, and tongue trauma).

Statistical analysis
Our primary outcome was the incidence of difficult laryngoscopy. According to a pilot study, we found that the incidence of difficult laryngoscopy in obese females is 80%. We used G power software (3.1.9.2) to calculate a sample size that detects an absolute risk reduction of 40% in the incidence of difficult laryngoscopy. A total number of 54 patients was calculated to have a study power of 80% and alpha error of 0.05. the number was increased to 60 patients to compensate for dropouts.

Statistical package for social science (SPSS) software, version 21 for Microsoft Windows (SPSS inc., Chicago, iL, USA) was used for data analysis. Categorical data were presented as frequencies (%) and analyzed using chi-squared test. Continuous data were checked for normality using the Shapiro-Wilk test and were presented as means (standard deviations) or medians (quartiles) as appropriate. Continuous data were analyzed using the unpaired t-test or the Mann Whitney test as appropriate. Repeated measures were analyzed using the two-way analysis of variance (ANOVA) for repeated measures with post-hoc pairwise comparisons using the Bonferroni test. A P value less than 0.05 was considered statistically significant.

Results

Sixty-five patients were screened for eligibility. Five patients were excluded for not meeting our inclusion criteria. Sixty patients were randomized in the study; all of them completed the intervention and were available for final analysis (Fig. 4). Demographic data and baseline characteristics were comparable between both groups (Table 1). The modified-ramped group showed lower incidence of difficult laryngoscopy (3% versus 47%, $p < 0001$), lower incidence of difficult mask ventilation (20% versus 83%, $p < 0.001$), shorter time for glottic visualization (13 ± 3 s versus 17 ± 2 s, $p < 0.001$), and shorter time for endotracheal tube insertion compared to the ramped position (Table 2). The Cormack-Lehane grade of laryngeal view was better in the modified-ramped position (Table 2); however, with cricoid pressure, most of the patients had adequate laryngeal visualization (Cormack-Lehane grade < III) (Table 2). None of the patients in the modified-ramped position needed head elevation to

improve the laryngeal view. None of our patients had significant hypoxemia nor airway trauma.

Discussion

We report that our modification of the ramped position improved the intubation conditions of obese females. This was demonstrated by the better laryngeal visualization, the less need of repositioning, and the shorter intubation time in the modified-ramped position compared to the ramped position.

The original ramped position, which is achieved by elevation of the patient's head whilst keeping the face in horizontal position, had been described to facilitate airway management of obese patients. In obese patients, there is increased fat deposition in the chest wall, especially in the back, which consequently increases the antero-posterior chest diameter. Therefore, application of the ordinary sniffing position, the recommended position of laryngoscopy, is usually difficult in obese patients. This high chest/head ratio in obese individuals would result in a lower head position when the patient lies flat; thus, the ramped position was proposed to overcome this problem. Collins et al. were the first authors who reported that the ramped position is superior to the sniffing position in morbidly obese patients in terms of

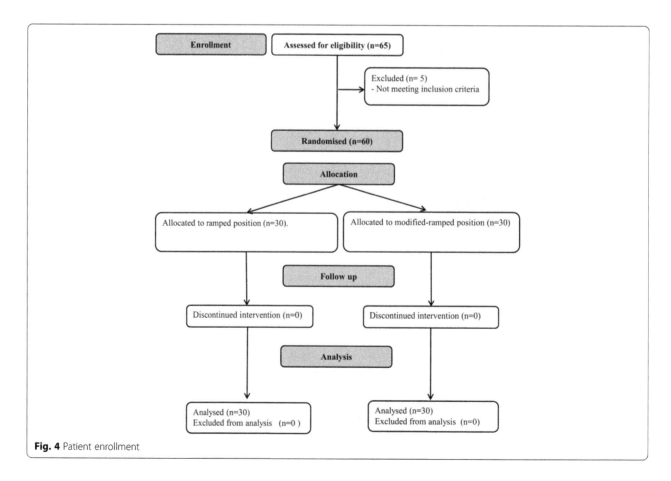

Fig. 4 Patient enrollment

Table 1 Baseline characteristics. Data are presented as mean (standard deviation), and frequency (%)

	Ramped group (n = 30)	Modified ramped group (n = 30)	P value
Age (years)	42 (13)	39 (9)	0.26
Body mass index (Kg/m^2)	41 (6)	43 (6)	0.4
Diabetes	4 (13%)	5 (17%)	1
Hypertension	6 (20%)	9 (30%)	0.55
Snoring	11 (37%)	9 (30%)	0.78
Mallampati score			
Grade I	3 (10%)	8 (27%)	0.35
Grade II	15 (50%)	10 (33%)	
Grade III	10 (33%)	10 (33%)	
Grade IV	2 (7%)	2 (7%)	

laryngeal view; however, they did not report a major difference in the difficulty of intubation [5]. Since then, the studies which compared the ramped position and the sniffing position showed relatively conflicting results. The ramped position was proved superior to the sniffing position in both obese, non-obese populations [11]; and in patients with expected difficult intubation [12]. Semler et al. had, surprisingly, reported different results which favored the sniffing position over the ramped position in 260 critically ill patients [6]. Therefore, further research had been suggested to reach the proper intubating position [7, 8].

In our patients, we introduced a novel modification on the ramped position by the aid of a special pillow. Our modification achieved more neck and head extension than that of the ramped position. This position was hypothesized to 1- Facilitate the insertion of laryngoscope into the oral cavity 2- Improve the mask ventilation. 3- Improve the grade of laryngeal view.

Insertion of the laryngoscope in the mouth cavity is usually difficult in obese females [9]. We reported that patients in modified-ramped position showed easier laryngoscopy and less need for patient reposition.

Table 2 Outcomes. Data are presented as mean (standard deviation), median (quartiles), and frequency (%)

	Ramped group (n = 30)	Modified ramped group (n = 30)	P value
Relatively difficult mask ventilation	25 (83%)*	6 (20%)	< 0.001
Difficult laryngoscopy	14 (47%)*	1 (3%)	< 0.001
Time till vocal cord visualization (seconds)	17 (2)*	12 (3)	< 0.001
Time till endotracheal tube insertion (seconds)	42 (3)*	33 (2)	< 0.001
Cormak-Lehane view without cricoid pressure	IIb (IIa-IIb) *	IIa (I-IIb)	0.01
Cormack-Lehane view with cricoid pressure	I (I-IIa) *	I (I-I)	0.03
Cormack-Lehane view without cricoid pressure			
I	5 (17%)	14 (47%)	0.04
II(a)	7 (24%)	8 (27%)	
II(b)	12 (40%)	5 (17%)	
III	6 (20%)	3 (10%)	
Cormack-Lehane view with cricoid pressure			
I	16 (53%)	24 (80%)	0.09
II(a)	11 (37%)	5 (17%)	
II(b)	3 (10%)	1 (3%)	
III			
Number of intubation trials	1 (1,1)	1 (1,1)	1
First end-tidal CO$_2$ reading (mmHg)	35.1 (4.4)	34.9 (3.9)	0.88

*denotes statistical significance (P < 0.05)

Performing neck extension in the modified-ramped position gave more space for the handle of the laryngoscope away from the sternum and the breast of the patient.

We reported that mask ventilation was easier in the modified-ramped position; this is most probably explained by the easier movement of the jaw when the neck is in extension; whilst, the accumulated fat in the neck and the lower face impaired the jaw movement when the head is in the horizontal plane in the ordinary ramped position. Moreover, when the physician pulls the patient jaw upwards with head in the tilted position, this moves the jaw in 2 directions (anterior and caudal); this would provide better airway patency than moving the jaw in 1 direction (anterior) only when the head in horizontal in the ramped position.

The impact of the patient position on the grade of laryngeal view is a principal factor during comparison of different positions. We had no data about the Cormack-Lehane grade in the modified-ramped position. Therefore, we suggested that manual mobilization of the head would be performed as a rescue maneuver in case of difficult visualization of the glottis; however, we found that, the laryngeal view was better in modified-ramped position and the planned rescue maneuver was not needed in any patient. Proper visualization of the laryngeal view is based in alignment of oral, pharyngeal, and laryngeal axes; this is classically achieved in the sniffing position. The use of the ramped position for improving the laryngeal visualization, although widely applied, is still controversial. The proper alignment of three airway axes was confirmed in the sniffing position using magnetic resonance imaging [4]; however, in the ramped position, the alignment of the three axes is only a theoretical assumption [5] without similar magnetic resonance imaging confirmation. Semler et al. had demonstrated that the ramped position might worsen the laryngoscopic view and increase the number of intubation attempts compared to the sniffing position [6].

Proper position of the head and the neck is an important step for successful laryngoscopy and endotracheal intubation. Airway management in obese patients is relatively challenging due to accumulated fat deposition in the airway that might impair adequate ventilation and visualization of the larynx; furthermore, insertion of the laryngoscope in the oral cavity might also be difficult due to accumulated fat in the anterior chest wall and breasts. Obese patients commonly have restrictive lung disorders which impair their tolerance to any delay in endotracheal intubation. We provided a novel modification for the ramped position which is easily achieved using a simple pillow which provided good space for the handle of the laryngoscope without impairment of the laryngeal visualization. The modified-ramped position would help to avoid the hazards of re-positioning of the

patient which is common in obese females; and would consequently avoid unwarranted delay in the endotracheal intubation process.

Our study had some limitations: 1- It is a single center study. 2- Our methodology did not enable blinding of the physician. 3- We investigated our approach in elective, stable patients. We need to confirm its benefits in emergency endotracheal intubation.

Conclusion

In conclusion, the modified-ramped position provided better intubating conditions, improved the laryngeal view and eliminated the need for repositioning of obese female patients during insertion of the laryngoscope.

Abbreviations
ANOVA: Analysis of variance; SPSS: Statistical package for social science

Acknowledgments
We would like to acknowledge all the residents and assistant lecturers in our department who helped in this work.

Authors' contributions
AH and TA: These authors helped in conception of the idea, study design, analysis of the data, and drafting the manuscript. HT, MMM, AGS, MHE, OH, AG, GAH, MM, SA: These authors helped in acquisition of data, and revising the manuscript. AA is the senior investigator and the group leader. This author revised the manuscript and supervised the whole research. All authors approved the manuscript and agreed to be accountable for all aspects of the work.

Author details
[1]Department of anesthesia and critical care medicine, Cairo university, Giza, Egypt. [2]Department of surgery, Cairo university, Giza, Egypt. [3]Department of anesthesia and critical care medicine, Beni suef university, Beni suef, Egypt.

References
1. Bannister FBMR. Direct laryngoscopy and tracheal intubation. Lancet. 1944;ii:651–4.
2. IW M. Endotracheal anesthesia. Am J Surg. 1936;34:450–5.
3. Rao SL, Kunselman AR, Schuler HG, DesHarnais S. Laryngoscopy and tracheal intubation in the head-elevated position in obese patients: a randomized, controlled, Equivalence Trial. Anesth Analg. 2008;107:1912–8.
4. Greenland KB, Edwards MJ, Hutton NJ. External auditory meatus-sternal notch relationship in adults in the sniffing position: a magnetic resonance imaging study. Br J Anaesth. 2010;104:268–9.
5. Collins JS, Lemmens HJM, Brodsky JB, Brock-Utne JG, Levitan RM. Laryngoscopy and morbid obesity: a comparison of the "sniff" and "ramped" positions. Obes Surg. 2004;14:1171–5.
6. Semler MW, Janz DR, Russell DW, Casey JD, Lentz RJ, Zouk AN, et al. A multicenter, randomized trial of ramped position vs sniffing position during endotracheal intubation of critically ill adults. Chest. 2017;152:712–22.
7. Rahiman SN, Keane M. Ramped position: what the "neck"! Chest [internet]. Am Coll Chest Physicians. 2018;153:339–48.
8. Vetrugno L, Orso D, Bove T. Ramped position, an uncertain future. Crit Care. 2018;22:6–7.
9. Mushambi MC, Kinsella SM, Popat M, Swales H, Ramaswamy KK, Winton AL, et al. Obstetric Anaesthetists' association and difficult airway society guidelines for the management of difficult and failed tracheal intubation in obstetrics. Anaesthesia. 2015;70:1286–306.
10. Koh LKD, Kong CF, Ip-Yam PC. The modified Cormack-Lehane score for the grading of direct laryngoscopy: evaluation in the Asian population. Anaesth Intensive Care. 2002;30:48–51.
11. Lebowitz PW, Shay H, Straker T, Rubin D, Bodner S. Shoulder and head elevation improves laryngoscopic view for tracheal intubation in nonobese as well as obese individuals. J Clin Anesth. 2012;24:104–8.
12. Lee J-H, Jung H-C, Shim J-H, Lee C. Comparison of the rate of successful endotracheal intubation between the "sniffing" and "ramped" positions in patients with an expected difficult intubation: a prospective randomized study. Korean J Anesthesiol. 2015;68:116.

7

Utility of oxygen insufflation through working channel during fiberoptic intubation in apneic patients

Go Un Roh[1], Joon Gwon Kang[1], Jung Youn Han[1] and Chul Ho Chang[2*]

Abstract

Background: Airway management is a part of routine anesthetic procedures; however, serious complications, including hypoxia and death, are known to occur in cases of difficult airways. Therefore, alternative techniques such as fiberoptic bronchoscope-assisted intubation (FOB intubation) should be considered, although this method requires more time and offers a limited visual field than does intubation with a direct laryngoscope. Oxygen insufflation through the working channel during FOB intubation could minimize the risk of desaturation and improve the visual field. Therefore, the aim of this prospective randomized controlled study was to evaluate the utility and safety of oxygen insufflation through the working channel during FOB intubation in apneic patients.

Methods: Thirty-six patients were randomly allocated to an N group (no oxygen insufflation) or an O group (oxygen insufflation). After preoxygenation, FOB intubation was performed with (O group) or without (N group) oxygen insufflation in apneic patients. The primary outcome was the velocity of decrease in the partial pressure of oxygen (PaO_2) during FOB intubation (V_{PaO2}, mmHg/sec) defined as the difference of PaO_2 before and after intubation divided by the time to intubation. The secondary outcomes included the success rate for FOB intubation, time to intubation, visual field during FOB intubation, findings of arterial blood gas analysis, and occurrence of FOB intubation-related complications.

Results: We found that V_{PaO2} was significantly greater in the N group than in the O group (1.0 ± 0.4 vs. 0.4 ± 0.4; $p < 0.001$), while the visual field was similar between groups. There were no significant intergroup differences in the secondary outcomes.

Conclusions: These findings suggest that oxygen insufflation through the working channel during FOB intubation aids in extending the apneic window during the procedure.

Keywords: Fiberoptic intubation, Apneic oxygenation, Oxygenation during intubation

* Correspondence: anezzang@yuhs.ac
[2]Department of Anesthesiology and Pain Medicine, and Anesthesia and Pain Research Institute, Yonsei University College of Medicine, Gangnam Severance Hospital, 211 Eonju-ro, Gangnam-gu, Seoul 06273, Korea

Background

Airway management is a part of essential anesthetic procedures. However, it becomes challenging in cases of difficult airways and may cause several complications, including airway trauma, hypoxia, and even death [1, 2]. Therefore, intubation techniques involving the use of fiberoptic bronchoscopes (FOBs) and videolaryngoscopes should be considered as alternative options [3, 4]. During FOB-assisted intubation (FOB intubation), superior visualization of anatomical structures is the key for successful intubation, and suction through the working channel of FOB is commonly performed for the clearance of secretions and blood and improvement of the visual field. Oxygen insufflation through this working channel during the procedure is also possible and recommended by some physicians [5–7]. Oxygen insufflation through the working channel during FOB intubation, which requires a longer time than does direct laryngoscopic intubation, can minimize the risk of desaturation in apneic patients [8]. In addition, oxygen flow at the end of FOB could help in the clearance of secretions and small structural barriers, resulting in improved visualization during the procedure [5, 9]. However, a few reports have documented rare but critical complications such as gastric rupture and pneumothorax [10–12]. Moreover, this technique is not recommended for pediatric patients or patients with significant airway edema [11]. Thus, oxygen insufflation through the working channel during FOB intubation has certain advantages and limitations. However, few studies have evaluated its utility and safety in clinical practice. Therefore, the aim of the present study was to evaluate the utility and safety of oxygen insufflation through the working channel during FOB intubation via measurement of the velocity of decrease in the partial pressure of oxygen (PaO_2) during the procedure (V_{PaO2}). In addition, the time to intubation, visual field, and occurrence of FOB intubation-related complications were investigated.

Methods

Patients

This prospective randomized controlled study was approved by the Institutional Review Board of Yonsei University Gangnam Severance Hospital (IRB No 3–2015-0218, NCT02625194, https://clinicaltrials.gov/ct2/show/NCT02625194?term=NCT02625194&rank=1). After the acquisition of written informed consent, 36 patients aged 20–60 years (American Society of Anesthesiolgists class I to III) who were scheduled for elective surgery under general endotracheal anesthesia with arterial cannulation at Yonsei University Gangnam Severance Hospital were included. The exclusion criteria included lung disease, anticipated difficult airway, inability to read or write, and

pregnancy. The randomization table at www.random.org was used to allocate patients to an N group (no oxygen insufflation) or an O group (oxygen insufflation) at ratio of 1:1.

Study design and procedure

After premedication with 0.02 mg/kg of midazolam and 0.004 mg/kg of glycopyrrolate in the preanesthesia care unit, patients were transferred to the operating room, where standard monitoring procedures, including electrocardiography, pulse oximetry, and noninvasive blood pressure measurement, were initiated. Vital signs, including the heart rate, systolic blood pressure, diastolic blood pressure, and peripheral oxygen saturation, were recorded before anesthesia induction. Preoxygenation with 100% oxygen using a facemask was performed for 5 min, following which anesthesia was induced with propofol 1.5 mg/kg, remifentanil 0.1 mcg/kg/min, and rocuronium 0.8 mg/kg. The radial artery was cannulated during manual ventilation. After 2 min of manual ventilation, arterial blood was collected and the facemask was removed for intubation (T1). The airway was opened by the jaw thrust maneuver, and endotracheal intubation was performed using a flexible FOB (Intubation fiberscope, 5.2 × 65 mm, Karl Stortz GmbH & CO, Germany) with a preloaded endotracheal tube. In the O group, 100% oxygen was administered at 5 L/min through the working channel. The N group did not receive oxygen insufflation. Intubation success was confirmed by bronchoscopy, following which arterial blood was collected before the initiation of ventilation (T2). The first end-tidal carbon dioxide value after the resumption of ventilation following intubation was recorded.

Study endpoints

The primary endpoint was V_{PaO2}, defined as the difference of PaO_2 between T1 and T2 divided by the time to intubation (mmHg/sec). Secondary endpoints included the FOB intubation success rate, time to intubation (from facemask removal until resumption of ventilation), visual field during FOB intubation (excellent, clear view of anatomical structures and no limitation; good, < 50% limitation in the view but no difficulty in intubation; poor, > 50% limitation in the view, resulting in significant difficulty in intubation; and impossible, inability to identify the anatomical structures and intubate), and occurrence of FOB intubation-related complications, including mucosal injury, abdominal distension, postoperative nausea and/or vomiting, and desaturation [peripheral capillary oxygen saturation (SpO_2) < 90%]. In addition, vital signs and pH, partial pressure of carbon dioxide ($PaCO_2$), and PaO_2 values were recorded for all patients.

Statistical analysis

Considering the findings of Rosenstock, who reported a mean V_{PaO2} of 0.9 mmHg/s with a standard deviation of 0.17, we found that 16 patients per group were required for detection of a 0.25 mmHg/s decrease in V_{PaO2} with a type 1 error and power of 0.05 and 80%, respectively [13]. Accordingly, a total of 18 patients per group were included after accounting for the withdrawal rate during study. All statistical analyses were performed using SPSS, version 18.0 (SPSS Inc., Chicago, IL, USA). For V_{PaO2}, Mann-Whitney U test was performed. Secondary endpoints including time to intubation, vital signs and arterial blood gas analysis data were also assessed with Mann-Whitney U test. Visual field and FOB intubation-related complications were analysed by Fisher's exact test. In comparing the patients' characteristics, continuous variables were assessed using Mann–Whitney U-test, while categorical variables were assessed using the chi-square test or Fisher's exact test. The results from Mann-Whitney U test were expressed as mean with standard deviation. The categorical data was presented as number. The Bonferroni method was used to compensate the error of multiple comparisons. A P-value of < 0.05 was considered statistically significant.

Results

In total, 36 patients were enrolled, 35 of whom completed the study. One patient in the N group was excluded because of malfunction of the arterial blood gas analysis machine (Fig. 1). The patients' baseline characteristics were not different between the two groups (Table 1). All patients were successfully intubated. Vital signs and pH, $PaCO_2$, PaO_2 and SaO_2 values also showed no significant intergroup differences throughout the procedure. The time to intubation was approximately 150 s in both groups. Although PaO_2 showed no significant intergroup differences at T1 and T2, the decrease in PaO_2 during FOB intubation was significantly greater in the N group than in the O group (139.4 ± 74.3 vs. 72.0 ± 67.7, $p = 0.012$). In addition, V_{PaO2} was significantly greater in the N group than in the O group (1.0 ± 0.4 vs. 0.4 ± 0.4, $p < 0.001$). An excellent visual field was obtained for 12 and 7 patients in the O and N groups, respectively, with no significant intergroup difference. None of the patients presented mucosal injury, abdominal distension, and desaturation. One patient in the O group exhibited postoperative nausea (Table 2).

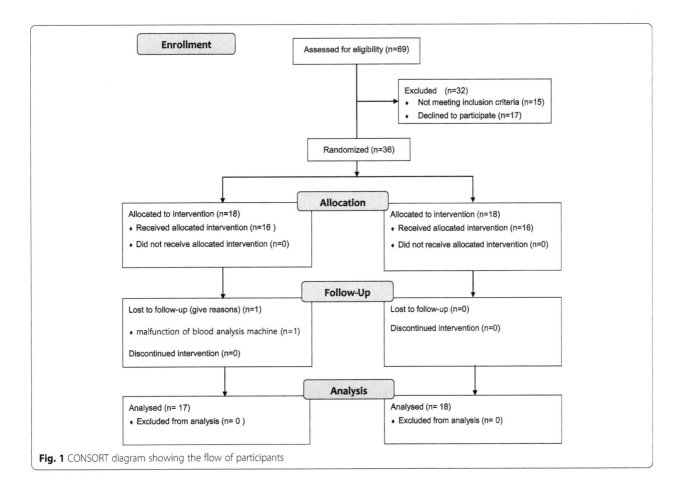

Fig. 1 CONSORT diagram showing the flow of participants

Table 1 Patients' Characteristics

	No Oxygen (n = 17)	Oxygen (n = 18)	P-value	Standardized differences
Age (year)	53.1 ± 15.7	59.1 ± 9.6	0.330	0.622
Sex (male, number)	5 (29.4%)	6 (33.3%)	0.803	0.083
Height (cm)	161.6 ± 10.7	162.4 ± 9.1	0.655	0.094
Weight (kg)	63.9 ± 12.5	66.1 ± 14.0	0.741	0.159
ASA Class			0.391	0.581
I	8 (47.1)	4 (22.2)		
II	8 (47.1)	12 (66.7)		
III	1 (5.9)	2 (11.1)		

Values are expressed as mean ± standard deviation or number
ASA American Society of Anesthesiologist

Discussion

In the present study assessing the utility of oxygen insufflation during FOB intubation, V_{PaO2} was significantly reduced when oxygen was insufflated through the working channel. However, patients with and without oxygen insufflation showed no significant differences in the intubation success rate, time to intubation, visual field, and occurrence of complications.

Despite recent advances in airway management devices such as videolaryngoscopes and supraglottic airways, FOB intubation is still considered the gold standard for difficult airway management [14, 15]. However, it requires a longer time than does intubation with a direct laryngoscope. In addition, secretions and bleeding in the airway obscure the airway anatomy and complicate intubation [3]. Therefore, methods to improve patient oxygenation after the induction of anesthesia can facilitate faster and safer FOB intubation.

Several studies have attempted to overcome the limitations of FOB intubation. A direct laryngoscope or Glide-Scope can assist the placement of FOB near the glottis and facilitate easy intubation [16–18]. In addition, supraglottic airways such as I-gel or LMA can be used as conduits for FOB intubation, providing a better route to the glottic inlet and, at the same time, ventilating the lungs during the procedure [19, 20]. However, these techniques require the use of additional devices and result in an increased time to intubation. Especially, they are inappropriate in patients with limited mouth opening [21]. Oxygen insufflation through the working channel during FOB intubation does not require extra time and devices. Oxygen insufflation through the working channel of FOB could alleviate both hypoxia and visual field impairment in children [5]. In our study, V_{PaO2} was 1.01 ± 0.39 mmHg/s in the N group, which was more than twice the value for the O group (0.42 ± 0.42 mmHg/s). If the hypoxia-free apnea time during FOB intubation is defined as the time from the discontinuation of mask ventilation at a PaO_2 of 500 mmHg to the achievement of 90% SpO_2 at a PaO_2 of 60 mmHg, under the assumption

that PaO_2 exhibits a linear decrease during apnea, the hypoxia-free apnea duration could be approximately 10 min longer in the O group than in the N group (1047.62 s vs. 435.64 s, respectively).

This calculation is based on a ventilatory mass flow, also known as apneic oxygenation. During regular breathing in an adult, oxygen and carbon dioxide are exchanged between the lungs and blood at a flow rate of 250 ml/min. During apnea, the carbon dioxide flow returning to the lungs is significantly reduced to 8–20 ml/min while the oxygen flow to the blood is maintained. Therefore, negative pressure is generated in the lungs according to the volume difference during oxygen and carbon dioxide exchange; this facilitates the movement of oxygen from the pharynx to the lungs [8, 22].

Apneic oxygenation could be applied in various clinical situations involving different types of devices, including nasal prongs, nasopharyngeal catheters, and tracheal or bronchial catheters. The first two are commonly used because they are practical [8]. Oxygenation with nasal prongs at 5 l/min during FOB intubation could lower the decrease in PaO_2 at 3 min during apnea [23]. In Teller's crossover study evaluating the influence of oxygen delivery via a nasopharyngeal catheter at 3 l/min, apnea was continued for 10 min or until SpO_2 decreased to 92%. None of the patients in the apneic oxygenation group showed an SpO2 of < 97% until 10 min. On the other hand, the mean apnea time in the control group was 6.8 min and the lowest SpO_2 value was 91% [24]. In present study, we used the working channel of FOB to continuously deliver oxygen as FOB moved toward the trachea. This increases the efficiency of oxygen delivery to the lungs and could be particularly useful for patients prone to desaturation during apnea, such as obese patients [25].

One limitation of apneic oxygenation is that it cannot efficiently remove carbon dioxide from the blood, resulting in an increase in the carbon dioxide level at a rate of 1.1–3.4 mmHg/min and, eventually, hypercarbia and acidosis [8]. Therefore, it should not be used in patients

Table 2 Primary and secondary endpoints

	No Oxygen ($n=17$)	Oxygen ($n=18$)	P-value
Heart rate (bpm)			
T1	75.1 ± 15.5	67.9 ± 10.4	0.291
T2	93.4 ± 15.9	87.2 ± 14.9	0.261
SBP (mmHg)			
T1	105.2 ± 21.7	106.1 ± 17.4	0.428
T2	142.4 ± 33.1	132.1 ± 27.5	0.391
DBP (mmHg)			
T1	57.8 ± 12.0	61.9 ± 14.5	0.437
T2	79.9 ± 19.6	77.8 ± 18.1	0.656
SpO_2 (%)			
T1	99.4 ± 0.7	99.4 ± 0.9	0.809
T2	99.0 ± 1.3	98.7 ± 1.2	0.376
pH			
T1	7.4 ± 0.1	7.4 ± 0.0	0.106
T2	7.3 ± 0.0	7.3 ± 0.0	0.373
SaO_2			
T1	99.9 ± 0.2	99.9 ± 0.1	0.929
T2	99.4 ± 1.2	99.6 ± 1.4	0.335
$PaCO_2$			
T1	37.6 ± 6.4	38.3 ± 6.1	0.552
T2	46.7 ± 6.6	47.5 ± 6.1	0.632
PaO_2 (mmHg)			
T1	415.0 ± 90.4	379.7 ± 72.3	0.137
T2	275.6 ± 94.9	307.8 ± 97.2	0.322
PaO_2 difference (mmHg)	139.4 ± 74.3	72.0 ± 67.7	0.012
Intubation time (sec)	145.5 ± 74.8	155.9 ± 70.1	0.632
$VPaO_2$ (mmHg/sec)	1.0 ± 0.4	0.4 ± 0.4	0.000
Visual field			0.183
Excellent	7	12	
Good	8	3	
Poor	2	3	
Complication			
PONV (N)	0	1	1.000

Values are expressed as mean ± standard deviation or number

T1, 2 min after manual ventilation with 100% oxygen, T2 after intubation confirmed with bronchoscopy, before ventilation resumed, SBP systolic blood pressure, DBP diastolic blood pressure, SpO_2 peripheral oxygen saturation, SaO_2 arterial oxygen saturation, $PaCO_2$ arterial partial pressure of carbon dioxide, PaO_2 arterial partial pressure of oxygen, PaO_2 difference difference of arterial partial pressure of oxygen between T1 and T2, $VPaO_2$ velocity of decrease in arterial partial pressure of oxygen, PONV postoperative nausea and vomiting

with a risk of hypercarbia-related complications. Of late, the use of a high flow nasal cannula has garnered attention in various clinical situations, and it can be effectively used for apneic oxygenation during intubation as well. Studies found that it could deliver a high concentration of oxygen, generate a positive airway pressure of approximately 7 cmH_2O, and slow down the increase in the carbon dioxide level during apneic oxygenation [22, 26]. In the present study, the increase in $PaCO_2$ during the apneic period was similar in the O and N groups.

With regard to the visual field, the number of patients with an excellent visual field was not significantly different between groups, although the number was higher in the O group. This result was inconsistent with those of previous reports, and there are a few possible explanations for the discrepancy. Unlike Rosen's study, which included pediatric patients with difficult airways and involved the use of smaller FOBs [5], the present study included adult patients without anticipated difficult airways and involved the use of FOBs with a larger diameter. Moreover, all patients were premedicated with glycopyrrolate in order to minimize secretions [3]. The visual field can be easily disrupted during awake FOB intubation because of patient movement and lens fogginess caused by spontaneous breathing [7]. However, we performed the study under anesthesia with complete muscle relaxation, so there were no disturbances during FOB intubation. Therefore, the intubation conditions were quite good, and the actual effect of oxygen insufflation may not have been as significant as expected.

The two groups in our study showed a comparable intubation success rate and time to intubation; this could be attributed to the lack of differences in the visual field quality. The optimal intubation conditions may be another factor that repressed the influence of oxygen on the intubation-related parameters. We believe that different results may be derived if the measurements were recorded in emergency situations involving patients with unanticipated difficult airways. Further studies should take this aspect into consideration and assess the usefulness of oxygen insufflation during FOB intubation in different clinical scenarios.

From our results, it is evident that oxygen insufflation through the working channel of FOB can reduce $VPaO_2$ during FOB intubation. Oxygen insufflation through the working channel of FOB can cause rare but serious complications such as gastric rupture and pneumothorax [10, 11, 27]. Oxygen can enter the trachea or esophagus during the procedure. If oxygen is delivered to the esophagus and stomach, it could cause nausea, vomiting [10, 12]. If FOB with oxygen insufflation enters the stomach, it could cause significant distension of the stomach and even rupture, because the maximal capacity of the stomach is approximately 1 l, and FOB could deliver approximately 2.5 l of oxygen in just 30 s, theoretically [10, 28]. However, according to Wong's review of several studies on nasal or nasopharyngeal apneic oxygenation, no complications related to pressure effects have been reported till date [8]. The esophagus is closed by a sphincter, and approximately 20 cmH_2O of pressure is required to open it [29]. According to a previous report using nasal high flow oxygen insufflation, the mean airway pressure was approximately 7 cmH_2O [26], which is considerably lower than the pressure required to open the esophageal sphincter. In the present study, none of the patients complained of vomiting or abdominal distension, and only one patient in group O developed postoperative nausea. Furthermore, there was no case of mucosal injury or desaturation during the procedure. This was probably due to the optimal intubation

conditions and the completion of intubation within 5 min, which is considered safe if the patient is preoxygenated [26].

This study has some limitations. First, FOB intubation was conducted under optimal conditions as described earlier. Therefore, the results cannot be applied to other clinical situations such as emergency difficult airway management. Second, our sample size was enough for $VPaO_2$ measurement but not adequate to assess the occurrence of complications, which are anyways rare.

Conclusions

In conclusion, our findings suggest that oxygen insufflation through the working channel of FOB can help in extending the apneic window after the induction of general anesthesia during FOB intubation, with minimal complications.

Abbreviations
FOB intubation: Fiberoptic bronchoscope-assisted intubation; FOB: Fiberoptic bronchoscope; PaO_2: Partial pressure of oxygen; V_{PaO2}: Velocity of decrease in the partial pressure of oxygen; $PaCO_2$: Partial pressure of carbon dioxide; SpO_2: Peripheral capillary oxygen saturation

Acknowledgements
Not applicable.

Authors' contributions
Conceptualization, C.H.C.; Methodology, G.U.R.; Validation, G.U.R. and C.H.C.; Formal Analysis, G.U.R and J.G.K.; Investigation, G.U.R. and C.H.C.; Resources, C.H.C; Data Curation, C.H.C.; Writing – Original Draft Preparation, G.U.R.; Writing – Review & Editing, C.H.C., G.U.R. and J.Y.H.; Visualization, G.U.R.; Supervision, C.H.C; Project Administration, J.Y.H. All authors read and approved the final manuscript.

Author details
[1]Department of Anesthesiology and Pain Medicine, CHA Bundang Medical Center, CHA University School of Medicine, 59 Yatap-ro, Bundang-gu, Seongnami-si, Gyeonggi-do 13496, Korea. [2]Department of Anesthesiology and Pain Medicine, and Anesthesia and Pain Research Institute, Yonsei University College of Medicine, Gangnam Severance Hospital, 211 Eonju-ro, Gangnam-gu, Seoul 06273, Korea.

References
1. Caplan RA, Posner KL, Ward RJ, Cheney FW. Adverse respiratory events in anesthesia: a closed claims analysis. Anesthesiology. 1990;72(5):828–33.
2. Hove LD, Steinmetz J, Christoffersen JK, Moller A, Nielsen J, Schmidt H. Analysis of deaths related to anesthesia in the period 1996-2004 from closed claims registered by the Danish patient insurance association. Anesthesiology. 2007;106(4):675–80.
3. Collins SR, Blank RS. Fiberoptic intubation: an overview and update. Respir Care. 2014;59(6):865–78 discussion 78-80.
4. Xue FS, Cheng Y, Li RP. Awake intubation with video laryngoscope and fiberoptic bronchoscope in difficult airway patients. Anesthesiology. 2013; 118(2):462–3.
5. Rosen DA, Rosen KR, Nahrwold ML. Another use for the suction port on the pediatric flexible bronchoscope. Anesthesiology. 1986;65(1):116.
6. Roberts JT. Preparing to use the flexible fiber-optic laryngoscope. J Clin Anesth. 1991;3(1):64–75.
7. Benumof JL. Management of the difficult adult airway. With special emphasis on awake tracheal intubation. Anesthesiology. 1991;75(6):1087–110.

8. Wong DT, Yee AJ, Leong SM, Chung F. The effectiveness of apneic oxygenation during tracheal intubation in various clinical settings: a narrative review. Can J Anaesth. 2017;64(4):416–27.
9. Bennett-Guerrero E, Stolp BW. Fiberoptic intubation. N Engl J Med. 2011; 365(6):574 author reply 5-6.
10. Chapman N. Gastric rupture and pneumoperitoneum caused by oxygen insufflation via a fiberoptic bronchoscope. Anesth Analg. 2008;106(5):1592.
11. Khan RM, Sharma PK, Kaul N. Barotrauma: a life-threatening complication of fiberoptic endotracheal intubation in a neonate. Paediatr Anaesth. 2010; 20(8):782–4.
12. Ho CM, Yin IW, Tsou KF, Chow LH, Tsai SK. Gastric rupture after awake fibreoptic intubation in a patient with laryngeal carcinoma. Br J Anaesth. 2005;94(6):856–8.
13. Rosenstock CV, Thogersen B, Afshari A, Christensen AL, Eriksen C, Gatke MR. Awake fiberoptic or awake video laryngoscopic tracheal intubation in patients with anticipated difficult airway management: a randomized clinical trial. Anesthesiology. 2012;116(6):1210–6.
14. Lohse J, Noppens R. Awake video laryngoscopy - an alternative to awake fiberoptic intubation? Anasthesiol Intensivmed Notfallmed Schmerzther. 2016;51(11–12):656–63.
15. Law JA, Morris IR, Brousseau PA, de la Ronde S, Milne AD. The incidence, success rate, and complications of awake tracheal intubation in 1,554 patients over 12 years: an historical cohort study. Can J Anaesth. 2015;62(7): 736–44.
16. Ara T, Mori G, Adachi E, Asai T, Okuda Y. Combined use of the GlideScope and fiberoptic bronchoscope for tracheal intubation in a patient with difficult airway. Masui. 2014;63(6):647–9.
17. Gu J, Xu K, Ning J, Yi B, Lu K. GlideScope-assisted fiberoptic bronchoscope intubation in a patient with severe rheumatoid arthritis. Acta Anaesthesiol Taiwanica. 2014;52(2):85–7.
18. Sharma D, Kim LJ, Ghodke B. Successful airway management with combined use of Glidescope videolaryngoscope and fiberoptic bronchoscope in a patient with Cowden syndrome. Anesthesiology. 2010; 113(1):253–5.
19. Kanda T, Kasai H, Sanefuji Y. Fiberoptic tracheal intubation through the supraglottic airway device air-Q in a patient with Shprintzen-Goldberg syndrome. Masui. 2013;62(8):942–5.
20. Arevalo-Ludena J, Arcas-Bellas JJ, Alvarez-Rementeria R, Alameda LE. Fiberoptic-guided intubation after insertion of the i-gel airway device in spontaneously breathing patients with difficult airway predicted: a prospective observational study. J Clin Anesth. 2016;35:287–92.
21. Moore A, Gregoire-Bertrand F, Massicotte N, Gauthier A, Lallo A, Ruel M, et al. I-gel versus LMA-Fastrach Supraglottic airway for flexible bronchoscope-guided tracheal intubation using a Parker (GlideRite) endotracheal tube: a randomized controlled trial. Anesth Analg. 2015;121(2): 430–6.
22. Patel A, Nouraei SA. Transnasal humidified rapid-insufflation Ventilatory exchange (THRIVE): a physiological method of increasing apnoea time in patients with difficult airways. Anaesthesia. 2015;70(3):323–9.
23. Lee SC. Improvement of gas exchange by apneic oxygenation with nasal prong during fiberoptic intubation in fully relaxed patients. J Korean Med Sci. 1998;13(6):582–6.
24. Teller LE, Alexander CM, Frumin MJ, Gross JB. Pharyngeal insufflation of oxygen prevents arterial desaturation during apnea. Anesthesiology. 1988; 69(6):980–2.
25. Ramachandran SK, Cosnowski A, Shanks A, Turner CR. Apneic oxygenation during prolonged laryngoscopy in obese patients: a randomized, controlled trial of nasal oxygen administration. J Clin Anesth. 2010;22(3):164–8.
26. Ritchie JE, Williams AB, Gerard C, Hockey H. Evaluation of a humidified nasal high-flow oxygen system, using oxygraphy, capnography and measurement of upper airway pressures. Anaesth Intensive Care. 2011;39(6):1103–10.
27. Ovassapian A, Mesnick PS. Oxygen insufflation through the fiberscope to assist intubation is not recommended. Anesthesiology. 1997;87(1):183–4.
28. Geliebter A, Hashim SA. Gastric capacity in normal, obese, and bulimic women. Physiol Behav. 2001;74(4–5):743–6.
29. Lawes EG, Campbell I, Mercer D. Inflation pressure, gastric insufflation and rapid sequence induction. Br J Anaesth. 1987;59(3):315–8 Lawes, E.G.; Campbell, I.; Mercer, D. Inflation pressure, gastric insufflation and rapid sequence induction. British journal of anaesthesia 1987, 59, 315–318.

8

Comparison of the new flexible tip bougie catheter and standard bougie stylet for tracheal intubation by anesthesiologists in different difficult airway scenarios

Kurt Ruetzler[1], Jacek Smereka[2], Cristian Abelairas-Gomez[3,4,5], Michael Frass[6], Marek Dabrowski[7], Szymon Bialka[8], Hanna Misiolek[8], Tadeusz Plusa[9], Oliver Robak[6], Olga Aniolek[10], Jerzy Robert Ladny[11], Damian Gorczyca[10], Sanchit Ahuja[12] and Lukasz Szarpak[10]*

Abstract

Background: Incidence of difficult endotracheal intubation ranges between 3 and 10%. Bougies have been recommended as an airway adjunct for difficult intubation, but reported success rates are variable. A new generation flexible tip bougie appears promising but was not investigated so far. We therefore compared the new flexible tip with a standard bougie in simulated normal and difficult airway scenarios, and used by experienced anesthesiologists.

Methods: We conducted a observational, randomized, cross-over simulation study. Following standardized training, experienced anesthesiologists performed endotracheal intubation using a Macintosh blade and one of the bougies in six different airway scenarios in a randomized sequence: normal airway, tongue edema, pharyngeal obstruction, manual cervical inline stabilization, cervical collar stabilization, cervical collar stabilization and pharyngeal obstruction. Overall success rate with a maximum of 3 intubation attempts was the primary endpoint. Secondary endpoints included number of intubation attempts, time to intubation and dental compression.

Results: Thirty-two anesthesiologist participated in this study between January 2019 and May 2019. Overall success rate was similar for the flexible tip bougie and the standard bougie. The flexible tip bougie tended to need less intubation attempts in more difficult airway scenarios. Time to intubation was less if using the flexible tip bougie compared to the standard bougie. Reduced severity of dental compression was noted for the flexible tip bougie in difficult airway scenarios except cervical collar stabilization.

(Continued on next page)

* Correspondence: lukasz.szarpak@gmail.com
[10]Polish Society of Disaster Medicine, Swieradowska 43 Str, 02-662 Warsaw, Poland

Comparison of the new flexible tip bougie catheter and standard bougie stylet for tracheal intubation...

51

(Continued from previous page)

Conclusion: In this simulation study of normal and difficult airways scenarios, overall success rate was similar for the flexible tip and standard bougie. Especially in more difficult airway scenarios, less intubation attempts, and less optimization maneuvers were needed if using the flexible tip bougie.

Keywords: Airway management, Endotracheal intubation, Medical simulation, Bougie catheter

Background

During induction of anesthesia, the estimated incidence of difficult endotracheal intubation ranges between 3 and 10%, depending on the definition used [1, 2]. Recent advances in airways adjuncts like the introduction of videolaryngoscopes into clinical practice have led to fewer life-threatening complications, however the risk of serious complications still remains. Despite protracted convalescent, the current definitions to predict difficult airway situations are inadequate and often times prove unchallenging [3, 4]. Conversely, unanticipated difficult airway scenarios occur when least expected and significantly lead to anesthesia-related morbidity. The majority of these scenarios arise due to poor visualization of laryngeal inlet - "epiglottis only view" ostensibly due to condition such as pharyngeal obstruction, obesity, limited cervical mobility etc. [5–7]. Situations in which glottic view is expected to improve by external laryngeal manipulation — a readily available airway adjunct device (commonly known as bougie) is recommended to assist tracheal intubation.

A recent study in the emergency care setting demonstrated, that the use of a bougie resulted in a higher first attempt success rate when compared to conventional endotracheal intubation [8]. Previous work also reported the utility of bougie in difficult airway scenarios (such as cervical spine injuries) with a reported success rate ranging between 74 to 99% [9–12]. The variable success rate of the standard bougie was most commonly attributed to the inability to insert the bougie through the hypopharynx and laryngeal inlet [13]. To overcome this limitation, a new generation flexible tip bougie is designed to flexibly navigate the distal tip and help facilitate precise insertion of the endotracheal tube — even in a hyper curve airway [14]. The flexible tip bougie has an integrated slider along the surface which moves the tip anterior and posterior while the pre-curved distal portion of shaft allows the angulation to provide anterior flexion. The flexible tip is held, inserted and used like a standard bougie, except the intubator has an additional ability to navigate the bougie tip.

Intuitively the new flexible tip bougie seems to be a valuable device but the efficacy has not been investigated in the difficult airway setting yet. We therefore conducted a randomized cross over study to evaluate the usefulness of this new device, and used by experienced anesthesiologists in several airway manikin scenarios. We hypothesized that the new flexible tip bougie would perform comparably to the standard bougie in the normal airway scenario. In the difficult airway (tongue edema, manual in-line stabilization, or cervical collar stabilization), we hypothesized that the new flexible tip bougie would prove superior to the standard bougie.

Methods

Study design

This was an observational, randomized, cross-over simulation study. The study protocol was approved by the Institutional Review Board (IRB) of the Polish Society of Disaster Medicine (Approval no: 21.11.2017.IRB), and registered in www.clinicaltrials.gov (identifier: NCT03733158).

Study participants

Following IRB approval and written informed consent, 32 experienced anesthesiologists with at least 2 years of clinical experience participated in this study. No anesthesiologist had any prior experience with the new flexible tip bougie, but each was experienced with the standard bougie and all had performed a minimum of 500 endotracheal intubations using the Macintosh laryngoscope.

Intubation devices

All intubation procedures were performed using a Macintosh blade size 3 (Heine Optotechnik, Herrsching, Germany) and one out of two bougies:

1. The standard bougie for difficult intubation (Sumi, Sulejówek, Poland);
2. The new flexible tip bougie (FMDSS Construct Medical, Hawthorn, Austria, Fig. 1).

Tracheal tubes (Portex, St. Paul, MN, USA) with an internal diameter of 7.5 mm were used for all intubations. Before each intubation attempt, the endotracheal tube and the manikin's airway were thoroughly lubricated using an airway lubricant for training manikins (Laerdal, Stavanger, Norway). A regular 20 cc syringe (B. Braun Melsungen AG, Hessen, Germany) was used for cuff inflation.

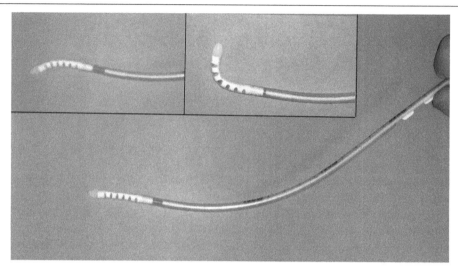

Fig. 1 The new Flexible tip bougie catheter

Study protocol

Each anesthesiologist participated a standardized 5 min lasting practical demonstration of the flexible tip bougie and the standard bougie by one of the investigators. Once completed, each anesthesiologist performed tracheal intubation with both devices in a Laerdal Airway Management Trainer (Laerdal, Stavanger, Norway) in 2 scenarios:

1. normal airway in the supine position
2. normal airway with the neck immobilized using a hard-cervical collar.

Afterwards, anesthesiologists performed tracheal intubation in a SimMan 3G simulator (Laerdal, Stavanger, Norway) in 6 different airway scenarios:

A) Normal airway;
B) Tongue edema;
C) Pharyngeal obstruction;
D) Manual cervical inline stabilization;
E) Cervical collar stabilization;
F) Cervical collar stabilization and pharyngeal obstruction.

Once anesthesiologists completed all intubations in all eight scenarios, they were asked to perform another endotracheal intubations on the Laerdal Airway Management Trainer with a normal airway using both devices. The intubation procedure was closely monitored by one of the investigators, to certify, that intubations using both devices were performed in an adequate manner. If needed, endotracheal intubations were repeated until both the anesthesiologist and the investigator were satisfied.

For the study, the SimMan 3G simulator (Laerdal, Stavanger, Norway) was placed on a hard, flat table to simulate an "in the bed" scenario. Anesthesiologists were instructed to intubate the manikin with one of the two devices, insufflate the cuff of the tube, attach a bag valve mask, and provide one breath to ventilate the lungs of the simulator for an overall of six different airway scenarios:

- Normal airway;
- Tongue edema;
- Pharyngeal obstruction;
- Manual cervical inline stabilization;
- Cervical collar stabilization;
- Cervical collar stabilization and pharyngeal obstruction.

Both, the sequence of the intubation devices and the six airway scenarios were randomized using the research randomizer (randomizer.org).

Measurements

The primary endpoint was the rate of successful placement of the tracheal tube in the trachea with a maximum of three intubation attempts. A failed intubation attempt was defined as an attempt in which the trachea was not intubated, or lasted longer than 120 s [15]..

The secondary endpoint was time required for successful tracheal intubation. The time for successful intubation, was defined as the time between insertion of the blade between the teeth until the manikin was successfully ventilated, confirmed by lung insufflation during bas-mask ventilation [15].

Number of intubation attempts, and number of optimization maneuvers required (re-adjustment of manikin's head position, and BURP -backward, upward, and rightward pressure to the larynx- maneuver performed by a researcher), served as additional secondary endpoints. All outcomes were assessed by one of the researchers. A researcher further scored the severity of dental compressions, which was assessed by the number of audible teeth clicks (0; 1; ≥2) with the Laerdal airway trainer, and by a grading of pressure of the teeth (none = 0; mild = 1; moderate/serve ≥2) on the SimMan 3G simulator. At the end of each scenario, each participant scored the ease of use of each intubation device on a visual analogue scale ranging from 0 (extremely easy) to 100 (extremely difficult).

Sample size
The sample size was calculated with the G*Power 3.1 software, and the two-tailed t test was applied (Cohen's d, 0.8; alpha error, 0.05; power, 0.95). We calculated that at least 28 participants would be required (paired, 2-sided). To minimize the impact of potentially data loss, we planned to enroll up to 32 anesthesiologists into this study.

Statistics
All statistical analyses were performed with statistical package STATISTICA 13.3EN (TIBCO Inc., Tulsa, OK, USA). The normal distribution of data was tested using the Kolmogorov-Smirnov test. Results obtained from each trial were compared using two-way repeated-measurements analysis of variance for intubation time. Fisher's exact test was used for the success rate. The participants' subjective opinions were compared with the use of the Stuart-Maxwell test. Data were presented as medians and interquartile range (IQR) or number and percentage (%). The α-error level for all analyses was set as $P < .05$.

Results
Between January 2019 and May 2019, a total of thirty-two anesthesiologists were recruited. The median clinical experience of the anesthesiologists was 3.5 years (Inter Quartile Range IQR; 2.5–5). Each anesthesiologist had previously performed at least 500 endotracheal intubations using the Macintosh laryngoscope, and none had any experience with the new flexible tip bougie, but with the standard bougie.

Scenario 1: Normal airway
All anesthesiologists successfully intubated the trachea with the first intubation attempt using both bougies (Table 1).

Scenario 2: tongue edema
Overall intubation success rate was 100% for both intubation devices. Successful intubation with the first intubation attempt was 22% with the bougie and 34% for the flexible tip bougie (Table 2). Use of the new flexible tip bougie was associated with less optimization maneuvers

Table 1 Data from intubation in Scenario A: Normal airway. Data are presented as median (IQR), or as number (percentage)

parameter	standard bougie	flexible tip bougie catheter	*p*-value
Overall success rate, %	32 (100%)	32 (100%)	NS
Duration of 1st intubation attempt, sec	27 (21.5–36)	25 (19–34)	NS
Number of intubation attempts (%)			
1	32 (100%)	32 (100%)	
2	0 (0%)	0 (0%)	
3	0 (0%)	0 (0%)	
Median (IQR)	1 (1–1)	1 (1–1)	NS
Number of optimization maneuvers (%)			
0	30 (94%)	31 (97%)	
1	2 (6%)	1 (3%)	
2	0 (0%)	0 (0%)	
Median (IQR)	0 (0–0)	0 (0–0)	NS
Severity of dental compression (%)			
0	14 (44%)	17 (53%)	
1	16 (50.0%)	15 (47%)	
2	2 (6%)	0 (0%)	
Median (IQR)	1 (0–1)	0 (0–1)	NS
Ease of use (1–100)	18 (10–21)	18 (10–19)	NS

NS Not statistically significant

and less dental compression compared to the standard bougie.

Scenario 3: pharyngeal obstruction

Anesthesiologists successfully intubated with the first intubation attempt with both bougies (Table 3). The use of new flexible tip bougie again caused less optimization maneuvers and less dental compression compared to the standard bougie.

Scenario 4: manual inline stabilization

Overall rate of successful was 100% in both devices (Table 4). Successful intubation with the first intubation attempt was 94% with the flexible tip bougie compared to 59% with the standard bougie (statistically not significant). The rate of optimization maneuvers and dental compression was less if used the flexible tip bougie compared to the standard bougie.

Scenario 5: cervical collar stabilization

Overall success rate was 100% with both bougies. First intubation attempt success rate was 81% for the standard bougie and 94% for the new flexible tip bougie (Table 5). Time to intubation was shorter with the new flexible tip bougie (37 s) compared to the standard bougie (46 s, $p = < 0.001$).

Scenario 6: cervical collar stabilization and pharyngeal obstruction

Overall success rate (100% vs. 94%, not significant) as well as first attempt success rate (72% vs 66%, not significant) was higher with the new flexible tip bougie compared to the standard bougie (Table 6). The new flexible tip bougie again caused less optimization maneuvers ($p = < 0.001$) and less dental compression ($p = 0.008$) compared to the standard bougie.

The new flexible tip bougie was assessed by the participating anesthesiologists to be easier to use in all difficult, but not in the normal airway scenario.

Discussion

The purpose of this manikin study was to compare the flexible tip bougie with the standard bougie as aids for endotracheal intubation, using simulated normal and difficult airway scenarios. During normal simulated airways scenarios, overall and first attempt success rates, number of intubation attempts, number of optimizing maneuvers and complications such as dental compression, and ease of use were similar for the flexible tip bougie and the standard bougie. This might be mostly based on the fact, that participating anesthesiologists were previously familiar with the standard bougie. This is also reassuring, that the new flexible tip bougie did not require additional previous extensive training to familiarize with the slightly different technique.

Table 2 Data from intubation in Scenario B: Tongue edema. Data are presented as median (IQR), or as number (percentage)

parameter	standard bougie	flexible tip bougie catheter	*p*-value
Overall success rate, %	32 (100%)	32 (100%)	NS
Duration of 1st intubation attempt, s	44 (35–73)	40 (30–55)	**0.046**
Number of intubation attempts (%)			
1	7 (22%)	11 (34%)	
2	17 (53%)	19 (59%)	
3	8 (25%)	2 (6%)	
Median (IQR)	2 (2–2.3)	2 (1–2)	NS
Number of optimization maneuvers (%)			
0	0 (0%)	6 (19%)	
1	7 (22%)	23 (72%)	
2	25 (78%)	3 (9%)	
Median (IQR)	2 (2–2)	1 (1–1)	**< 0.001**
Severity of dental compression (%)			
0	2 (6%)	4 (13%)	
1	1 (3%)	10 (31%)	
2	29 (91%)	18 (56%)	
Median (IQR)	2 (2–2)	2 (1–2)	**0.024**
Ease of use (1–100)	56 (41–67)	45 (40–57)	**0.038**

NS Not statistically significant

Table 3 Data from intubation in Scenario C: Pharyngeal obstruction. Data are presented as median (IQR), or as number (percentage)

parameter	standard bougie	flexible tip bougie catheter	*p*-value
Overall success rate, %	32 (100%)	32 (100%)	NS
Duration of 1st intubation attempt, s	29 (23.5–36)	24 (20.5–32)	**0.010**
Number of intubation attempts (%)			
1	32 (100%)	32 (100%)	
2	0 (0%)	0 (0%)	
3	0 (0%)	0 (0%)	
Median (IQR)	1 (1–1)	1 (1–1)	NS
Number of optimization maneuvers (%)			
0	19 (59%)	30 (94%)	
1	13 (41%)	2 (6%)	
2	0 (0%)	0 (0%)	
Median (IQR)	0 (0–1)	0 (0–0)	**0.018**
Severity of dental compression (%)			
0	7 (22%)	15 (47%)	
1	9 (28%)	13 (41%)	
2	16 (50%)	4 (12%)	
Median (IQR)	1.5 (1–2)	1 (0–1)	**0.004**
Ease of use (1–100)	34 (22–41)	32 (20–39)	NS

NS Not statistically significant

Table 4 Data from intubation in Scenario D: Manual cervical inline stabilization. Data are presented as median (IQR), or as number (percentage)

parameter	standard bougie	flexible tip bougie catheter	*p*-value
Overall success rate, %	32 (100%)	32 (100%)	NS
Duration of 1st intubation attempt, s	34 (30–48)	29 (25–34)	**0.001**
Number of intubation attempts (%)			
1	27 (84%)	30 (94%)	
2	5 (16%)	2 (6%)	
3	0 (0%)	0 (0%)	
Median (IQR)	1 (1–1)	1 (1–1)	NS
Number of optimization maneuvers (%)			
0	10 (31%)	12 (37%)	
1	15 (47%)	19 (59%)	
2	7 (22%)	1 (3%)	
Median (IQR)	1 (0–1)	1 (0–1)	NS
Severity of dental compression (%)			
0	0 (0%)	6 (19%)	
1	12 (37%)	15 (47%)	
2	20 (62%)	11 (34%)	
Median (IQR)	2 (1–2)	1 (1–2)	**0.015**
Ease of use (1–100)	61 (40–72)	53 (38–69)	**0.013**

NS Not statistically significant

Table 5 Data from intubation in Scenario E: Cervical collar stabilization. Data are presented as median (IQR), or as number (percentage)

parameter	standard bougie	flexible tip bougie catheter	*p*-value
Overall success rate, %	32 (100%)	32 (100%)	NS
Duration of 1st intubation attempt, s	46 (38–53)	37 (31.5–46)	**< 0.001**
Number of intubation attempts (%)			
1	26 (81%)	30 (94%)	
2	5 (16%)	1 (3%)	
3	1 (3%)	1 (3%)	
Median (IQR)	1 (1–1)	1 (1–1)	NS
Number of optimization maneuvers (%)			
0	9 (28%)	12 (37%)	
1	15 (47%)	17 (53%)	
2	8 (25%)	3 (9%)	
Median (IQR)	1 (0–1.3)	1 (0–1)	NS
Severity of dental compression (%)			
0	0 (0%)	4 (12%)	
1	9 (28%)	13 (41%)	
2	23 (72%)	15 (47%)	
Median (IQR)	2 (1–2)	1 (1–2)	NS
Ease of use (1–100)	72 (53–79)	60 (45–71)	**0.014**

NS Not statistically significant

Table 6 Data from intubation in Scenario F: Cervical collar stabilization and pharyngeal obstruction. Data are presented as median (IQR), or as number (percentage)

parameter	standard bougie	flexible tip bougie catheter	*p*-value
Overall success rate, %	30 (94%)	32 (100%)	NS
Duration of 1st intubation attempt, s	53 (44–73)	44 (35–59)	**0.002**
Number of intubation attempts (%)			
1	21 (66%)	24 (72%)	
2	10 (31%)	6 (19%)	
3	1 (3%)	3 (9%)	
Median (IQR)	1 (1–2)	1 (1–1.3)	NS
Number of optimization maneuvers (%)			
0	3 (9%)	10 (31%)	
1	8 (25%)	19 (59%)	
2	21 (66%)	3 (9%)	
Median (IQR)	2 (1–2)	1 (0–1)	**< 0.001**
Severity of dental compression (%)			
0	0 (0%)	7 (22%)	
1	6 (19%)	10 (31%)	
2	26 (81%)	15 (47%)	
Median (IQR)	2 (2–2)	1 (1–2)	**0.008**
Ease of use (1–100)	83 (72–90)	69 (54–77)	**< 0.001**

NS Not statistically significant

Generally, bougies are advocated to facilitate intubations, when external manipulation seemed to improve glottic visualization [14]. The prime advantage of flexible tip bougie — ability to negotiate hyper acute curves — was therefore further tested by creating a simulated scenario of difficult intubation. Flexible tip bougie was able to achieve comparable overall success rate with reduced number of intubation attempts and optimization maneuver. We further investigated the two different bougie's in predicted difficult intubation scenarios such as cervical spine immobilization. Importantly, we observed a trend whereby the use flexible tip bougie appears to be superior to standard bougie with comparable success rates, reduced number of intubation attempts and time to endotracheal intubation. Advantages of decreased cervical movements and high first-time success rate of tracheal intubation have been described previously [16]. The application of manual in-line stabilization and cervical collar are known to worsen glottic visualization by at least one grade – thereby significantly impede intubation further leading to difficult laryngoscopy, increased hypoxia times and poor outcomes [11, 17]. Finally, a more complex scenario was created where we combined the cervical collar stabilization and pharyngeal obstruction together, and found improved overall success rate with the flexible tip bougie, earlier intubation by 9 s with number of optimization attempts restricted to 0–1 in the majority. The reduced time to intubation in cervical immobilization scenarios indicate that navigation with the flexible tip bougie is less time consuming compared to the standard bougie.

A recent study in the emergency room setting compared the standard bougie with an endotracheal tube equipped with a stylet and reported, that using a bougie resulted in higher first attempt intubation success rate and similar time to intubation (36 vs. 38 s, not significant) [8]. Another comparative manikin study evaluated the standard bougie and a fiberoptic stylet in difficult airways scenario and reported comparable mean time to successful intubation (31 vs 45 s, not significant) [18]. Previous studies further reported increased first pass success rate by standard bougie in simulated settings [6, 11, 19].

We noticed a decreased rate of dental compressions with the flexible tip bougie in difficult scenarios, except cervical collar scenario. Previous work suggests that the strain is not affected by the level of experience or training or number of previous intubations, however it varies widely across intubators and the severity may be reduced by the application of alcohol protective pads [20]. In our study, reduced strain may be attributed due to improved maneuverability of flexible tip bougie.

Standard bougies are commonly used as a rescue device for unexpected difficult intubations, most likely due to poor glottic visualization. Maneuvers such as "rotations" – signs like "clicks" and "hold up" are considered assurances of tracheal intubation [21, 22]. In such scenarios, the maneuverability of the flexible tip bougie can be utilized in conjunction with video laryngoscopes, to finally achieve endotracheal intubation— under indirect visualization [23, 24]. Although further research is needed with the flexible tip bougie, we expect that the utilization of flexible tip bougie with video laryngoscope may be helpful in difficult airways situations. Additionally, flexible tip bougie can be manipulated to rotate with a one-handed integrated slider, however excessive rotational force and additional help from a bystander is needed to achieve free rotation with standard bougie [25].

Our analysis should be interpreted with several limitations. It is worth noting that our study is a preliminary manikin study, the results of which are often times difficult to extrapolate to humans. Time to perform intubation is usually quicker in simulated models and the manikin does not fully reproduce laryngoscopic conditions in real patients. Anyhow, a reduction of a few seconds in any manner doesn't seem to be clinically relevant. Although not investigated in this study, the endotracheal tube may encounter resistance when railroaded over the bougie, and therefore makes intubation over the bougie more difficult [26, 27]. Airway perforation and soft tissue damage are important clinical concerns, although there is limited published evidence to support [28]. Based on the nature of this research, it was impossible to blind neither the intubators nor the assessing researchers. We included only experienced anesthesiologists which may be partly responsible for the high success rates, and faster time to intubation. However, results of this study are difficult to generalize to physicians with variable level of experience. We also did not standardize the techniques for using the bougies. There might be a small variety of techniques used in this study, which is mostly due to the fact, that all anesthesiologists had previous clinical experience with the standard bougie. Interestingly, although not having any previous experience with the flexible tip bougie, anesthesiologists achieved a high success rate of intubation, indicating a fast learning curve with the new device. However, this needs to be proven in less experienced providers. Finally, intubation using a bougie is considered a rescue technique for unexpected difficult intubations. Although also investigated in this manikin study, routine use of bougies in expected difficult intubations is currently not recommended.

CONLUSIONS

The newly introduced flexible tip bougie offered similar overall and first attempt success rates in normal airway scenarios compared to the standard bougie. In more difficult airway scenarios, the flexible tip bougie was associated with similar overall success rates, but less intubation attempts, less adjustment maneuvers, less dental compression, and assessment of easier to use compared to standard bougie. It appears that the innovative flexible tip bougie might a valuable airway adjunct for difficult intubations. Further research in the human clinical setting is indicated to confirm these findings and possibly address the limitations of this study.

Abbreviations
IRB: Institutional Review Board; NCT: National Clinical Trial number; BURP: Backward, upward, and rightward pressure to the larynx- maneuver; IQR: Inter Quartile Range

Acknowledgements
We are grateful to all the persons who participated in this study. Study was supported by the ERC Research NET and the Polish Society of Disaster Medicine.

Authors' contributions
JS, MD, DD, OA, SB and LS recruited the participants, collected the data, performed preliminary data analysis and drafted the manuscript. KR, LS, MS and TP performed detailed statistical analysis and prepared the Fig. HM, SA, TP, OR, MF, KR and LS participated in the discussion and improved the manuscript. JS, HM, KR, CAG and LS made substantial contributions to the original idea and design, analyses and interpretation of data as well as revising the manuscript. LS is the corresponding author and is responsible for the finalization of the manuscript. All authors have read and approved the final manuscript.

Author details
[1]Departments of Outcomes Research and General Anesthesia, Cleveland Clinic, Anesthesiology Institute, Cleveland, OH, USA. [2]Department of Emergency Medical Service, Wroclaw Medical University, Wroclaw, Poland. [3]CLINURSID Research Group, University of Santiago de Compostela, Santiago de Compostela, Spain. [4]Faculty of Education, University Santiago de Compostela, Santiago de Compostela, Spain. [5]Institute of Research of Santiago (IDIS) and SAMID-II Network, Santiago de Compostela, Spain. [6]Department of Internal Medicine I, Medical University of Vienna, Vienna, Austria. [7]Chair and Department of Medical Education, Poznan University of Medical Sciences, Poznan, Poland. [8]Department of Anaesthesiology and Critical Care, School of Medicine with Division of Dentistry in Zabrze, Medical University of Silesia, Zabrze, Poland. [9]Medical Faculty, Lazarski University, Warsaw, Poland. [10]Polish Society of Disaster Medicine, Swieradowska 43 Str, 02-662 Warsaw, Poland. [11]Department of Emergency Medicine, Medical University Bialystok, Bialystok, Poland. [12]Department of Anesthesia, Henry Ford Health System, Detroit, MI, USA.

References
1. Crosby ET, Cooper RM, Douglas MJ, et al. The unanticipated difficult airway with recommendations for management. Can J Anaesth. 1998;45(8):757–76.
2. Ruetzler K, Guzzella SE, Tscholl DW, et al. Blind intubation through self-pressurized, disposable Supraglottic airway laryngeal intubation masks: an international, multicenter, Prospective Cohort Study. Anesthesiology. 2017; 127(2):307–16. https://doi.org/10.1097/ALN.0000000000001710.
3. Law JA, Broemling N, Cooper RM, et al. The difficult airway with recommendations for management--part 1--difficult tracheal intubation encountered in an unconscious/induced patient. Can J Anaesth. 2013; 60(11):1089–118. https://doi.org/10.1007/s12630-013-0019-3.
4. Palczynski P, Bialka S, Misiolek H, et al. Thyromental height test as a new method for prediction of difficult intubation with double lumen tube. PLoS One. 2018;13(9):e0201944. https://doi.org/10.1371/journal.pone.0201944.
5. Rose DK, Cohen MM. The incidence of airway problems depends on the definition used. Can J Anaesth. 1996;43(1):30–4.
6. Gataure PS, Vaughan RS, Latto IP. Simulated difficult intubation. Comparison of the gum elastic bougie and the stylet. Anaesthesia. 1996;51(10):935–8.
7. Saasouh W, Laffey K, Turan A, et al. Degree of obesity is not associated with more than one intubation attempt: a large Centre experience. Br J Anaesth. 2018;120(5):1110–6. https://doi.org/10.1016/j.bja.2018.01.019.
8. Driver BE, Prekker ME, Klein LR, et al. Effect of use of a Bougie vs endotracheal tube and Stylet on first-attempt intubation success among patients with difficult airways undergoing emergency intubation: a randomized clinical trial comparison of intubation techniques in patients with difficult airways comparison of intubation techniques in patients with difficult airways. JAMA. 2018;319(21):2179–89. https://doi.org/10.1001/jama.2018.6496.
9. Green DW. Gum elastic bougie and simulated difficult intubation. Anaesthesia. 2003;58(4):391–2.
10. Evans A, Morris S, Petterson J, Hall JE. A comparison of the seeing optical Stylet and the gum elastic bougie in simulated difficult tracheal intubation: a manikin study. Anaesthesia. 2006;61(5):478–81.
11. Nolan JP, Wilson ME. Orotracheal intubation in patients with potential cervical spine injuries. An indication for the gum elastic bougie. Anaesthesia. 1993;48(7):630–3.
12. Jabre P, Combes X, Leroux B, et al. Use of gum elastic bougie for prehospital difficult intubation. Am J Emerg Med. 2005;23(4):552–5.
13. Shah KH, Kwong B, Hazan A, Batista R, Newman DH, Wiener D. Difficulties with gum elastic bougie intubation in an academic emergency department. J Emerg Med. 2011;41(4):429–34. https://doi.org/10.1016/j.jemermed.2010.05.005.
14. Latto IP, Stacey M, Mecklenburgh J, Vaughan RS. Survey of the use of the gum elastic bougie in clinical practice. Anaesthesia. 2002;57(4):379–84.
15. Ruetzler K, Roessler B, Potura L, et al. Performance and skill retention of intubation by paramedics using seven different airway devices--a manikin study. Resuscitation. 2011;82(5):593–7. https://doi.org/10.1016/j.resuscitation.2011.01.008.
16. Austin N, Krishnamoorthy V, Dagal A. Airway management in cervical spine injury. Int J Crit Illn Inj Sci. 2014;4(1):50–6. https://doi.org/10.4103/2229-5151.128013.
17. Manoach S, Paladino L. Manual in-line stabilization for acute airway management of suspected cervical spine injury: historical review and current questions. Ann Emerg Med. 2007;50(3):236–45.
18. Kovacs G, Law JA, McCrossin C, Vu M, Leblanc D, Gao J. A comparison of a fiberoptic stylet and a bougie as adjuncts to direct laryngoscopy in a manikin-simulated difficult airway. Ann Emerg Med. 2007;50(6):676–85.
19. Nolan JP, Wilson ME. An evaluation of the gum elastic bougie. Intubation times and incidence of sore throat. Anaesthesia. 1992;47(10):878–81.
20. Engoren M, Rochlen LR, Diehl MV, et al. Mechanical strain to maxillary incisors during direct laryngoscopy. BMC Anesthesiol. 2017;17(1):151. https://doi.org/10.1186/s12871-017-0442-z.
21. Kidd JF, Dyson A, Latto IP. Successful difficult intubation. Use of the gum elastic bougie. Anaesthesia. 1988;43(6):437–8.
22. Weisenberg M, Warters RD, Medalion B, Szmuk P, Roth Y, Ezri T. Endotracheal intubation with a gum-elastic bougie in unanticipated difficult direct laryngoscopy: comparison of a blind technique versus indirect laryngoscopy with a laryngeal mirror. Anesth Analg. 2002;95(4):1090–3.
23. Takenaka IMD, Aoyama KMD, Iwagaki TMD, et al. Approach combining the airway scope and the Bougie for minimizing movement of the cervical spine during endotracheal intubation. Anesthesiology. 2009;110(6):1335–40. https://doi.org/10.1097/ALN.0b013e31819fb44a.
24. Booth AWG, Wyssusek KH, Lee PK, Pelecanos AM, Sturgess D, van Zundert AAJ. Evaluation of the D-FLECT®; deflectable-tip bougie in a manikin with a simulated difficult airway. Br J Anaesth. 2018;121(5):1180–2. https://doi.org/10.1016/j.bja.2018.08.006.
25. Takenaka I, Aoyama K, Iwagaki T, Takenaka Y. Bougies as an aid for endotracheal intubation with the airway scope: bench and manikin comparison studies. BMC Anesthesiol. 2017;17(1):133. https://doi.org/10.1186/s12871-017-0424-1.
26. Marson BA, Anderson E, Wilkes AR, Hodzovic I. Bougie-related airway trauma: dangers of the hold-up sign. Anaesthesia. 2014;69(3):219–23. https://doi.org/10.1111/anae.12534.
27. Pande A, Ramachandran R, Rewari V. Bougie-associated bronchial injury complicated by a nephropleural fistula after percutaneous nephrolithotomy: a tale of two complications. BMJ Case Rep. 2018:bcr-2017-223969. https://doi.org/10.1136/bcr-2017-223969.
28. Kadry M, Popat M. Pharyngeal wall perforation--an unusual complication of blind intubation with a gum elastic bougie. Anaesthesia. 1999;54(4):404–5.

9

Supraglottic jet oxygenation and ventilation assisted fiberoptic intubation in a paralyzed patient with morbid obesity and obstructive sleep apnea

Hansheng Liang[1], Yuantao Hou[1], Huafeng Wei[2] and Yi Feng[1]* ⓘ

Abstract

Background: Hypoxia is a major concern and cause of morbidity or mortality during tracheal intubation after anesthesia induction in a pathological obese patient with obstructive sleep apnea (OSA). We introduce a case using Supraglottic jet oxygenation and ventilation (SJOV) to promote oxygenation/ventilation during fiberoptic intubation in a paralyzed patient with morbid obesity and OSA.

Case presentation: A 46-year-old man weighting 176 kg with BMI 53.7 kg/m2 was scheduled for gastric volume reduction surgery to reduce body weight under general anesthesia. SpO2 decreased during induction, and two hand pressured mask ventilation partial failed. We then placed WEI Nasal Jet Tube (WNJ) in the patient's right nostril to provide SJOV. Then fiberoptic bronchoscopy guided endotracheal intubation was performed via mouth approach, and vital signs were stable. The operation was successfully completed after 3 h. Patient recovered smoothly in hospital for 8 days and did not have any recall inside the operating room.

Conclusion: SJOV via WNJ could effectively maintain adequate oxygenation/ventilation during long time fiberoptic intubation in an apnea patient with morbid obesity and OSA after partial failure of two hand pressured mask ventilation, without obvious complications. This may provide a new effective approach for difficult airway management in these patients.

Keywords: Supraglottic, Jet ventilation, Oxygenation, Obesity, OSA, Fiberoptic bronchoscope, Intubation, Difficult airway

Background

The pathological difficult airway usually place patients in danger during general anesthesia induction [1], which may result in a high percentage of airway-related morbidity and mortality [2, 3]. Hypoxia is a major concern and cause of morbidity or mortality during tracheal intubation after anesthesia induction in a pathological obese patient with obstructive sleep apnea (OSA) [4–6]. A new approach to promote oxygenation/ventilation has been described during various difficult airway managements (*Peng J,Xie P,Wu CN,Wei HF,et al.*) [1, 7–11] and under propofol anesthesia (*Su DS,BJA 2017*), especially

in obese patient. We introduce a case using Supraglottic jet oxygenation and ventilation (SJOV) to promote oxygenation/ventilation during fiberoptic intubation in a paralyzed patient with morbid obesity and OSA.

Case presentation

A 46-year-old man weighting 176 kg with BMI 53.7 kg/m2 was scheduled for gastric volume reduction surgery to reduce body weight under general anesthesia. The patient was diagnosed of obstructive sleep apnea (OSA) 3 years ago, without treatment. Airway inspection showed short neck with circumference of 51 cm, limited neck extension due to its thick fat and the Mallampatti score-III. The patient felt tired preoperatively because of his sleep deprivation secondary to OSA. He was very

* Correspondence: fengyimzk@163.com
[1]Department of Anesthesiology, Peking University People' s Hospital, Beijing 100044, China

nervous and refused to consent for awake fiberoptic intubation under sedation.

We elected to perform tracheal intubation after anesthesia induction but keeping patient's spontaneous breathing to avoid hypoxia, with initial direct laryngoscopy using video laryngoscope, and back up with fiberoptic intubation and then laryngeal mask airway (LMA). Bispectral index (BIS) was used to monitor anesthesia depth.

Vital signs showed Bp 142/79 mmHg, HR 88 bpm, SpO2 96%, RR 22 bpm before anesthesia induction. Midazolam 3 mg and sufentanil 10 μg was given intravenously to reach BIS at 62 for sedation. Thereafter, intravenous 100 mg propofol was given and BIS fell to 51. Mask pressurized ventilation could be performed to maintain SpO2 100% with patient under continuous target controlled infusion (TCI) at propofol 3μg/mL.Direct laryngoscope with video laryngoscope was tried twice but failed because of the invisible glottis obstructed by Huge epiglottis (Grace IIb view). SpO2 fell to 75% at the end of second laryngoscopy. Two hand pressurized mask ventilation was initiated and became difficult, although SpO2 could be maintained around 88% with following vital signs: BP 133/73 mmHg, HR 86 bpm, normal sinus rhythm, BIS 57.We then placed WEI Nasal Jet Tube (WNJ), (Well Lead Medical Equipment Ltd., Guangzhou, China. Production batch number: 20140901) (Fig. 1) in the patient's right nostril to provide SJOV. The jet catheter of the WNJ was connected to an automatical jet ventilator-TKR-400 (Well Lead Medical Equipment Ltd.,Guangzhou, China.) with following working parameters: driving pressure (DP) 35 psi, respiratory rate (RR): 55 bpm, I/E ratio 1:3.SpO2 began to rise again and reached 100% at 1 min after initiation of SJOV. Thoracic

cage moved ups and downs during SJOV indication of both oxygenation and ventilation. We then administered intravenous rocuranium 60 mg, TCI propofol 4μg/mL and controlled ventilation was achieved using SJOV. Fiberoptic bronchoscopy guided endotracheal intubation was performed via mouth approach. Fiberoptic intubation was difficult due to hypertrophy of the patient's tongue and epiglottis but eventually succeded 5 min later. The vital signs at the end of successful intubation were as followings: SpO2 100%,BP 125/64 mmHg, HR 71 bpm, sinus rhythm, BIS 45.PetCO2 was not monitored during fiberoptic intubation due to the both Ports being not consistent and hurry to raise oxygenation. However,instant blood gas analysis showed pH 7.36, PaO2 124 mmHg and PaCO2 49 mmHg. Total time of SJOV via WNJ was about 7 min. No obvious barotrauma, nose bleeding etc.,was seen at the end of intubation.

The operation was successfully completed after 3 h. The patient was transferred to the ICU and was extubated in ICU without event. Patient recovered smoothly in hospital for 8 days and did not have any recall inside the operating room.

Discussion and conclusion

This case clearly demonstrated the SJOV via WNJ could effectively maintain adequate oxygenation/ventilation during long time fiberoptic intubation in an apnea patient with morbid obesity and OSA after partial failure of two hand pressured mask ventilation, without obvious complications. This may provide a new effective approach for difficult airway management in these patients.

According to the world health organization (WHO) standards established 1989, body mass index (BMI) ≥28

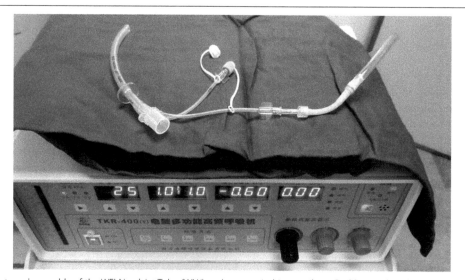

Fig. 1 Components and assembly of the WEI Nasal Jet Tube (WNJ) and automatical jet ventilator: $P_{et}CO_2$ = end tidal CO_2 pressure (Compliance with ethical standards: The automatical jet ventilator-TKR-400 and WNJT upon examination and approval by the company, pictures can be used)

is defined as obesity, BMI≥40 is defined as morbid obesity [12]. Adipose tissue accumulated in pharyngeal can make patient's pharyngeal cavity narrow and make the oropharyngeal muscles and soft tissue collapse, obstructing the airway [12, 13]. Obviously, this increases the patient's workload of breathing and reducing functional residual capacity, causing ventilation/perfusion mismatch,eventually hypoxia and intolerance of hypoxia [14]. The incidence of difficult intubation in morbid obesity patients during general anesthesia induction undergoing abdominal surgery can be as high as 24% [15], and the awake intubation may be required in about 8% of patients [15]. The potential upper respiratory tract obstruction in OSA patient contribute to its high perioperative complication rate at about 19.6% [16]. The incidence of failed intubation in OSA patients is10 times higher than normal [17], while the incidence of intubation failure about patients with morbid obesity and OSA increases to 100 times [17, 18]. We discussed awake intubation with this patient on pre-anesthesia visit, but the patient was nervous and could not be comforted and refused the plan. In addition, the patient's large neck circumference makes it difficult to identify the cricothyroid membrane. Since we underestimated the difficulty of this patient's airway, and this patient was very nervous and unwilling to be stimulated, we did not choose awake intubation or awake look. Even though this case was an unanticipated difficult airway, we were able to maintain and improve oxygenation using WEI nasal jet tube for supraglottic jet oxygenation and ventilation,because we have some experiences applying this device on obese patients. We have completed a randomized controlled study(Registration number, ChiCTR 1,800,017,028) of supraglottic jet ventilation to improve oxygenation in obesity patients, and the results revealed that Nasal Jet tube could prevent patients suffering from desaturation during propofol-remifentanil protocol undergoing hysteroscopy. We are in the process of writing a paper.

The most important features of supraglottic airway is most characteristic of the patient with pathological obesity and OSA is serious airway collapse after anesthesia due to hypertrophy of the patient's tongue,epiglottis and supraglottic muscles [19]. Airway collapse make supraglottic airway narrower, making the air flow of the mask pressurized ventilation difficult to pass the narrow area [20]. WNJ can pass the narrow airway and support the collapse and resolve the ventilation problem. WNJ is designed to be soft to void injury of nasal mucosa damage and bleeding. The evaluation of nasal cavity and the use of the lubricant also ease its insertion and minimizing nose bleeding. In our case, nasal jet tube maintained this patient's oxygenation. According to the "Difficult Airway Society 2015 guidelines for management of unanticipated difficult intubation in adults" [21],

muscle relaxant can make tracheal intubation easier, and prevent laryngospasm, so we administered rocuronium. Succinylcholine should be a better choice in this case, but we don't have it in our department. With quick and short-acting effect, rocuronium could exert muscle relaxant effect 60 s after administration, which is equivalent with succinylcholine.

The capacity of tolerance to hypoxia in pathological obese patients with OSA is reduced significantly. It is critical in this case to have an effective method to maintain the patient's oxygenation during intubation because of the shorter Oxygen Saturation Falling Time (OSFT) [22]. The definition of OSFT is the time of the patient's SpO2 dropped to 90% after full oxygenation 100% oxygen inhaled and removed nitrogen [22, 23]. The obese patient's OSFT is only 163 s due to the increased oxygen consumption and the changes in the airway described above,but the average of a normal adult is 526 s [22–24]. So it is almost impossible to complete this fiberoptic intubation without maintaining effective oxygenation using SJOV via WNJ for 7 min in this anesthetized and paralyzed morbid obese patient with OSA. This patient didn't reach "can't intubate and can't ventilate"(CICV) so that LMA placement was not tried, nor did the emergent tracheotomy was considered.

In combination with previous publications [1, 7–11], It seems that SJOV has following advantages compared to the transtracheal jet ventilation (TTJV) recommended by American Society of Anesthesiologists (ASA) guidelines for the management of difficult airway. First,SJOV via WNJ is less invasive than TTJV which may increase the incidence of barotrauma barotrauma [7, 19]. Secondly, it usually take longer time to perform effective TTJV than placement of WNJ in the nose and could be very difficult to achieve successful TTJV in obese patient with thick neck. Thirdly, it is convenient to monitor ventilation using the built-in port for PetCO2 monitoring in WNJ. Forth and most importantly, SJOV maintain the open feature of airway during jet ventilation, minimizing or preventing the severe barotrauma, often seen during the use of TTJV, especially in emergent difficult airway management [1].

In summary, SJOV via WNJ seems to be an effective new approach to maintain adequate oxygenation/ventilation during difficult airway management in an apnea patient with morbid obesity and OSA.

Abbreviations
ASA: American Society of Anesthesiologists; BIS: Bispectral index; BMI: Body mass index; CICV: Can't intubate and can't ventilate; DP: Driving pressure; LMA: Laryngeal mask airway; OSA: Obstructive sleep apnea; OSFT: Oxygen Saturation Falling Time; SJOV: Supraglottic jet oxygenation and ventilation; TCI: Target controlled infusion; TTJV: Transtracheal jet ventilation; WHO: World health organization; WNJ: WEI Nasal Jet Tube

Acknowledgements
Not applicable.

Author details
[1]Department of Anesthesiology, Peking University People's Hospital, Beijing 100044, China. [2]Department of Anesthesiology and Critical Care, Hospital of the University of Pennsylvania, Philadelphia, PA 19104, USA.

References
1. Peng J, Ye J, Wei H, et al. Supraglottic jet ventilation in difficult airway management. J Emerg Med. 2012;43(2):382–90.
2. Fritzsche K, Osmers A. Anesthetic management in laryngotracheal surgery. High-frequency jet ventilation as strategy forventilation during general anesthesia. HNO. 2011;59(9):931–41.
3. Leiter R, Aliverti A, Frykholm P, et al. Comparison of superimposed high-frequency jet ventilation with conventional jet ventilation for laryngeal surgery. Br J Anaesth. 2012;108(4):690–7.
4. Ross-Anderson DJ, Ferguson C, Patel A. Transtracheal jet ventilation in 50 patients with severe airway compromise and stridor. Br J Anaesth. 2011; 106(1):140–4.
5. Ihra GC, Tsai CJ, Kimberger O. Intrinsic positive end-expiratory pressure at various frequencies of supraglottic jet ventilation in a model of dynamic upper airway obstruction. Anesth Analg. 2010;111(3):703–6.
6. Cobas MA, Martin ND, Barkin HB. Two lost airways and one unexpected problem: undiagnosed tracheal stenosis in a morbidly obese patient. J Clin Anesth. 2016;35:225–7.
7. Li Q, Xie P, Wei H, et al. Supraglottic jet oxygenation and ventilation saved a patient with 'cannot intubate and cannot ventilate' emergency difficult airway. J Anesth. 2017;31(1):144–7.
8. Wu CN, Ma WH, Wei JQ, et al. Laryngoscope and a new tracheal tube assist Lightwand intubation in difficult airways due to unstable cervical spine. PLoSOne. 2015;10:202–31.
9. Wei HF. A new tracheal tube and methods to facilitate ventilation and placement in emergency airway management. Resuscitation. 2006;70:438–44.
10. Yang ZY, Meng Q, Xu YH, Wang JW, Yu DS, Wei HF. Supraglottic jet oxygenation and ventilation during colonoscopy under monitored anesthesia care: a controlled randomized clinical trial. Eur Rev Med Pharmacol Sci. 2016;20:1168–73.
11. Dziewit JA, Wei H. Supraglottic jet ventilation assists intubation in a Marfan's syndrome patient with a difficult airway. J Clin Anesth. 2011;23:407–9.
12. Mushambi MC, Kinsella SM, Popat M, et al. Obstetric Anaesthetists' Association and Difficult Airway Society guidelines for the management of difficult and failed tracheal intubation in obstetrics. Anaesthesia. 2015;70(11): 1286–306.
13. Troop C. The difficult airway and or obesity and the importance of positioning. Br J Anaesth. 2016;117(5):674–5.
14. Dohrn N, Sommer T, Larsen JF, et al. Difficult Tracheal Intubation in Obese Gastric Bypass patients. Obes Surg. 2016;26(11):2640–7.
15. Whalen FX, Gajieo T, Hompson GB, et al. The effects ofthe alveolar recruitment maneuver and positive end-expiratory pressure on arterial oxygenation during laparoscopie bariatrie surgery. Anesth Analg. 2006; 102(1):298–305.
16. Corso RM, Cattano D, Maitan S, et al. Post analysis simulated correlation of the El-Ganzouri airway difficulty score with difficult airway. Braz J Anesthesiol. 2016;66(3):298–303.
17. Stierer TL, Wfiight C, George A, et al. Risk assessment of obstructive sleep apnea in a population of patients undergoing ambulatory surgery. J Clin Sleep Med. 2010;6(5):467–72.
18. Gupata RM, Parvizl J. Postoperative complication in patients with obstructive sleep apnea syndrome undergoing hip or knee replacement:a case-control study. Mayo Clin Proc. 2001;76(9):897–904.
19. Sato S, Sato Y, Isono S, et al. Mask Ventilation during Induction of General Anesthesia: Influences of Obstructive Sleep Apnea. Anesthesiology. 2017; 126(1):28–38.
20. Domi R, Laho H. Anesthetic challenges in the obese patient. J Anesth. 2012; 26(5):758–65.
21. Frerk C, Mitchell VS, McNarry AF, et al. Difficult airway society 2015 guidelines for management of unanticipated difficult intubation in adults. Br J Anaesth. 2015;115(6):827–48.
22. Gray EL, McKenzie DK, Eckert DJ. Obstructive Sleep Apnea without Obesity Is Common and Difficult to Treat: Evidence for a Distinct Pathophysiological Phenotype. J Clin Sleep Med. 2017;13(1):81–8.
23. Sprung J, Whalley DG, Faleone T. The effects of tidal volume and respiratory rate on oxygenation and respiratory mechanics during laparoseopy in morbidly obese patient. Anesth Analg. 2003;97(1):268–74.
24. Reinius H, Jonsson L, Gustafsson S, et al. Prevention of ateleetasis in morbidly obese patients during general anesthesia and paralysis:a computerized tomography study. Anesthesiology. 2009;111(5):979–87.

10

Laryngeal mask airway reduces incidence of post-operative sore throat after thyroid surgery compared with endotracheal tube

Yahong Gong, Xiaohan Xu, Jin Wang, Lu Che, Weijia Wang and Jie Yi[*]

Abstract

Background: Sore throat is a remarkable complication after thyroid surgery with endotracheal tube (ETT). Many studies revealed that laryngeal mask airway (LMA) might reduce the incidence and severity of postoperative sore throat. However, little is known about the use of a flexible reinforced LMA (FLMA) in thyroid surgery. The purpose of this study was to explore the potential benefits of FLMA compared with ETT on postoperative sore throat.

Methods: In this prospective, single-blinded, randomized, controlled trial, ninety-six patients aged 20–80 years, scheduled for elective radical thyroidectomy under general anesthesia were enrolled. They were randomly divided into ETT group and FLMA group. All the included patients received total intravenous anesthesia (with propofol, fentanyl and rocuronium) and controlled mechanical ventilation during the surgery. Cuff pressure of ETT and FLMA were strictly controlled. Incidence and severity of postoperative sore throat, numbness and hoarseness at 1, 24, and 48 h after surgery was evaluated and compared between the two groups. Incidence and severity of buckling during extubation and the hemodynamic profile during intubation were also recorded and compared.

Results: The incidence of sore throat and hoarseness was significantly lower in FLMA group than those in ETT group at 1 h, 24 h and 48 h postoperatively, as well as the severity of sore throat. Compared to ETT group, there was a significantly lower incidence of buckling during extubation and less fluctuation of HR and BP at 1 min and 3 min after intubation in FLMA group.

Conclusions: Patients undergoing thyroid surgery with FLMA had less postoperative laryngopharyngeal symptoms when compared with ETT. The use of FLMA also achieved less buckling during extubation and better hemodynamic profiles during intubation.

Keywords: Sore throat, Thyroid surgery, Postoperative, Endotracheal tube, Flexible laryngeal mask airway

* Correspondence: easyue@163.com
Department of Anesthesiology, Peking Union Medical College Hospital
(PUMCH), 1 Shuai Fuyuan, Wangfujing Street, Dongcheng District, Beijing
100730, China

Background

Sore throat is a common complication after general anesthesia with endotracheal tube (ETT) [1]. Incidence of moderate to severe sore throat varies from 15 to 62% [1–5]. In the case of thyroid surgery, an even higher incidence of approximately 68.4% was reported [6–8]. Postoperative sore throat could last 2 to 3 days, and could be a real concern for patients and causes distress and anxiety during the recovery [9], thus may need additional attention from doctors and nurses. This problem would be even more prominent in ambulatory and overnight stay thyroid surgery. Many studies suggested that laryngeal mask airway may reduce potential damage to the vocal cord and thus prevent postoperative laryngopharyngeal symptoms [10]. In 1991, Greatorex et al. firstly published their experience of using LMA in thyroid surgery [11]. However, little information has been reported about the use of a flexible reinforced LMA (FLMA) during thyroidectomy and the incidence of postoperative laryngopharyngeal discomfort. With the clinical goal of reducing the incidence of postoperative sore throat, the aim of this study was to explore the potential benefits of FLMA compared with ETT on postoperative sore throat.

Methods

Subjects

This single-blinded, parallel, controlled trial with equal randomization was approved by the Institutional Review Board of Peking Union Medical College Hospital (PUMCH) (IRB No. S-631) and registered in Chinese Clinical Trial Registry (ChiCTR-IOR-15006602) on May 23th, 2015. Informed consent was obtained from all individual participants included in the study. The study protocol adhered to CONSORT guidelines.

Nighty-six patients with American Society of Anesthesiology Physical Status Classification (ASA)I-II, aged 20–80 years, scheduled for elective radical thyroidectomy under general anesthesia from May 26th 2015 to April 2016 were enrolled. Exclusion criteria were: preoperative sore throat, hoarseness, dysphagia, high risk of regurgitation or aspiration, obesity (body mass index, BMI > 30 kg/m^2), symptoms of upper respiratory infection within 2 weeks before surgery, previous surgeries of the oral cavity or pharynx, and estimated surgery time > 4 h. All the patients scheduled for thyroid surgery received laryngofiberscope preoperatively to evaluate the function of vocal cord. Cases without definitive identification of recurrent laryngeal nerve or with mechanical or thermal injury of recurrent laryngeal nerve during surgery were also excluded.

Study design

The admitted patients were randomly assigned to ETT group (ETT group, $n = 48$) or flexible reinforced LMA group (LMA group, $n = 48$) by a computer-generated table of random numbers immediately prior to surgery. No restriction was used for randomization. The random numbers for assignment were sealed in opaque envelopes, which could only be opened by the anesthesia providers.

The study was conducted in the operating rooms in Peking Union Medical College Hospital in Beijing, China. In ETT group, patients were intubated with a high-volume, low-pressure-cuff plain endotracheal tube (Covidien, Mexico). In order to control the possible bias, smaller sized ETTs (size 7.0 for female patients and 7.5 for male) were chosen for our patients, which were reported to be associated with a lower incidence of sore throat [6]. The cuff of ETT was inflated with room air, and cuff pressure was strictly adjusted to 25cmH$_2$O with a handheld aneroid manometer (VBM, Einsteinstr, Germany). In LMA group, a flexible reinforced LMA (LMA Flexible™, Laryngeal Mask Company Limited, Seychelles, Singapore) was used according to the patient's body weight (BW) (size 3 (BW < 50 kg), 4 (BW 50–70 kg), or 5 (BW > 70 kg)). The cuff of flexible reinforced LMA was fully deflated before insertion. After lubrication of the posterior surface with water-based jelly, FLMA was inserted with digital intraoral manipulation. Cuff pressure of FLMA was adjusted to 40cmH$_2$O with manometer. Proper position was confirmed by a visualization of more than half vocal cords through bronchoscopy.

The patients, data collectors and outcome assessors were blinded to the group assignment. In order to ensure patients' safety, the anesthesiologist in charge of the anesthesia was not blinded to the group assignment. ETT and FLMA were placed by two experienced anesthesiologists who had successfully inserted ETT for over 300 times in thyroid surgeries and ETT for over 300 times in other surgeries. All the surgeries were carried out by one surgical team.

Anesthesia management

On arrival at the operating room, all the patients received midazolam 0.03 mg·kg-1 as a premedication. Intraoperative monitoring included electrocardiography, noninvasive blood pressure, pulse oximetry (SpO$_2$), capnograpy (EtCO$_2$), gas analysis, tidal volume, airway pressure and bispectral index (BIS). Anesthesia was induced with target-controlled infusion of propofol (at effect-site concentration of 3–3.5 μg/ml) and bolus injection of fentanyl 2 μg/kg and rocuronium 0.6 mg/kg.

During the operation, anesthesia was maintained with intermittent bolus injection of fentanyl and target controlled infusions (TCI) of propofol using Graseby 3500 Anaesthesia Syringe Pump - Diprifusor (Smiths-medical, UK). The systolic blood pressure fluctuation was maintained within 15% of baseline and BIS value between 40 and 60 (Aspect XP, space Lab, USA). Propofol infusion was discontinued around 10 min before the end of surgery and neostigmine 6 mg was given to antagonize the residual muscle relaxant. FLMA/

ETT was extracted when the patient could follow voice commands and EtCO$_2$ was bellow 45 mmHg on spontaneous respiration. None of the patients received additional analgesics in PACU or wards during postoperative 48 h.

Data collection

The primary end point was the incidence and severity of postoperative sore throat. Secondary end points were: (1) the incidence and severity of buckling during extubation, (2) postoperative numbness and hoarseness, (3) hemodynamic profiles. Laryngopharyngeal symptoms were evaluated at 1, 24, and 48 h after surgery by three anesthesiologists who were blinded to the treatment group of the patient. Sore throat was assessed using a visual analog scale (VAS, 0 = none, 10 = most severe). Numbness was evaluated according to patients' self-report. Hoarseness was assessed based on whether there were changes of the voice to harsh or strained. The scale used to evaluate the severity of buckling during extubation was a three-graded scale: 0 = None, 1 = Mild buckling (once/twice cough without head lifting-off the bed and lasting less than 15 s), 2 = Severe buckling (cough more than twice with head lifting-off the bed or lasting longer than 15 s). In addition, the diastolic blood pressure (DBP), systolic blood pressure (SBP) and heart rate (HR) [12] were recorded the time before, at 1 min, 3 min and 5 min after endotracheal intubation/insertion of LMA.

Statistical analysis

Previous study showed that the incidence of sore throat at 6 h after thyroid surgery was 84% for the control group [5]. If a 30% decrease in the incidence of sore throat was considered clinically significant, power analysis program (G* power 3.1) calculated that 35 patients per group were needed for a power of 80% and an error of 0.05. Considering a 10% dropout rate, 38 patients for each group were necessary. SPSS software (version 13.0; SPSS, Inc., Chicago, IL, USA) was used for data analysis. Continuous normally and non-normally distributed data was described as mean ± standard deviation and median [13], respectively. Between-group demographic data with normal distribution was analyzed with unpaired t-test or Chi Square test, if appropriate. Hemodynamic data at each time point was compared by one-way ANOVA. The incidences of sore throat, hoarseness, numbness and buckling were analyzed using Fisher's exact test. The Mann–Whitney U test was used to compare the severity of sore throat. A two-sided p-value < 0.05 was considered statistically significant.

Results

Demographic characteristics

A total of 90 patients from May 2015 to April 2016 were included in the final analysis. One patient from ETT group was excluded since surgery time lasted longer than 4 h. Three patients (2 from ETT group and 1 from LMA group) were excluded during the study period due to a change in the operation plan. Another two patients (from LMA group) were excluded because of loss of follow up (Fig. 1). Demographic characteristics are presented in Table 1. There were no differences between

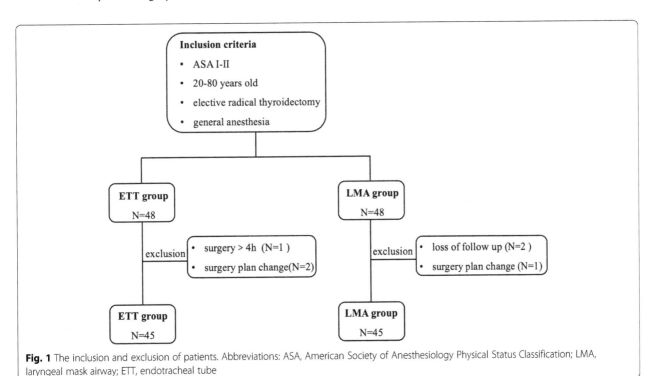

Fig. 1 The inclusion and exclusion of patients. Abbreviations: ASA, American Society of Anesthesiology Physical Status Classification; LMA, laryngeal mask airway; ETT, endotracheal tube

Table 1 Demographic data

	Group ETT (n = 45)	Group LMA (n = 45)	p-value
Age (yrs)	42.1 ± 10.9	42.7 ± 10.6	0.777
Male/Female (n)	9/36	8/37	0.788
Body Weight (kg)	64.1 ± 10.2	65.5 ± 13.3	0.580
Body Height (cm)	164.7 ± 5.7	165.1 ± 7.3	0.711
Operative time (min)	48.20 ± 21.45	54.00 ± 21.63	0.205

Values are means ± SDs or number of patients. Between-group demographic data with normal distribution was analyzed with unpaired t-test or Chi Square test, if appropriate. A two-sided p-value < 0.05 was considered statistically significant
Abbreviations: ETT endotracheal tube, FLMA flexible laryngeal mask airway

the groups regarding age, gender, body weight, height and duration of surgery.

Postoperative laryngopharyngeal symptoms

The incidence of sore throat was significantly lower in group LMA than in the group ETT at 1 h (48.9% vs 68.9%, $p < 0.001$), 24 h (37.8% vs 51.1%, $p = 0.012$) and 48 h (6.7% vs 24.4%, $p = 0.023$) postoperatively (Table 2). The incidence of hoarseness was also significantly less in the group LMA than in the group ETT at 1, 24 and 48 h postoperatively (8.9% vs. 57.8%, $p < 0.001$; 6.7% vs. 28.9%, $p < 0.001$; 0% vs. 13.3%, $p = 0.002$) (Table 2). Postoperative numbness was comparable in two groups (Table 2). The severity of sore throat in the group LMA was significantly lower than in the group ETT at 1 h (0[0–4] vs. 2 [0–7], $p = 0.006$) and 48 h (0 [0–1] vs. 0 [0–2] at 48 h, $p = 0.017$) after surgery (Table 3). VAS score of sore throat was higher in the group ETT than in the group LMA at 24 h after surgery, but the difference was not significant.

Table 2 Postoperative laryngopharyngeal symptoms

	Group ETT (n = 45)	Group LMA (n = 45)	p-value
Sore throat			
PO 1 h	31 (68.9%)	22 (48.9%)	< 0.001*
PO 24 h	23 (51.1%)	17 (37.8%)	0.012*
PO 48 h	11 (24.4%)	3 (6.7%)	0.023*
Hoarseness			
PO 1 h	26 (57.8%)	4 (8.9%)	< 0.001*
PO 24 h	13 (28.9%)	3 (6.7%)	< 0.001*
PO 48 h	6 (13.3%)	0 (0%)	0.002*
Numbness			
PO 1 h	1 (2.2%)	3 (6.7%)	0.738
PO 24 h	1 (2.2%)	0 (0%)	0.085
PO 48 h	0 (0%)	0 (0%)	NA

Values are expressed as number of patients (percentage). The incidences of sore throat, hoarseness and numbness were analyzed using Fisher's exact test. A two-sided p-value < 0.05 was considered statistically significant. * p<0.005
Abbreviations: ETT endotracheal tube, FLMA flexible laryngeal mask airway, PO post-operative, NA not applicable

Table 3 Severity of sore throat

	Group LMA (n = 45)	Group ETT (n = 45)	p-value
PO 1 h	0 (0–4)	2 (0–7)	0.006
PO 24 h	0 (0–3)	1 (0–5)	0.07
PO 48 h	0 (0–1)	0 (0–2)	0.017*

Values are presented as median (range). VAS, 0 none, 10 most severe. The Mann–Whitney U test was used to compare the severity of sore throat. A two-sided p-value < 0.05 was considered statistically significant. * p<0.005
Abbreviations: ETT endotracheal tube, FLMA flexible laryngeal mask airway, PO post-operative

Hemodynamic profiles and buckling

Baseline and pre-intubation HR, SBP and DBP were comparable between the two groups, but the values were significantly lower in Group LMA than in Group ETT at 1 min and 3 min after endotracheal intubation or insertion of FLMA (Fig. 2). There was a significantly lower incidence of buckling during extubation in the group LMA compared to the group ETT ($p < 0.001$, Table 4).

Discussion

The results of this study showed that compared with the endotracheal tube, the use of a flexible LMA during thyroidectomy decreased the incidence and severity of postoperative laryngopharyngeal symptoms, including sore throat and hoarseness. Furthermore, flexible LMA achieved better hemodynamic profile during intubation and less buckling during extubation.

Many studies have shown that the incidence of sore throat was higher after thyroid surgery when compared to general cases that did not involve neck surgery. This problem may be attributed to tracheal mucosal trauma, laryngeal edema, vocal cord hematoma or bilateral vocal cords palsy [12–14].

As a supraglottic device, LMA is positioned superior to the larynx and thus can cause less tracheal injury [15]. The use of LMA in general anesthesia could lower the incidence of postoperative sore throat than an ETT [16]. Although LMA may be dislocated during thyroidectomy due to neck hyperextension and surgical manipulation, the successful use of FLMA in head and neck surgeries [16, 17] and gained more and more popularity because it may protect the airway with less postoperative airway morbidity [18–20]. However, information about its use in thyroidectomy and the incidence of postoperative laryngopharyngeal discomfort is rare. Jung-Hee Ryu et al. [9] reported that an FLMA placed during thyroidectomy decreased the incidence and severity of postoperative laryngopharyngeal symptoms [21]. However, the reported incidence of sore throat in Jung-Hee Ryu's study (97–100%) was significantly higher than that in other studies (68.4%), and the sample size was not large. Thereby we aimed to revalidate the hypothesis that FLMA was superior to ETT in reducing postoperative sore throat.

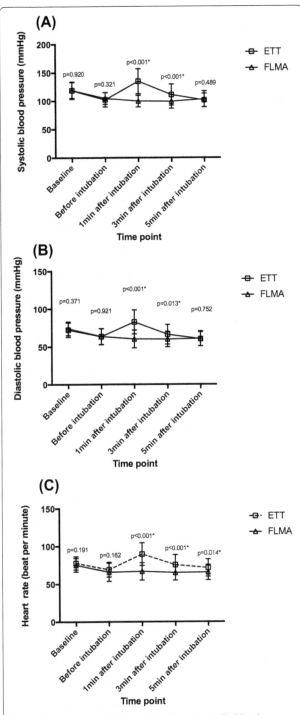

Fig. 2 Hemodynamic Profiles and Buckling. **a** systolic blood pressure changes during intubation, **b** diastolic blood pressure changes during intubation, **c** heart rate changes during intubation. Data between FLMA and ETT group at each time point was compared by one-way ANOVA and a $p < 0.05$ was considered to be statistically significant. *$p < 0.05$. Abbreviations: FLMA, reinforced laryngeal mask airway; ETT, endotracheal tube

Table 4 Incidence of buckling during extubation

	Group LMA ($n = 45$)	Group ETT ($n = 45$)	p-value
Buckling			
0	43 (95.6%)	16 (35.6%)	< 0.001*
1	2 (4.4%)	17 (37.8%)	
2	0 (0.0%)	12 (26.7%)	

Values are presented as number (percentage). The incidences of buckling were analyzed using Fisher's exact test. A two-sided p-value < 0.05 was considered statistically significant. * $p<0.005$
Abbreviations: *ETT* endotracheal tube, *FLMA* flexible laryngeal mask airway

The causes for postoperative laryngopharyngeal discomfort were complicated. Several prospective clinical trials aimed to illustrate the risk factors for postoperative sore throat. Tracheal-tube size was considered to be a strong risk factor by different researchers [1, 6, 8]. The application of topical lignocaine gel to the ETT cuff may also affect the general incidence of sore throat, although its effect is controversial [8, 22]. In order to strictly control those potential confounding factors, a relatively smaller ETT was chosen and topical oxybuprocaine gel was applied to the ETT cuff in our study. Previous studies reported that higher cuff pressure of LMA might be associated with higher incidence of sore throat [23, 24], so the cuff pressure of flexible LMA was limited to 40 mmHg in our study to rule out the injury caused by overinflated cuff. Hisham AN. et al. suggested that extent of surgical procedure were also significant contributing factors affecting the postoperative recovery [8]. Therefore, we only recruited patients with thyroid cancer underdoing radical thyroidectomy, and all the surgeries were carried out by one surgeon group. Finally, analgesia methods may also have impacts on the laryngopharyngeal symptoms. A recent study indicated that high-dose intraoperative remifentanil infusion is associated with increased incidence of postoperative sore throat [25]. To minimizing such confounding effects, patients included in our study received standard intraoperative pain management strategy and no additional analgesics were given postoperatively.

The reasons why LMA is superior to ETT in reducing laryngopharyngeal discomfort may also be multifactorial. First, the movement of the ETT during positioning or traction on the trachea in thyroidectomy is an important attributor. This type of injury could be avoided with the use of flexible LMA. Second, the extent of surgical traction could be reduced because the mild leakage around LMA during manipulation may alert the surgeon of the excessive traction. Therefore, the operation may be more meticulous with an LMA airway. Less traction and gentler manipulation may result in less inflammation and edema in surgical area, and thereby less postoperative sore throat. However, this hypothesis needs further validation.

Our study was limited in the following aspects. First, the air seal of LMA was satisfactory in radial thyroidectomy in our study. However, the safety of LMA should be prudently evaluated if estimated surgery time is longer than 4 h. Second, since the anesthesia and operations were performed by experienced physicians, our conclusions might be less applicable in medical centers lacking specialized staff. Furthermore, the benefits for FLMA over ETT could be due to a more careful manipulation and less tissue injury from surgical team for the concern of FLMA displacement. Third, considering that hoarseness was assessed only by the change of voice, it could be more accurate if vocal chord evaluation or recurrent laryngeal nerve stimulation was used. Finally, recurrent laryngeal nerve injury is an obviously more serious complication of thyroid surgery than temporary postoperative sore throat and hoarseness, thus should be avoided by using an endotracheal tube with an electrode, which can help monitor of the function of recurrent laryngeal nerve. Therefore, LMA is not an appropriate choice in patients at high risk of nerve injury.

Our study provides clues for further research. First, considering the rapid developments of supraglottic device, the performance of other types of supraglottic device in thyroid surgeries can be investigated in the future. Second, the laryngopharyngeal symptoms after postoperative 48 h can also be further studied, since sore throat and hoarseness may last for 4 days or more.

Conclusions

In conclusion, patients undergoing thyroid surgery with FLMA had less postoperative laryngopharyngeal symptoms, when compared with ETT. The use of FLMA also achieved less buckling during extubation and better hemodynamic profiles during intubation.

Abbreviations
ASA: American Society of Anesthesiology Physical Status Classification; BIS: Bispectral index; BMI: Body mass index; BW: Body weight; DBP: Diastolic blood pressure; EtCO$_2$: Capnograpy; ETT: Endotracheal tube; FLMA: Flexible reinforced laryngeal mask airway; HR: Heart rate; LMA: Laryngeal mask airway; PUMCH: Peking Union Medical College Hospital; SBP: Systolic blood pressure; SpO$_2$: Pulse oximetry; TCI: Target controlled infusions; VAS: Visual analog scale

Acknowledgements
Not applicable.

Authors' contributions
YG conducted the study, analyzed the data and composed the article. XX analyzed the data, prepared the figure and revised the manuscript. JW helped with registration. LC and WW helped revise the manuscript. JY helped design and conduct the study. All authors read and approved the final manuscript.

References
1. Jensen PJ, Hommelgaard P, Sondergaard P, et al. Sore throat after operation: influence of tracheal intubation, intracuff pressure and type of cuff. Br J Anaesth. 1982;54(4):453–7.
2. Eidi M, Seyed Toutounchi SJ, Kolahduzan K, et al. Comparing the effect of dexamethasone before and after tracheal intubation on sore throat after Tympanoplasty surgery: a randomized controlled trial. Iran J Otorhinolaryngol. 2014;26(75):89–98.
3. Biro P, Seifert B, Pasch T. Complaints of sore throat after tracheal intubation: a prospective evaluation. Eur J Anaesthesiol. 2005;22(4):307–11.
4. Sanou J, Ilboudo D, Rouamba A, et al. Sore throat after tracheal intubation. Cahiers d'anesthesiologie. 1996;44(3):203–6.
5. Thomas DV. Hoarseness and sore throat after tracheal intubation. Small tubes prevent. Anaesthesia. 1993;48(4):355–6.
6. McHardy FE, Chung F. Postoperative sore throat: cause, prevention and treatment. Anaesthesia. 1999;54(5):444–53.
7. Martis C, Athanassiades S. Post-thyroidectomy laryngeal edema. A survey of fifty-four cases. Am J Surg. 1971;122(1):58–60.
8. Hisham AN, Roshilla H, Amri N, et al. Post-thyroidectomy sore throat following endotracheal intubation. ANZ J Surg. 2001;71(11):669–71.
9. Ryu JH, Yom CK, Park DJ, et al. Prospective randomized controlled trial on the use of flexible reinforced laryngeal mask airway (LMA) during total thyroidectomy: effects on postoperative laryngopharyngeal symptoms. World J Surg. 2014;38(2):378–84.
10. Premachandra DJ. Application of the laryngeal mask airway to thyroid surgery and the preservation of the recurrent laryngeal nerve. Ann R Coll Surg Engl. 1992;74(3):226.
11. Greatorex RA, Denny NM. Application of the laryngeal mask airway to thyroid surgery and the preservation of the recurrent laryngeal nerve. Ann R Coll Surg Engl. 1992;74(3):225–6.
12. Lombardi CP, Raffaelli M, D'Alatri L, Marchese MR, Rigante M, Paludetti G, Bellantone R. Voice and swallowing changes after thyroidectomy in patients without inferior laryngeal nerve injuries. Surgery. 2006;140:1026–32. https://doi.org/10.1016/j.surg.2006.08.008.
13. Soylu L, Ozbas S, Uslu HY, Kocak S. The evaluation of the causes of subjective voice disturbances after thyroid surgery. Am J Surg. 2007;194:317–22.
14. Stojadinovic A, Shaha AR, Orlikoff RF, Nissan A, Kornak MF, Singh B, Boyle JO, Shah JP, Brennan MF, Kraus DH. Prospective functional voice assessment in patients undergoing thyroid surgery. Ann Surg. 2002;236:823–32.
15. Yu SH, Beirne OR. Laryngeal mask airways have a lower risk of airway complications compared with endotracheal intubation: a systematic review. J Oral Maxillofac Surg. 2010;68:2359–76.
16. Martin-Castro C, Montero A. Flexible laryngeal mask as an alternative to reinforced tracheal tube for upper chest, head and neck oncoplastic surgery. Eur J Anaesthesiol. 2008;25:261–6.
17. Quinn AC, Samaan A, McAteer EM, Moss E, Vucevic M. The reinforced laryngeal mask airway for dento-alveolar surgery. Br J Anaesth. 1996;77:185–8.
18. Webster AC, Morley-Forster PK, Janzen V, Watson J, Dain SL, Taves D, Dantzer D. Anesthesia for intranasal surgery: a comparison between tracheal intubation and the flexible rein- forced laryngeal mask airway. Anesth Analg. 1999;88:421–5.
19. Williams PJ, Bailey PM. Comparison of the reinforced laryngeal mask airway and tracheal intubation for adenotonsil- lectomy. Br J Anaesth. 1993;70:30–3.
20. Brimacombe J. The advantages of the LMA over the tracheal tube or facemask: a meta-analysis. Can J Anaesth. 1995;42:1017–23.
21. Kumar C, Mishra A. Prospective randomized controlled trial on the use of flexible reinforced laryngeal mask airway (LMA) during Total thyroidectomy: effects on postoperative Laryngopharyngeal symptoms: reply. World J Surg. 2014;39(3):810.
22. Suma KV, Bhaskar KU. Prevention of post intubation sore throat by inflating endotracheal tube cuff with alkalinized lignocaine. Indian J Public Health Res Dev. 2015;6(4):200.
23. Gross. The influence of laryngeal mask airway (LMA) cuff pressure on postoperative sore throat: 19AP3–1. Eur J Anaesthesiol. 2010;27(47):250.
24. Kang JE, Oh CS, Choi JW, et al. Postoperative Pharyngolaryngeal adverse events with laryngeal mask airway (LMA supreme) in laparoscopic surgical procedures with cuff pressure limiting 25 cmH2O: prospective, blind, and randomised study. Sci World J. 2014;2014(1):709801.
25. Park JH, Lee YC, Lee J, et al. The influence of high-dose intraoperative remifentanil on postoperative sore throat: a prospective randomized study: a CONSORT compliant article. Medicine (Baltimore). 2018;97(50):e13510.

11

Comparison of standard versus 90° rotation technique for LMA Flexible™ insertion

Bon-Wook Koo[1], Ah-Young Oh[1,2]* ⓘ, Jung-Won Hwang[1], Hyo-Seok Na[1] and Seong-Won Min[2,3]

Abstract

Background: Insertion of a flexible laryngeal mask airway (LMA Flexible) is known to be more difficult than that of a conventional laryngeal mask airway. The 90° rotation technique can improve the success rate with a conventional laryngeal mask airway but its effect with the LMA Flexible remains unknown. We assessed whether the 90° rotation technique increased the first-attempt success rate of LMA Flexible insertion versus the standard technique.

Methods: In total, 129 female patients undergoing breast surgery were analyzed. The primary endpoint was success at the first attempt. The insertion time, number of trials, number of manipulations required, and oropharyngeal leak pressure were also evaluated. Heart rate and mean blood pressure were recorded 1 min before and 1 min after insertion. Blood staining on the LMA Flexible after removal and postoperative sore throat were checked.

Results: The first-attempt success rates were comparable between the groups (93% vs. 98.3%, $P = .20$). The insertion time, number of trials and manipulations, hemodynamic variables, and complications, such as blood staining and sore throat, did not differ between the groups.

Conclusions: The 90° rotation technique is a good alternative to the standard technique for insertion of the LMA Flexible.

Keywords: LMA flexible

Background

The roles of supraglottic airways in anesthesia and airway management are increasing and are emphasized [1–4]. It is known that perioperative respiratory adverse events, such as laryngospasm, bronchospasm, sore throat, postoperative hoarse voice, and coughing, are decreased with the use of supraglottic airway compared to endotracheal tube [1–3]. The practice guidelines for management of the difficult airway by ASA also emphasize the role of supraglottic airway and recommends to always consider its use in the management of difficult airway [4].

The flexible laryngeal mask airway, LMA Flexible (Teleflex Co., Westmeath, Ireland), has a unique design, allowing the tube to be moved out of the surgical field without displacement of the cuff or loss of a seal. It also allows the tube complete flexibility and resistance to compression, such that the head and neck can be turned without dislodging the mask. The manufacturer recommends its use in head and neck surgery instead of tracheal intubation, such as bilateral myringotomy tubes, rhinoplasty, nasal sinus surgery, adenoidectomy, and tonsillectomy. Regarding the ease of insertion of the LMA Flexible, controversy exists. Some authors stated that it is more difficult to insert because the elasticity of its shaft makes it difficult to insert. They proposed tools to improve insertion of the LMA Flexible, such as a modified Magill forcep, a stylet, the Bosworth introducer, and the spatula introducer [5–8]. However, similar ease of

* Correspondence: oay1@snubh.org

[1]Department of Anesthesiology and Pain Medicine, Seoul National University Bundang Hospital, 137-82 Gumi-ro, Bundang-gu, Sungnam-si, Gyeonggi-do 463-707, South Korea

[2]Department of Anesthesiology and Pain Medicine, Seoul National University College of Medicine, Seoul, South Korea

insertion of the LMA Flexible is also reported [9]. 100% success rate of insertion of the LMA Flexible at the first attempt with the use of stadard insertion technique was also reported [10].

The 90° rotation technique was first described by Hwang et al. and involves the following steps: the entire cuff of the LMA is inserted inside the mouth, rotated counter-clockwise through 90° and advanced until the resistance of the hypopharynx is felt [11]. The use of this method is known to increase the success rate of insertion and decrease the incidence of blood staining of the LMA and sore throat compared to standard technique when inserting a Proseal LMA and i-gel [11–15]. The 90° rotation technique has the advantage over the previously reported methods that it does not require a separate tool and reduces pharyngeal mucosal trauma.

It is unknown whether this method increases the success rate of LMA Flexible insertion. Thus, we evaluated whether the 90° rotation technique increased the success rate of the LMA Flexible insertion compared to the standard insertion method.

Methods

This prospective randomized study was approved by the Seoul National University Bundang Hospital Institutional Review Board (B-1409/265–005) and was registered at ClinicalTrials.gov (NCT 03028896). Written informed consent was obtained from all participants.

In total, 129 female patients aged 18–65 years, with an ASA physical class I–II and who were scheduled for elective breast surgery under general anesthesia using the LMA Flexible, were recruited to the study. Exclusion criteria were a known difficult airway, mouth opening less than 2.5 cm, limited extension of the neck, recent sore throat, and gastro-oesophageal reflux disease. Patients were randomised into two groups by a nurse who was not involved in the rest of the study using computer-generated random numbers (Random Allocation Software, ver. 2.0). Premedication with midazolam 0.03 mg kg^{-1} I.V. was performed in the reception area. Anesthesia was induced with I.V. propofol 1.5 mg kg^{-1}, alfentanil 5 µg kg^{-1}, and rocuronium 0.5 mg kg^{-1}, and was maintained with inhaled desflurane. Insertion of the LMA Flexible was performed by a single anesthesiologist who had experience with more than 500 cases with the standard technique. A size 3 LMA Flexible for patients weighing 50–70 kg and a size 4 LMA Flexible for those weighing 70–100 kg, were used. The standard method followed the manufacturer's instructions [16]. In the neck-flexed-and-head-extended position, holding the mask like a pen and with the index finger placed anteriorly at the junction of the cuff and tube, the mask was pushed backwards, maintaining pressure against the palate until resistance was felt. The 90° rotation method

was the same as in previous reports: after insertion of the entire cuff inside the mouth, the LMA Flexible was rotated anticlockwise through 90° and advanced through the right side of the tongue until resistance was felt, and was then then turned back in the hypopharynx [11–14]. In both methods, insertion of the LMA Flexible was done with the cuff deflated, and followed by re-inflation to 60 cmH$_2$O using a manometer. Effective ventilation was indexed by a square-wave capnograph trace and no audible leak during manual ventilation at peak airway pressures $\geq$10 cmH$_2$O. If ventilation was ineffective, manipulations like jaw thrust, chin lift, and extension and flexion of the neck were allowed. If ventilation was still ineffective, re-insertion was tried up to three times. The insertion time was defined as time from mouth passage of the device to effective ventilation after inflation of the cuff. The oropharyngeal leak pressure was checked by hearing the leak sound at mouth using stethoscope while watching the pressure gauge of the ventilator and manually inflating the bag at a fresh gas flow of 5 L min^{-1} with the pop-off valve closed. The number of insertion attempts, number of manipulations needed during insertion, and insertion time were recorded. Heart rate and mean arterial pressure (MAP) were checked 1 min before and after LMA Flexible insertion.

At the end of surgery, the LMA Flexible was removed after confirming the return of spontaneous ventilation and consciousness. A nurse blinded to the patient group checked for blood staining of the LMA Flexible after removal. Sore throat was rated on a numerical rating scale (NRS; 0–10) by asking to patients a standard questionnaire before discharge from the post-anesthetic care unit (PACU). A score of more than 4 points on the NRS was considered to indicate a sore throat.

Statistics

The primary outcome was the success rate of first-attempt insertion of the LMA Flexible, which was confirmed by successful ventilation. Secondary outcome variables were insertion time, the number of trials and manipulations required for proper positioning, oropharyngeal leak pressure, and postoperative complications, such as blood staining of the mask and sore throat. The sample size was calculated on the basis of a previous study reporting the success rate of first-attempt insertion of the LMA Flexible to be 81% [17]. We assumed the success rate of the rotation technique would be 97% [13]. Thus, 59 patients per group would be needed to detect the difference with a power of 80% and type 1 error of 0.05. Considering a 10% drop-out rate, we recruited 66 patients per group. Patients' characteristics, insertion time, and air leak pressure were compared using Student's t-test after the Kolmogorov-Smirnov test. Success rates, blood staining of the LMA flexible, and sore throat were compared using χ^2 and Fisher's exact test. Repeated-measures analysis of variance was used to evaluate the effect on haemodynamic changes after LMA Flexible insertion. Data are presented as mean (± SD), median (Range), or number of patients (proportion). A P value < 0.05 was considered to indicate statistical significance.

Results

In total, 132 patients were enrolled. One patient did not meet the inclusion criteria and three were excluded after randomisation, leaving 129 patients to be analysed. The standard and the rotation groups finally included 63 and 66 patients, respectively (Fig. 1). Patient characteristics did not differ between the groups (Table 1).

The first-attempt success rate was not significantly different between the groups (59/63, 93.7% vs. 65/66, 98.5%, $P = 0.20$). The LMA Flexible was inserted successfully at the first attempt in almost all patients except for four in the standard group and one in the rotation group. The insertion time (10.5 ± 4.7 vs. 9.7 ± 4.7, $P = 0.58$), number of

trials and manipulations required for proper positioning (2/63, 3.2% vs. 1/66, 1.5%, $P = 0.61$), and air leak pressure (19.8 ± 4.9 vs. 20.5 ± 4.2, $P = 0.38$) also showed no significant difference between the groups (Table 2). MAP and heart rate 1 min before and after the insertion of the LMA did not differ between the groups. Blood staining on the LMA Flexible after removal (1/63, 1.6% vs. 3/66, 4.5%, $P = 0.33$), and the incidence (6/63, 9.5% vs. 12/66, 18.2%, $P = 0.21$) and degree [NRS 3 [1–8] vs. 3.5 [1–7], $P = 0.16$] of sore throat checked in the PACU before discharge, were also not different between the groups (Table 3).

Discussion

A 90° rotation technique for insertion of LMA was first proposed by Hwang et al. for the ProSeal LMA. They showed that the rotation technique was more successful than the standard technique and was associated with less pharyngeal mucosal trauma. They explained that this was because the lateral edge of the LMA reduced resistance between the LMA and the posterior pharyngeal wall [11]. We would add that another advantage of the

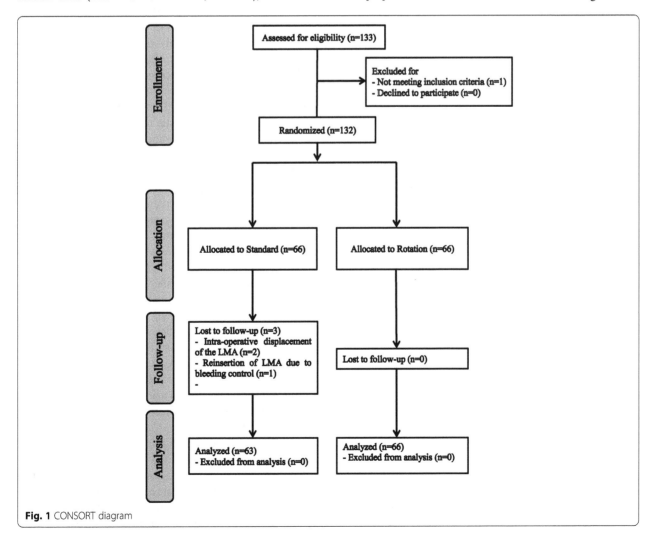

Fig. 1 CONSORT diagram

Table 1 Patient characteristics

	Standard (n = 63)	Rotation (n = 66)	p-value
Age (years)	42.1 ± 10.2	47.4 ± 11.4	0.09
Height (cm)	160 ± 6.1	159.2 ± 5.6	0.99
BMI (kg/m²)	22.4 ± 2.8	23.3 ± 3.5	0.57
ASA (I/II)	59/5	46/20	0.13

Values are number of patients, mean ± SD. *BMI* body mass index, *ASA* American Society of Anesthesiologists

90° rotation technique is that insertion of the operator's fingers into the patient's mouth is not necessary. The value of this advantage would be greater when the patient is awake and the possibility of biting exists. In subsequent studies, they showed that rotation technique was superior to the standard technique in various size of ProSeal LMA including children, with or without the use of neuromuscular blockers, and also in i-gel [12–14].

In this study, the first attempt success rate for insertion of the LMA Flexible was not significantly different between the two methods used. This is different from findings of previous studies reporting superiority of the 90° rotation technique compared to standard method. However, this was not because the 90° rotation technique was ineffective but because the success rate of both methods was high enough. Indeed, the first attempt success rate of rotation group was 98.5%, which is comparable to previously reported ones of 97–100%. In contrast, the first attempt success rate of 95.3% of standard group is higher than those reported previously with ProSeal LMA or i-gel. This is also higher than previously reported first-attempt success rate for the LMA Flexible of 81.5–90% [17, 18]. One study reported that use of a laryngoscope increased the first-attempt success rate from 81.5 to 96.3% [17]. There has been recognition that

Table 2 Intraoperative variables

	Standard (n = 63)	Rotation (n = 66)	P-value
Success rate (n, %)			
First attempt	59 (93.7)	65 (98.5)	0.2
Second attempt	3 (4.8)	1 (1.5)	0.36
Third attempt	1 (1.6)	0 (0)	0.49
Manipulations required (n, %)	2 (3.2)	1 (1.5)	0.61
Neck extension	0	1	
push in LMA	1	0	
cuff pressure adjustment	1	0	
Insertion time (sec)	10.5 ± 4.7	9.7 ± 4.7	0.58
Air leak pressure (cmH₂O)	19.8 ± 4.9	20.5 ± 4.2	0.38
Operation time (min)	51.7 ± 26.5	57.3 ± 29.4	0.26
Anesthesia time (min)	71.4 ± 26.8	77.8 ± 30.2	0.21

Values are number of patients (%), mean ± SD. *LMA* laryngeal mask airway

Table 3 Hemodynamic variables and complications

	Standard (n = 63)	Rotation (n = 66)	P-value
MAP (mmHg)			
Before insertion	65.5 ± 13.4	63.3 ± 10.9	0.31
After insertion	61.1 ± 12.7	63.7 ± 14.7	0.29
Heart Rate (beats/min)			
Before insertion	73.7 ± 14.3	70.4 ± 12.0	0.16
After insertion	73.0 ± 17.2	70.1 ± 11.5	0.27
Blood staining (n, %)	1 (1.6)	3 (4.5)	0.33
Sore throat at PACU (NRS)	3 (1–8)	3.5 (1–7)	0.16
Sore throat (NRS > 4) (n) %	6 (9.5)	12 (18.2)	0.21

Values are number of patients (%), mean ± SD, or median (range). *MAP* mean arterial pressure, *PACU* post-anesthetic care unit, *NRS* numerical rating scale (0–10)

insertion of the LMA Flexible is more difficult than that of other LMAs, because it is difficult to transmit force along the flexible shaft [5–8]. They reported that the use of an extra-tool; such as a modified Magill forcep, a stylet, the Bosworth introducer, and the spatula introducer; would facilitate the insertion of the LMA Flexible. However, these methods not only require an extra-tool but also be a reason of trauma to the larynx. The benefits of the 90° rotation technique compared to those methods are no need for an extra-tool and decrease of laryngeal trauma. In our study, we did not find the LMA Flexible more difficult to insert versus other LMAs using either the conventional or 90° rotation technique. One reason for our relatively high success rate at the first attempt might have been the use of a neuromuscular blocker in our patients. Previous studies reported that use of neuromuscular blockers increased the pharyngeal space and improved the efficacy and success of insertion [19, 20]. Another reason may have been that we only included young female patients and excluded patients with the possibility of a difficult airway. We used an LMA that was one size smaller than the manufacturer's recommendations and this might also have affected the first-attempt success rate. We chose this smaller-sized LMA based on previous studies showing decreased mucosal injury and postoperative sore throat with the use of a smaller-sized LMA [21, 22]. We could find a previous study reporting classic and rotatory methods being comparable in paediatric patients using classic LMA. However, they used 180° rotation which is differ from our 90° rotation method [23].

Postoperative sore throat is a common complication after general anesthesia and the reported incidence is up to 35% with use of the supraglottic airways [17, 24]. The overall incidence of sore throat in our patients was 13.9%, which was relatively low compared with previous reports. In addition, the degree of sore throat was not severe with the median (range) NRS of 3 [1–8] and 3.5 [1–7] in each groups. The most important factors for the development of sore throat after insertion into the supraglottic airways are trauma during device insertion and a high intracuff pressure. However, most of the insertions in our patients were quick and smooth, as shown by the short insertion time of around only 10 s in both groups. We also controlled the intra-cuff pressure to < 60 cmH$_2$O using a manometer. These factors might be related to our relatively low incidence of postoperative sore throat. Female gender and younger age are also risk factors for postoperative sore throat and these factors might have been associated with our results, where all of our patients were relatively young female patients undergoing breast surgery [25].

This study had some limitations. First, double blinding was not possible because we could not disguise the insertion method. Second, most of our patients were relatively healthy, young, females and we excluded those with suspected difficult airways. Thus, it is unclear whether our results would generalise to the general population, including men, the elderly, and difficult airway patients. In a previous report studying more than 15,000 patients anesthetized using LMA, male sex and increased body mass index were independent risk factors for failed LMA, which was defined as and airway event requiring LMA removal and tracheal intubation [26]. The incidence of postoperative sore throat was higher in females compared to males after the use of LAM [27]. Third, a single investigator who was an expert in the use of LMA placed all LMA. This also limits generalizability of the finding of this study and additionally and might have affected the high incidence of the first attempt success rate of both methods in this study. Fourth, we used a neuromuscular blocker before insertion of the LMA Flexible and this might have affected the insertion conditions. Fifth, we did not use objective monitors such as bispectral index (BIS) monitor or nerve stimulator and cannot rule out the possibility of difference in depth of anesthesia or neuromuscular blockade among the patients. The last, we did not confirm the proper position of LMA using fiberoptic bronchoscopy and used clinical assessment of proper ventilation only. We checked the proper positioning of the LMA by a clinical indicator, such as an oropharyngeal leak pressure. If the position of the LMA is improper, it cannot seal the pharynx well, and the leakage of air will occur at lower pressure. This indicator has been widely used as an indicator of proper position of the LMA [28, 29]. However, caution is needed when comparing our data with those assessed proper positioning of LMA with direct visualization.

Conclusions

The 90°rotation technique was as effective as the standard method for insertion of the LMA Flexible in female patients undergoing breast surgery. Complications, such as blood staining and sore throat, were also comparable. The 90°rotation technique seems to be a good alternative to the standard method when using the LMA Flexible.

Abbreviations

ASA: American Society of Anesthesiologists; BMI: Body mass index; IV: Intravenous; LMA: Laryngeal mask airway; MAP: Mean arterial pressure; NRS: Numerical rating scale; PACU: Post-anesthetic care unit; SD: Standard deviation

Acknowledgments

All authors disclose no sponsorship or financial support in relation to this research.

Authors' contributions

BWK: data collection; AYO: study design, interpretation of data, write the manuscript; JWH: help in the study design and writing the manuscript; Hyo-Seok: data collection: SWM: analysis and interpretation of data; all authors read and approved the final manuscript.

Author details

[1]Department of Anesthesiology and Pain Medicine, Seoul National University Bundang Hospital, 137-82 Gumi-ro, Bundang-gu, Sungnam-si, Gyeonggi-do 463-707, South Korea. [2]Department of Anesthesiology and Pain Medicine, Seoul National University College of Medicine, Seoul, South Korea. [3]Department of Anesthesiology and Pain Medicine, Boramae Hospital, Seoul, South Korea.

References

1. Drake-Brockman TF, Ramgolam A, Zhang G, Hall GL, von Ungern-Sternberg BS. The effect of endotracheal tubes versus laryngeal mask airways on perioperative respiratory adverse events in infants: a randomised controlled trial. Lancet. 2017; 389:701–8.
2. Yu SH, Beirne OR. Laryngeal mask airways have a lower risk of airway complications compared with endotracheal intubation: a systematic review. J Oral Maxil Surg. 2010;68:2359–76.
3. Patki A. Laryngeal mask airway vs the endotracheal tube in paediatric airway management: a meta-analysis of prospective randomised controlled trials. Indian J Anaesth. 2011;55:537–41.
4. Apfelbaum JL, Hagberg CA, Caplan RA, et al. Practice guidelines for management of the difficult airway: an updated report by the American Society of Anesthesiologists Task Force on Management of the Difficult Airway. Anesthesiology. 2013;118:251–70.
5. Welsh BE. Use of a modified Magill's forceps to place a flexible laryngeal mask. Anaesthesia. 1995;50:1002–3.
6. Shimoda O, Yoshitake A. Stylet for reinforced laryngeal mask airway. Anaesthesia. 2002;57:1140–1.
7. Bosworth A, Jago RH. The Bosworth introducer for use with the flexible reinforced laryngeal mask airway. Anaesthesia. 1997;52:281–2.
8. Kil HK, Koo BN, Park JH, Kim WO. The spatula introducer for insertion of the flexible reinforced laryngeal mask airway (RLMA). Can J Anaesth. 2005;52:117–8.
9. Brimacombe J, Keller C. Comparison of the flexible and standard laryngeal mask airways. Can J Anaesth. 1999;46:558–63.
10. Keller C, Brimacombe J. The influence of head and neck position on oropharyngeal leak pressure and cuff position with the flexible and standard laryngeal mask airway. Anesth Analg. 1999;88:913–6.
11. Hwang JW, Park HP, Lim YJ, Do SH, Lee SC, Jeon YT. Comparison of two insertion techniques of ProSeal laryngeal mask airway: standard versus 90-degree rotation. Anesthesiology. 2009;110:905–7.
12. Jeon YT, Na HS, Park SH, et al. Insertion of the ProSeal laryngeal mask airway is more successful with the 90 degrees rotation technique. Can J Anaesth. 2010;57:211–5.

13. Kim HC, Yoo DH, Kim HJ, Jeon YT, Hwang JW, Park HP. A prospective randomised comparison of two insertion methods for i-gel placement in anaesthetised paralysed patients: standard vs rotational technique. Anaesthesia. 2014;69:729–34.

14. Yun MJ, Hwang JW, Park SH, et al. The 90 degrees rotation technique improves the ease of insertion of the ProSeal laryngeal mask airway in children. Can J Anaesth. 2011;58:379–83.

15. Dhulkhed PV, Khyadi SV, Jamale PB, Dhulkhed VK. A prospective randomised clinical trial for the comparison of two techniques for the insertion of Proseal laryngeal mask airway in adults-index finger insertion technique versus 90 degrees rotation technique. Turk J Anaesthesiol Reanim. 2017;45: 98–102.

16. Instruction for use-LMA Classic™, LMA Flexible™, LMA Flexible™ Single Use & LMA Unique™. Ireland: Teleflex Medical, 2013.

17. Choo CY, Koay CK, Yoong CS. A randomised controlled trial comparing two insertion techniques for the laryngeal mask airway flexible in patients undergoing dental surgery. Anaesthesia. 2012;67:986–90.

18. Flynn P, Ahmed FB, Mitchell V, Patel A, Clarke S. A randomised comparison of the single use LMA flexible with the reusable LMA flexible in paediatric dental day-case patients. Anaesthesia. 2007;62:1281–4.

19. Kuna ST. Respiratory-related activation and mechanical effects of the pharyngeal constrictor muscles. Respir Physiol. 2000;119:155–61.

20. Fujiwara A, Komasawa N, Nishihara I, et al. Muscle relaxant effects on insertion efficacy of the laryngeal mask ProSeal((R)) in anesthetized patients: a prospective randomized controlled trial. J Anesth. 2015;29:580–4.

21. Grady DM, McHardy F, Wong J, Jin F, Tong D, Chung F. Pharyngolaryngeal morbidity with the laryngeal mask airway in spontaneously breathing patients: does size matter? Anesthesiology. 2001;94:760–6.

22. Kim MH, Hwang JW, Kim ES, Han SH, Jeon YT, Lee SM. Comparison of the size 3 and size 4 ProSeal laryngeal mask airway in anesthetized, non-paralyzed women: a randomized controlled trial. J Anesth. 2015;29:256–62.

23. Aghdashi MM, Hasanloei MAV, Abbasivash R, Shokohi S, Gharrehvaran S. Comparison of the success rate of laryngeal mask airway insertion in classic & rotatory methods in pediatric patients undergoing general anesthesia. Anesth Pain Med. 2017;7:e38899.

24. L'Hermite J, Dubout E, Bouvet S, et al. Sore throat following three adult supraglottic airway devices: a randomised controlled trial. Eur J Anaesthesiol. 2017;34:417–24.

25. El-Boghdadly K, Bailey CR, Wiles MD. Postoperative sore throat: a systematic review. Anaesthesia. 2016;71:706–17.

26. Ramachandran SK, Mathis MR, Tremper KK, Shanks AM, Kheterpal S. Predictors and clinical outcomes from failed laryngeal mask airway unique: a study of 15,795 patients. Anesthesiology. 2012;116:1217–26.

27. Jaensson M, Gupta A, Nilsson U. Gender differences in sore throat and hoarseness following endotracheal tube or laryngeal mask airway: a prospective study. BMC Anesthesiol. 2014;14:56.

28. Keller C, Puhringer F, Brimacombe JR. Influence of cuff volume on oropharyngeal leak pressure and fibreoptic position with the laryngeal mask airway. Br J Anaesth. 1998;81:186–7.

29. Qamarul Hoda M, Samad K, Ullah H. ProSeal versus classic laryngeal mask airway (LMA) for positive pressure ventilation in adults undergoing elective surgery. Cochrane Database Syst Rev. 2017;7:CD009026.

12

Ossification of the cervical anterior longitudinal ligament is an underdiagnosed cause of difficult airway

Min Xu[1], Yue Liu[1], Jing Yang[1]*⊙, Hao Liu[2] and Chen Ding[2]

Abstract

Background: Ossification of the anterior longitudinal ligament (OALL) of the cervical spine is a common, but rarely symptomatic, condition mostly observed in the geriatric population. Although the condition usually requires no intervention, it could lead to a difficult airway and compromise the patient's safety.

Case presentation: Here, we describe the case of a 50-year-old man with cervical myelopathy and OALL that resulted in difficult endotracheal intubation after induction of anesthesia. Radiography and magnetic resonance imaging findings showed OALL, with prominent osteophytes involving four cervical vertebrae, a bulge in the posterior pharyngeal wall, and a narrow pharyngeal space. Airtraq® laryngoscope-assisted intubation was accomplished with rapid induction under sevoflurane-inhaled anesthesia.

Conclusion: Anesthesiologists should understand that OALL of the cervical spine could cause a difficult airway. However, it is difficult to recognize asymptomatic OALL on the basis of routine airway evaluation guidelines. For susceptible populations, a thorough evaluation of the airway, based on imaging studies and a history of compression symptoms, should be considered whenever possible. In case of unanticipated difficult intubation, anesthesiologists should refer to guidelines for unanticipated difficult airway management and identify OALL of the cervical spine as the cause.

Keywords: Ossification of the anterior longitudinal ligament, Difficult airway, Anesthesia

Background

Diffuse idiopathic skeletal hyperplasia (DISH), also named as "Forestier's disease," is a rare idiopathic spinal disease characterized by a "flowing" ossification of the anterior longitudinal ligament (OALL) of the spine with an unknown etiology [1]. OALL of the cervical spine is common in patients over the age of 50 years, with a prevalence of approximately 15–20% in the elderly [2, 3]. Although

usually asymptomatic, in rare cases, osteophytes caused by OALL of the cervical spine can encroach the digestive tract and airway, leading to swallowing and respiratory problems [4]. Regardless of the presence of symptoms, patients are at risk of developing a difficult airway after anesthesia induction due to cervical OALL [5, 6]. Here, we describe the case of a 50-year-old man with OALL of the cervical spine who underwent cervical surgery with difficult endotracheal intubation after anesthesia. Airtraq® laryngoscope-assisted intubation was accomplished under rapid induction. We also discuss our case in relation to a case-based literature review.

* Correspondence: hxyangjing@qq.com
[1]Department of Anesthesiology, West China Hospital, Sichuan University, No.37 Guo Xue Ave, Chengdu, Sichuan 610041, PR China

Case presentation

A 50-year-old man (height, 165 cm; weight, 66 kg) who complained of numb hands and experienced unsteadiness while walking was diagnosed with C3–C4 intervertebral disc herniation and C3–C6 OALL. He was scheduled to undergo C3–C6 anterior cervical osteophyte resection, C3–C4 anterior discectomy, spinal canal decompression combined with interbody fusion, internal fixation, and C4–C5/C5–C6 artificial cervical disc replacement. The patient had a 30-year history of smoking and had never undergone a surgery. The preoperative evaluation showed an American Society of Anesthesiologists class II and a normal airway. The inter-incisor distance was 48 mm, which was measured using a ruler with the patient sitting in the neutral position with his mouth maximally open. The thyromental distance was 60 mm, which was measured between the prominence of the thyroid cartilage and the bony point of the chin with the head maximally extended on the neck. The patient exhibited a Mallampati Class II airway. He did not present with any limitation in neck movements (the range of neck motion included the "chin-to-chest" distance and the full extension of the head), esophageal and airway obstruction, or hoarseness. A lateral cervical spine radiograph showed a "beak-like" osteophyte in front of the C4 vertebra, which protruded forward significantly (Fig. 1). In addition, a lateral magnetic resonance image (MRI) of the cervical spine

showed that the "beak-like" osteophyte compressed the esophagus and airway, while the protruding C3–C4 disc compressed the spinal cord (Fig. 2). Although there was no clinical evidences nor signs, the patient's image finding revealed that he would have a difficult airway (at the time of ventilation and/or intubation). The patient refused our suggested awake intubation, and, therefore, we chose succinylcholine for rapid induction to prevent intubation failure and wake the patient up in time. Moreover, we prepared a fiber-bronchoscope, video laryngoscope, and small-sized endotracheal tube. The patient provided written consent for publication of this report.

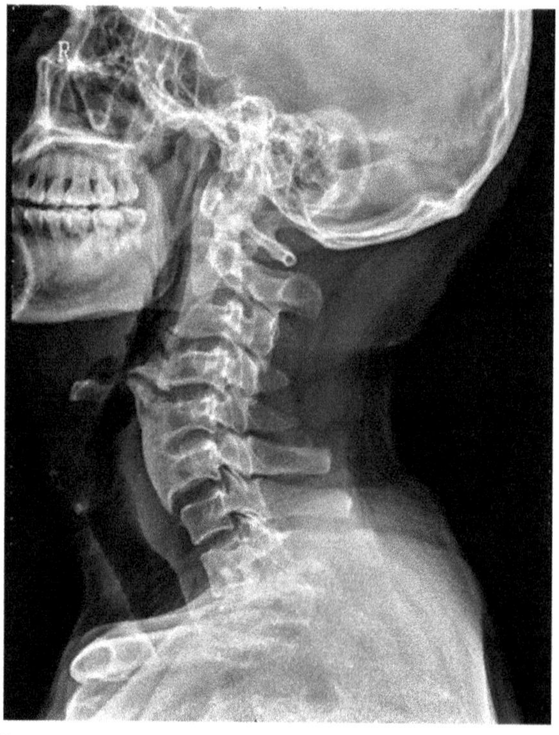

After entering the operating room, the patient was carefully placed in the sniffing position and the cervical hyperextension position without any discomfort. His vital signs were normal. After pre-oxygenation and gradual induction of anesthesia through inhalation of sevoflurane, the patient was deeply sedated with spontaneous breathing. No airway obstruction (airway obstruction score [AOS], 1) was observed, and mask ventilation was easy (Han's Mask ventilation score, 2). After spraying the throat with 2% lidocaine and administering succinylcholine and propofol, we performed direct laryngoscopy using a Macintosh blade ("adult large" size, 150 mm), which facilitated a Cormack-Lehane grade IV view. Vision was obscured by a mass approximately 1 cm in diameter in the posterior pharyngeal wall with a smooth mucosal surface. The Airtraq® video laryngoscope (Prodol Meditec, Bizkaia, Spain) was subsequently used and

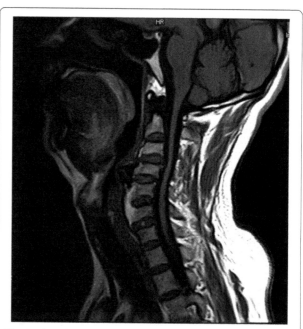

Fig. 1 A lateral cervical spine radiograph displayed osteophyte from C3 to C6. "Beak-like" osteophyte in front of the C4 vertebrae significantly protruded forward

Fig. 2 A lateral cervical spine MRI displayed osteophyte from C3 to C6. "Beak-like" osteophyte in front edges of the C4-C5 vertebrae protruded forward and compressed the esophagus and airway, and the post-protruding C3–4 disc compressed the spinal cord

provided a Cormack-Lehane grade II view. Finally, successful intubation was achieved, although only the posterior margin of the glottic structure was visualized.

The location of the 7.5# enforced endotracheal tube was confirmed by a normal ETCO$_2$, and symmetrical breathing sounds were heard from the lungs. The catheter depth was 22 cm from the central incisor. The endotracheal tube reached across the "beak-like" osteophyte in front of the C4–C5 vertebrae in the preoperative cervical spine radiograph (Fig. 3a). The "beak-like" osteophyte appeared resected in the postoperative cervical spine radiograph (Fig. 3b). The operation was successfully completed and lasted approximately 4 h. Then, the patient was transferred to the intensive care unit with the endotracheal tube retained in case of airway obstruction induced by postoperative laryngeal and tracheal edema. He was extubated after 1 day and discharged without any complications after 11 days of treatment. At the time of discharge, there was no numbness in the hands or walking instability. Moreover, there were no complications during a 12-month follow-up period after the surgery.

Literature review

We systematically searched PubMed, EMBASE, and the Cochrane Library for records dated from inception to February 2020 and identified articles reporting anesthetic techniques for difficult airway in patients with OALL of the cervical spine. A comprehensive search strategy was employed using relevant search terms selected from the Medical Subject Headings, EmTree, and Entry terms. The search terms were as follows: (Hyperostosis, Diffuse Idiopathic Skeletal OR Diffuse Idiopathic Skeletal Hyperostosis OR Vertebral Ankylosing Hyperostosis OR Forestier's Disease OR Forestier Rotes Disease OR Forestier Disease OR Calcification of Anterior Longitudinal Ligament OR calcific anterior longitudinal ligament OR Anterior Longitudinal Ligament Calcification OR Anterior Longitudinal Ligament Ossification OR Ossification of Anterior Longitudinal Ligament OR OALL OR cervical osteophytes OR cervical osteophytosis) AND (airway management OR difficult intubation OR difficult laryngoscopy OR difficult airway OR failed tracheal intubation OR difficult tracheal intubation). The search language was limited to English, and a total of 70 articles were retrieved. After removing duplicates, a total of 59 titles and abstracts were screened for eligibility. Of these, 34 full-text articles were evaluated, and 23 papers were potential candidates. One article was excluded because the full text could not be found [7], leaving 22 articles (summarized in Table 1) [5, 6, 8–27]. The excluded articles are presented in the appendix.

A total of 23 patients with OALL of the cervical had a difficult airway. Only two patients were women [11, 13], and only one patient was younger than 50 years [13]. Previous epidemiological studies have suggested that the prevalence of OALL increases with age, and the morbidity rate was found to be significantly higher for men than for women [28]. Among the patients included, the most commonly involved cervical vertebrae were C3–C4, followed by C4–C5 and C5–C6, leading to dysphagia and airway obstruction, possibly due to excessive activity. Six patients had no symptoms before intubation [5, 6, 10, 12, 14, 21], and the rest of the patients had symptoms such as dysphagia, dysphonia, dyspnea, airway obstruction, or restricted motion of the neck [8, 9, 11, 13, 15–20, 22–27]. Awake

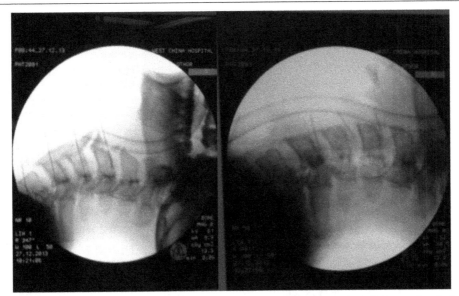

Fig. 3 Preoperative and postoperative cervical spine radiography: endotracheal tube got across the "beak-like" osteophyte in front edges of the C4, C5 vertebrae before operation (left, a) and the beak-like osteophyte has disappeared after operation (right, b)

Table 1 Review of anesthetic techniques reported for patients with OALL of the cervical

Author and (year)	Age	Sex	Anesthesia Method	Intubation tube	Symptom	Osteophyte
Lee (1979) [5]	73	M	awake intubation	direct laryngoscope with Miller blade	asymptomatic	C5-C7
Gorback (1991) [8]	61	M	rapid induction	bullard laryngoscope	restricted motion of the head and neck	NA
Crosby (1993) [6]	71	M	rapid induction	direct laryngoscope	asymptomatic	C5-C6
Togashi (1993) [9]	59	M	rapid induction	direct laryngoscopy	restricted motion of the neck	C5-C7
Broadway (1994) [10]	72	F	NA	laryngeal mask airway	asymptomatic	C3-C4
Ranasinghe (1994) [11]	72	F	awake intubation	fiberscope	dysphagia,	C2-C4
Aziz (1995) [12]	68	M	sedation and analgesia	facemask airway	asymptomatic	C3-C5
Palmer(2000) [13]	48	F	awake intubation.	intubating laryngeal mask and fiberscope	dysphagia and restricted motion of the neck	C3
Bougak (2004) [14]	62	M	awake intubation.	fiberscope	asymptomatic	C3-C7
Naik (2004) [15]	55	M	awake intubation	fiberscope	restricted motion of the neck, dysphagia, obstructive sleep apnea, and dysphagia	C2-C6
Cesur (2005) [16]	57	M	rapid induction	direct laryngoscopy with Magill's forceps	restricted motion of the neck	C2-C3
Ozkalkanli (2006) [17]	68	M	rapid induction	direct laryngoscope	restricted motion of the neck, dysphagia, dysphonia, and dyspnea	C2-C5
Montinaro (2006) [18]	67	M	NA	optical fibers	dysphagia, dysphonia	C3-C5
Satomoto (2007) [19]	67	M	NA	direct laryngoscope with the bougie guidance	dysphagia	NA
Baxi (2010) [20]	54	M	awake intubation	fiberoptic bronchoscope	dysphagia	C2-C3, C6-C7, T1
Thompson (2010) [21]	65	M	rapid induction	laryngeal mask airway and fibreoptic bronchoscope	asymptomatic	C3-C7
Eipe (2013) [22]	69	M	awake intubation	fiberoptic bronchoscope	dysphagia	C3-C5
Iida (2015) [23]	82	M	rapid induction	direct laryngoscope	dysphagia, aspiration pneumonia	C2-C4, C6-C7
Iida (2015) [23]	69	M	awake intubation	fibreoptic	restricted motion of the neck	C2-C3
Alsalmi (2018) [24]	66	M	awake intubation	fiberoptic bronchoscope	dysphagia, odynophagia, hoarseness	C3-C7
Gosavi (2018) [25]	62	M	awake intubation	fiberoptic bronchoscope	restricted motion of the neck, dysphagia, odynophagia	C2-C7
Garcia Zamorano (2019) [26]	85	M	sedation	fiberoptic bronchoscope	acute airway obstruction	C2-C5
Yoshimatsu (2019) [27]	80	M	NA	fiberoptic bronchoscope	sudden-onset upper airway obstruction, dysphonia, restricted motion of the neck	C2-C7

OALL Ossification of the anterior longitudinal ligament, *NA* Not available

intubation was chosen for 10 patients [5, 11, 13–15, 20, 22–25], and rapid induction was chosen for 7 patients [6, 8, 9, 16, 17, 21, 23]; fiberscope-assisted intubation was cited as the optimal choice in 13 articles [11, 13–15, 18, 20–27]; other cases favored the direct laryngoscope [5, 6, 9, 16, 17, 19, 23] or the intubating laryngeal mask [13, 21]. A small-sized endotracheal tube was selected for 4 patients [6, 17, 25, 27], while a nasotracheal tube was selected for 2 patients [11, 22]. The majority of patients required multiple endotracheal intubation attempts, and four patients could not undergo the surgery because of intubation failure [5, 14, 15, 18]. A laryngeal mask airway was used in one patient [10], a facemask airway was used

in one patient [12], and thyrocricoid puncture and retrograde intubation were attempted in one patient [16]. We also identified nine cases of emergency tracheotomies due to sudden upper airway obstruction induced by OALL of the cervical spine [18, 28–35].

Discussion and conclusion

Our literature review revealed that a difficult airway can be found in symptomatic [7, 8, 10, 12, 14–19, 21–26] and asymptomatic [5, 6, 10, 12, 14, 21] patients with OALL of the cervical spine who require surgery. Therefore, this possibility should be considered by anesthesiologists treating symptomatic patients with OALL and, as presented in this case report, those with cervical disease combined with asymptomatic OALL. Our radiography and MRI findings revealed OALL of the cervical spine, with prominent osteophytes involving four cervical vertebrae in combination with a bulge in the posterior throat wall, and a narrow pharyngeal space. This, with the inability to visualize the glottis, resulted in a difficult airway. The imaging data could suggest that the patient was at risk for difficult intubation. A postmortem study revealed that hypertrophic osteophytes were present in the cervical spines of 21 out of 75 asymptomatic patients (28%) during autopsy [36]. Cervical spine radiography is not routinely performed when patients with asymptomatic OALL of the cervical spine requires the performance of other surgeries or when symptomatic patients conceal their condition before surgery. Furthermore, it is difficult to recognize the risk of difficult intubation in such patients, despite routine preoperative evaluations for anesthesia. Therefore, to prevent challenges faced during an unanticipated difficult intubation, anesthesiologists should consider the possibility of a difficult airway in symptomatic and asymptomatic patients with OALL of the cervical spine.

Although appropriate guidelines are available for the management of unanticipated difficult intubation [37], unexpected difficult airways continue to concern anesthesiologists and endanger patients. According to our literature search, an unexpected difficult airway induced by OALL of the cervical spine leads to termination of the operation [5, 14, 15, 18]. In one case of a distorted airway caused by osteophytes, fiberoptic nasal intubation was extremely difficult, and an emergency tracheotomy had to be performed [11]. Therefore, to ensure the patient's safety, difficult airways induced by OALL of the cervical spine should be identified before surgery.

A critical question is how can we predict the possibility of a difficult airway induced by OALL of the cervical spine? Although radiological evaluation may be useful in assessing the risk of difficult intubation, it is still not recommended because OALL of the cervical spine is a relatively common condition that is only occasionally associated with difficult intubation [14]. Currently, the etiology and pathogenesis of OALL remain unclear, but this condition is strongly associated with frequently diagnosed metabolic abnormalities and joint degeneration [1]. In addition, it may be related to increased cervical motion or trauma. A recommendation to screen patients with risk factors, which should make the anesthesiologist suspect a difficult airway, should be entertained. Our literature review noted that men were more commonly affected than women, the disease was rare in patients younger than 50 years, and the incidents became more common as the age was advanced [38]. Patients with obesity, hypertension, diabetes, dyslipidemia, hyperuricemia, neck injury, cervical surgery history, osteoarthritis,

ossification of the posterior longitudinal ligament and Forestier's disease, or DISH were more likely to have cervical OALL [39, 40]. In these cases, cervical radiography and a detailed evaluation of the range of neck motion and swallowing function should be emphasized. Additionally, more effective clinical evaluation methods should be determined.

Moreover, our literature review found that in patients with OALL of the cervical spine with an anticipated difficult intubation, a fiberoptic bronchoscope-assisted awake intubation was the optimal method of intubation. The methods of intubation in patients with OALL of the cervical spine are summarized in Fig. 4. In general, a difficult airway was caused by limitations in cervical mobility and airway obstruction caused by OALL. Normally, the larger the osteophytes, the more evident the clinical presentations, and a difficult airway induced by osteophytes could also cause more severe symptoms. Therefore, routine radiological evaluation is important to determine the airway status in patients with OALL of the cervical spine and should be emphasized during preoperative anesthesia visits, especially for patients with airway obstructions, hoarseness, or other symptoms. It is beneficial to evaluate the degree of ossification and its impact on the surrounding tissue to identify the risk of a difficult intubation. Then, the physicians can strategize and arrange for the appropriate equipment. We recommend a fast-difficult airway evaluation in patients with potentially difficult ventilation/difficult intubation [41]. In brief, patients should gradually be sedated with sevoflurane, and the adequacy of manual mask ventilation during spontaneous breathing should be assessed at various sedation levels. Awake intubation with the Airtraq® video-laryngoscope or fiberoptic bronchoscope can be applied in cases with inadequate mask ventilation and severe airway obstruction. When adequate mask ventilation is retained and the vocal cords are visible, the patient can be intubated under general anesthesia.

When asymptomatic patients with OALL face an unanticipated difficult intubation, anesthesiologists should be aware of the possibility of a difficult airway due to OALL of the cervical spine and should follow the unanticipated difficult airway guidelines. Most importantly, adequate ventilation should be maintained through oropharyngeal, nasopharyngeal, or laryngeal mask airways. Then, the intubation equipment can be chosen after an airway assessment, using a direct laryngoscope, such as the UE® and the Airtraq® video laryngoscopes or a fiberoptic bronchoscope. In particular, a laryngoscopy using Airtraq® may alter the Cormack-Lehane score from III or IV to I or II. An emergency tracheotomy or thyrocricoid puncture can be performed where necessary.

In conclusion, it is important for anesthesiologists and spine surgeons to be aware and be prepared for the

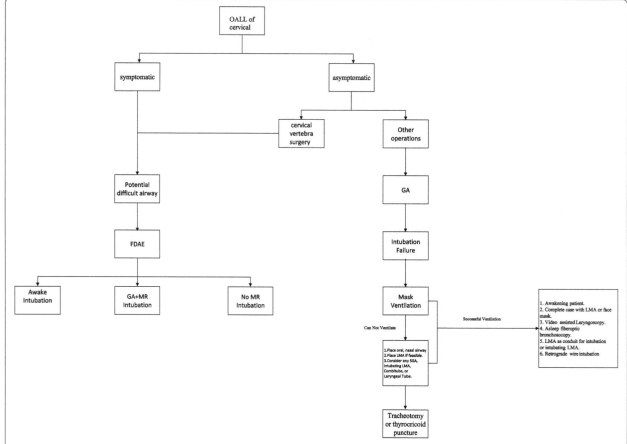

Fig. 4 A summary of intubation methods in patients with OALL of the cervical. FADE, fast difficult airway evaluation; GA, general anesthesia; MR, muscle relaxants; LMA, laryngeal mask airway

possibility of a difficult airway induced by OALL of the cervical spine. In case of an unanticipated difficult intubation, the anesthesiologist should be able to refer to the unanticipated difficult airway guidelines and identify OALL of the cervical spine as the cause of the difficult airway.

Abbreviations
OALL: Ossification of the anterior longitudinal ligament; MRI: Magnetic resonance imaging

Acknowledgements
Not applicable.

Authors' contributions
MX and YL analyzed and interpreted the patient data, handled the manuscript.
JY helped conceive and design the study. HL and CD revised the manuscript. All authors read and approved the final manuscript.

Author details
[1]Department of Anesthesiology, West China Hospital, Sichuan University, No.37 Guo Xue Ave, Chengdu, Sichuan 610041, PR China. [2]Department of Orthopedics, West China Hospital, Sichuan University, No.37 Guo Xue Ave, Chengdu, Sichuan 610041, PR China.

References
1. Ohara Y. Ossification of the ligaments in the cervical spine, including ossification of the anterior longitudinal ligament, ossification of the posterior longitudinal ligament, and ossification of the ligamentum flavum. Neurosurg Clin N Am. 2018;29(1):63–8.
2. Forestier J, Rotes-Querol J. Senile ankylosing hyperostosis of the spine. Ann Rheum Dis. 1950;9(4):321–30.
3. Forestier J, Lagier R. Ankylosing hyperostosis of the spine. Clin Orthop Relat Res. 1971;74:65–83.
4. Saito T, Wajima Z, Kato N, Shitara T, Inoue T, Ogawa R. Management of anesthesia in patients with the potential for difficult intubation due to ossification of anterior longitudinal ligament (OALL). Masui. 2006;55(10):1257–9.
5. Lee HC, Andree RA. Cervical spondylosis and difficult intubation. Anesth Analg. 1979;58(5):434–5.
6. Crosby ET, Grahovac S. Diffuse idiopathic skeletal hyperostosis: an unusual cause of difficult intubation. Can J Anaesth. 1993;40(1):54–8.
7. Thapa D, Sinha PK, Gombar S, Gombar KK, Palta S, Sen I. Large anterior cervical osteophytes: a cause for laryngeal "BURP" failure and difficult intubation - a case report. J Anesth Clin Pharmacol. 2002;18(3):320–2.
8. Gorback MS. Management of the challenging airway with the Bullard laryngoscope. J Clin Anesth. 1991;3(6):473–7.
9. Togashi H, Hirabayashi Y, Mitsuhata H, Saitoh K, Shimizu R. The beveled tracheal tube orifice abutted on the tracheal wall in a patient with Forestier's disease. Anesthesiology. 1993;79(6):1452–3.
10. Broadway JW. Forestier's disease (ankylosing hyperostosis): a cause for difficult intubation. Anaesthesia. 1994;49(10):919–20.
11. Ranasinghe DN, Calder I. Large cervical osteophyte--another cause of difficult flexible fibreoptic intubation. Anaesthesia. 1994;49(6):512–4.

12. Aziz ES, Thompson AR, Baer S. Difficult laryngeal mask insertion in a patient with Forestier's disease. Anaesthesia. 1995;50(4):370.

13. Palmer JH, Ball DR. Awake tracheal intubation with the intubating laryngeal mask in a patient with diffuse idiopathic skeletal hyperostosis. Anaesthesia. 2000;55(1):70–4.

14. Bougaki M, Sawamura S, Matsushita F, Hanaoka K. Difficult intubation due to ossification of the anterior longitudinal ligament. Anaesthesia. 2004;59(3):303–4.

15. Naik B, Lobato EB, Sulek CA. Dysphagia, obstructive sleep apnea, and difficult fiberoptic intubation secondary to diffuse idiopathic skeletal hyperostosis. Anesthesiology. 2004;100(5):1311–2.

16. Cesur M, Alici HA, Erdem AF. An unusual cause of difficult intubation in a patient with a large cervical anterior osteophyte: a case report. Acta Anaesthesiol Scand. 2005;49(2):264–6.

17. Ozkalkanli MY, Katircioglu K, Ozkalkanli DT, Savaci S. Airway management of a patient with Forestier's disease. J Anesth. 2006;20(4):304–6.

18. Montinaro A, D'Agostino A, Punzi F, Cantisani PL. Cervical anterior hyperostosis: a rare cause of dysphagia. Report of 3 cases. J Neurosurg Sci. 2006;50(3):75–7.

19. Satomoto M, Adachi YU, Sato S. Safe intubation with a gum-elastic bougie in a patient with Forestier's disease. J Anesth. 2007;21(4):519–20.

20. Baxi V, Gaiwal S. Diffuse idiopathic skeletal hyperostosis of cervical spine - an unusual cause of difficult flexible fiber optic intubation. Saudi J Anaesth. 2010;4(1):17–9.

21. Thompson C, Moga R, Crosby ET. Failed videolaryngoscope intubation in a patient with diffuse idiopathic skeletal hyperostosis and spinal cord injury. Can J Anaesth. 2010;57(7):679–82.

22. Eipe N, Fossey S, Kingwell SP. Airway management in cervical spine ankylosing spondylitis: between a rock and a hard place. Indian J Anaesth. 2013;57(6):592–5.

23. Iida M, Tanabe K, Dohi S, Iida H. Airway management for patients with ossification of the anterior longitudinal ligament of the cervical spine. JA Clin Rep. 2015;1(1):11.

24. Alsalmi S, Bugdadi A, Alkhayri A, Fichten A, Peltier J. Urgent anterior cervical osteophytectomy for an asymptomatic cervical hyperostosis to overcome failed intubation. Cureus. 2018;10(3):e2400.

25. Gosavi K, Dey P, Swami S. Airway management in case of diffuse idiopathic skeletal hyperostosis. Asian J Neurosurg. 2018;13(4):1260–3.

26. Garcia Zamorano S, Garcia Del Valle YMS, Andueza Artal A, Robles Angel P, Gijon HN. Acute airway obstruction in a patient with forestier disease. Case report Rev Esp Anestesiol Reanim. 2019;66(5):292–5.

27. Yoshimatsu Y, Tobino K, Maeda K, et al. Management of airway obstruction due to diffuse idiopathic skeletal hyperostosis in the cervical spine: a case report and literature review. Intern Med. 2019;58(2):271–6.

28. Caminos CB, Cenoz IZ, Louis CJ, Otano TB, Esain BF, Perez de Ciriza MT. Forestier disease: an unusual cause of upper airway obstruction. Am J Emerg Med. 2008;26(9):1072.e1071–3.

29. Demuynck K, Van Calenbergh F, Goffin J, Verschakelen J, Demedts M, Van de Woestijne K. Upper airway obstruction caused by a cervical osteophyte. Chest. 1995;108(1):283–4.

30. Matan AJ, Hsu J, Fredrickson BA. Management of respiratory compromise caused by cervical osteophytes: a case report and review of the literature. Spine J. 2002;2(6):456–9.

31. Lin HW, Quesnel AM, Holman AS, Curry WT Jr, Rho MB. Hypertrophic anterior cervical osteophytes causing dysphagia and airway obstruction. Ann Otol Rhinol Laryngol. 2009;118(10):703–7.

32. Varsak YK, Eryilmaz MA, Arbag H. Dysphagia and airway obstruction due to large cervical osteophyte in a patient with ankylosing spondylitis. J Craniofac Surg. 2014;25(4):1402–3.

33. Bird JH, Biggs TC, Karkos PD, Repanos C. Diffuse idiopathic skeletal hyperostosis as an acute airway presentation requiring urgent tracheostomy. Am J Emerg Med. 2015;33(5):737.e731–2.

34. Hoey AW, Dusu K, Gane S. Diffuse idiopathic skeletal hyperostosis (DISH): an unusual cause of airway obstruction. BMJ Case Rep. 2017;2017: bcr2017219635.

35. Psychogios G, Jering M, Zenk J. Cervical hyperostosis leading to dyspnea, aspiration and dysphagia: strategies to improve patient management. Front Surg. 2018;5:33.

36. Boachie-Adjei O, Bullough PG. Incidence of ankylosing hyperostosis of the spine (Forestier's disease) at autopsy. Spine. 1987;12(8):739–43.

37. Frerk C, Mitchell VS, McNarry AF, et al. Difficult airway society 2015 guidelines for management of unanticipated difficult intubation in adults. Br J Anaesth. 2015;115(6):827–48.

38. Resnick D. Degenerative diseases of the vertebral column. Radiology. 1985; 156(1):3–14.

39. Denko CW, Malemud CJ. Body mass index and blood glucose: correlations with serum insulin, growth hormone, and insulin-like growth factor-1 levels in patients with diffuse idiopathic skeletal hyperostosis (DISH). Rheumatol Int. 2006;26(4):292–7.

40. Kiss C, Szilagyi M, Paksy A, Poor G. Risk factors for diffuse idiopathic skeletal hyperostosis: a case-control study. Rheumatology (Oxford). 2002;41(1):27–30.

41. Wang JM, Ma EL, Wu QP, Tian M, Sun YY, Lin J, et al. Effectiveness and safety of a novel approach for management of patients with potential difficult mask ventilation and tracheal intubation: a multi-center randomized trial. Chin Med J. 2018;131(6):631–7.

13

Flexible fibreoptic intubation in swine – improvement for resident training and animal safety alike

Robert Ruemmler*![ORCID], Alexander Ziebart, Thomas Ott, Dagmar Dirvonskis and Erik Kristoffer Hartmann

Abstract

Background: Efficient airway management to facilitate tracheal intubation encompasses essential skills in anaesthesiologic and intensive care. The application of flexible fibreoptic intubation in patients with difficult airways has been identified as the recommended method in various international guidelines. However, providing the opportunity to adequately train residents can be challenging. Using large animals for practice during ongoing studies could help to improve this situation, but there is no recent data on fibreoptic intubation in swine available.

Methods: Thirty male German landrace pigs were anesthetized, instrumented and randomized into two groups. The animals were either intubated conventionally using direct laryngoscopy or a single-use flexible video-endoscope. The intervention was carried out by providers with 3 months experience in conventional intubation of pigs and a brief introduction into endoscopy. Intubation attempts were supervised and aborted, when SpO2 dropped below 93%. After three failed attempts, an experienced supervisor intervened and performed the intubation. Intubation times and attempts were recorded and analysed.

Results: Flexible fibreoptic intubation showed a significantly higher success rate in first attempt endotracheal tube placement (75% vs. 47%) with less attempts overall (1.3 ± 0.6 vs. 2.1 ± 1.3, $P = 0.043$). Conventional intubation was faster (42 s ± 6 s vs. 67 s ± 10s, $P < 0.001$), but showed a higher complication rate and more desaturation episodes during the trial.

Conclusions: Flexible fibreoptic intubation in swine is feasible and appears to be a safer and more accessible method for inexperienced users to learn. This could not only improve resident training options in hospitals with animal research facilities but might also prevent airway complications and needless animal suffering.

Keywords: Airway management, Animal safety, Difficult airway, Fibreoptic intubation, Resident training

Background

The efficient and safe airway management is one of the most important and outcome-relevant anaesthesiologic skills and directly affects perioperative mortality [1–4]. Flexible fibreoptic intubation (FFI) is recommended in national guidelines in the condition of an anticipated difficult airway [5–7] as well as a method amongst others in the unanticipated difficult airway [3, 5, 6] in order to safely facilitate tracheal tube placement in humans.

By comparison, while actual lung physiology is similar to humans and is regularly used for translational research in anaesthesiologic experiments [8], the airway management of swine can be challenging due to special anatomic properties on the orotracheal level [9–11]. The rate of encountered airway problems, resulting mortality or negative experimental effects in swine has not been sufficiently

* Correspondence: Robert.ruemmler@email.de
Department of Anaesthesiology, Medical Centre of the Johannes Gutenberg-University, Langenbeckstrasse 1, 55131 Mainz, Germany

reported but is frequently mentioned [12–14]. Accordingly, in terms of clinical assessment, swine may inhere an anticipated difficult airway, thus warranting the search for alternative strategies to secure tracheal tube placement. Subsequently, FFI could be a promising option to preserve positive trial outcomes without unnecessary animal losses.

However, the adequate establishment and maintenance of crucial technical skills concerning FFI often poses organisational and structural problems in the reality of clinical practice and hospital environments [15, 16]. Although the use of large animal models has been suggested and was rated superior to manikin-based simulations [17], no further prospective examinations in the field have been conducted since and porcine models are not implemented in standard training protocols to date.

In this prospective randomized pilot trial, we evaluated the feasibility and effectiveness of video-enhanced FFI by inexperienced providers in swine compared to conventional intubation (CI), while simultaneously assessing complication rates during orotracheal intubation. We hypothesized that the use of FFI would show a higher success rate and therefore provide a safer tracheal access than direct laryngoscopy. Specifically, we assessed intubation attempts necessary as well as the time needed to successfully secure the airway. Additionally, we discuss whether porcine models can be used as a training tool for FFI and the maintenance of proficiency in this technique.

Methods
Anaesthesia
The study was approved by the State and Institutional Animal Care Committee (Landesuntersuchungsamt Rheinland-Pfalz, Koblenz, Germany, approval no. G16–1-042) with an additional approval (Issue date: 8/28/2019) for the dual use of the animals in this protocol. Thirty male German landrace pigs (12–16 weeks, 28-35 kg) were acquired from a local farm and received pre-transport sedation via an intramuscular injection of azaperone ($2 \, mg \, kg^{-1}$) and ketamine ($4 \, mg \, kg^{-1}$). Once in our Large Animal Research Facility, anaesthesia was induced via an ear cannula (22G) by injecting fentanyl ($4 \, \mu g \, kg^{-1}$), propofol ($4 \, mg \, kg^{-1}$) and atracurium ($0.5 \, mg \, kg^{-1}$) as described before [18]. During the whole experiment, anaesthesia was maintained via continuous infusion of propofol ($5\text{-}10 \, mg \, kg^{-1} \, h^{-1}$) and fentanyl ($8\text{-}12 \, \mu g \, kg^{-1} \, h^{-1}$) as well as a balanced electrolyte infusion ($5 \, ml \, kg^{-1} \, h^{-1}$). The animals were transferred into a supine position and mechanically ventilated with a custom ventilation nose cone [19] using an intensive care respirator (Engstroem care station, GE healthcare, Munich; tidal volume 6-8 ml/kg, peak inspiratory pressure of $40 cmH_2O$, positive end expiratory pressure of $5 cmH_2O$). Adequate ventilation was confirmed by capnography,

peripheral oxygen saturation and auscultation of the thorax.

Intervention/ measurements
After 4 min of mask ventilation, the epiglottis of the swine was mobilized from the soft palate by the supervisor (Fig. 1) using a Macintosh blade (size 4) as well as a tube guiding rod and performing a careful scooping motion from the right piriform recess to the left along the soft palate. After the dislodgement was visually confirmed, the animals were randomized into two groups:

CI group (conventional intubation): Animals were intubated via direct laryngoscopy using a MacIntosh blade (size #4, large) and a standard tracheal tube (TT, internal diameter (ID) 7.0 mm).

FFI group (flexible fibreoptic intubation): Animals were intubated using a single-use endoscope with video monitoring (Ambu aScope regular and Ambu aView,

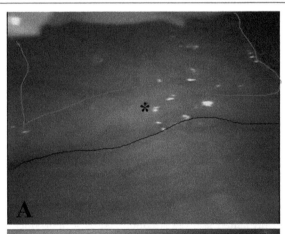
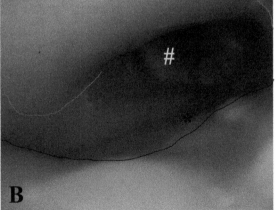

Fig. 1 Porcine laryngeal anatomy in supine position before (**a**) and after mobilisation of the epiglottis (**b**). Before mobilisation, the epiglottis (red line) is fixated behind transitional tissue between the hard palate (black line) and the soft palate (*). After mobilisation, the epiglottis usually stays slightly ventrally dislodged and the larynx (green #) can easily be identified

Ambu GmbH, Bad Nauheim, Germany) using a standard TT (ID 7.0 mm).

An exemplary video of FFI taken during the trial is available in the supplemental material of this article. As participants we used 3rd year medical students who had undergone basic training in animal handling in the university's Translational Animal Research Center and were approved by the State and Institutional Animal Care Committee. The participants had been introduced to large animal experiments and conventional intubation (mean of performed CIs: 4.5) for 3 months prior to the trial. A short explanation and standardized introduction to the FFI device was performed by the supervisor before the first use. None of the participants had used a flexible video-endoscope before or seen a FFI over a video monitor.

Intubation times were measured using a stopwatch beginning with the particular instrument entering the snout of the animal and were stopped when the connected ventilator revealed the first adequate capnography curve. Intubation attempts were aborted, when oxygen saturation dropped below 93% and animals were then mask ventilated again for 3 minutes until saturation recovered before the next try. Number of attempts until successful intubation of the trachea were counted. First pass success was noted separately. After a third unsuccessful attempt, an experienced supervisor performed the intubation.

After the intervention, the animals were ventilated, allowed to recover for 30 min and were then assigned to the primary research projects of our facility in order not to needlessly sacrifice them and adhere to ARRIVE and 3R guidelines.

Statistics

The presented study was conducted as a pilot since no adequate data on the topic could be consulted to perform a sample size calculation. Statistical analyses were performed using the Mann-Whitney-U test via GraphPad Prism 8 software (GraphPad Software Inc., La Jolla, CA, USA) assuming a non-normal distribution. Data are presented as mean (standard deviation). P-values < 0.05 were considered significant.

Results

All 30 animals survived the intervention in good health and no problems were encountered at any time during mask ventilation, even if tracheal intubation proved difficult. Accordingly, all animals were available for the respective primary research project without any restrictions. In the FFI group, a higher first pass success rate (75% vs. 47%) and significantly less intubation attempts were protocolled than in the CI group (1.3 ± 0.6 vs. 2.1 ± 1.3, $P = 0.043$, Fig. 2). Intervention by a supervisor to perform tracheal intubation was necessary twice in the CI group, whereas no interventions were necessary in the FFI group. Successful intubation attempts were significantly shorter in the CI group than in the FFI group ($42 s \pm 6 s$ vs. $67 s \pm 10s$, $P < 0.001$, Fig. 2). Intubations were performed by a total of four participants with two supervisors assessing the data and controlling the experiments. No correlations over time regarding improved performances of the individual students could be detected.

Discussion

This study shows that FFI can be performed with a higher success rate and a better first pass success in inexperienced providers than conventional intubation by a MacIntosh blade in swine. It is the first trial to prospectively evaluate the potential benefits towards airway management using FFI in an experimental design in swine that support FFI as a reasonable method for

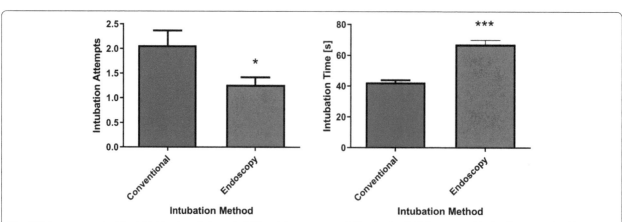

Fig. 2 Data assessment of the trial. Number of attempts (left) and time to successful intubation (right) compared by intubation method ($n = 15$ per group). With the endoscopic technique, significantly less intubation attempts were necessary (*: $P = 0.043$). Successful video-endoscopic intubation took more time per attempt until adequate ventilation was completely established (***:$P < 0.001$) but showed less desaturation episodes. Statistical analyses were performed using the Mann-Whitney U test

intubation. Furthermore, a practical and efficient approach to student and resident training at the same time is described and evaluated. Our results suggest significantly less problems with the establishment of a secure airway when provided with a FFI device compared to CI. This effect proved significant in inexperienced providers as shown by the limited amount of attempts needed to place a tracheal tube. Simultaneously, first pass success rate was distinctly increased when a FFI device was used, suggesting less stress for the animal, less hypoxic episodes during induction and, subsequently, less potentially confounding factors tainting research results.

FFI required a longer intubation time when compared to CI. However, this had no clinically relevant effect. The described prolongation was most likely due to device handling, coordination with the video monitor as well as the time needed to verify tube positioning, since ventilation in our experimental setup could not be initiated before the endoscope had been removed from the tube. A longer time to intubation using endoscopic devices is common when compared to CI in humans [20, 21]. However, the time to intubation using FFI significantly improves through training and expertise [21, 22]. Furthermore, a shorter time to ventilation by FFI is possible by using respiratory adapters to facilitate ventilation during endoscopy [23].

Teaching and training health care providers to adequately apply flexible endoscopes for intubation purposes is technically challenging, expensive and time-consuming [16, 20]. Manikins as well as virtual reality simulators are reliable training methods for FFI and can facilitate skill maintenance [15, 24]. In inexperienced providers, reported times until successful FFI compass 80 s [24] up to 260 s [15], whereas success rates are cited from 50% before training and 80% after virtual reality training [24]. On the one hand, this data is based on different study designs and obviously cannot be compared with the porcine model. On the other hand, there is a trend that swine can be intubated more quickly using FFI than the airway models currently used.

One common training opportunity in clinical routine for residents is the awake FFI in patients with anticipated difficult airway. This collective is found in ear-nose-throat and maxillofacial surgery to a higher degree than in other surgical disciplines [25]. However, various national guidelines considerably differ concerning the indication of awake FFI. Moreover, local protocols and clinical routine often does not foster FFI. Thus, structured and sufficient training programs have to rely on manikins and other models as well [22]. Animal models are perceived as more realistic compared to manikins, suggesting benefits during resident training [17]. Our model could not only provide the opportunity to perform airway management training, but, in contrast to clinical approaches, more than one

provider could also be trained on the same animal subsequently and repeat the procedure multiple times, offering a more efficient way to gain proficiency in device handling. Additionally, the use of a video monitor allows a supervisor to directly teach the procedure, thus potentially improving the experience even further. Single-use bronchoscopes, as shown in our trial, can also be used repeatedly to decrease material costs. Alternatively, following our own protocol, an established research facility could schedule regular short intubation trainings during the induction of their animals with the possibility to further use the animal for protocol purposes as needed afterwards. This obviously depends on experimental setups and possible confounding effects on specific studies but might be valid in some cases. Since this would decrease animal numbers by dual-use in research and education, institutional approval to respective protocol addenda should not be problematic.

Using endoscopic techniques for tracheal intubation in animals is sophisticated and rarely used, but reports in rodents [26], ruminants [27], swine [17] and more exotic animals [28] have been previously published. Interestingly, the last - and to the best of our knowledge - only published scientific use of FFI in swine was 30 years ago by Forbes et al., who not only proved feasibility, but concluded that training with a live porcine model was more realistic and had a greater clinical benefit for students and residents [17]. Unfortunately, the topic was never properly examined again, although porcine models have become an invaluable asset in translational research, especially of systemic diseases like sepsis and ARDS [29, 30] and are regularly established at university hospitals and research facilities. Most of these models usually rely on tracheal intubation [10, 12, 31], although some either resort to surgical airways, i.e. tracheostomy [32, 33], or supraglottic devices [34, 35]. However, tracheal intubation of pigs can be difficult and success depends on experience, expertise and correct preparation [12, 19]. Laryngeal anatomy of supine piglets can be challenging due to a hypermobile larynx, a long snout, deep perilaryngeal recesses and a long epiglottis that usually blocks direct access to the airway in sedated animals [9, 10]. The significantly longer oral cavity compared to humans can make it hard to visualize the epiglottis, which is long, U-shaped and often lodged on the soft palate. However, from the authors' experience, it is usually feasible to use conventional laryngoscopes (size 4) for adequate visualization and then mobilize the lodged epiglottis with a guide rod by carefully inserting it along the soft palate in the right or left piriform recess and then perform a scooping motion to the opposite side to mobilize it. Once mobilized, as long as the animal is not repositioned, the epiglottis usually does not lodge again and intubation and visualization should be easily feasible.

Complications and mortality associated with intubation in pigs have not been comprehensively described yet, but difficult airway management is regularly mentioned [9–11]. This includes the loss of research animals during induction [13, 14] suggesting underreporting and maybe the basis of a general confounder of animal airway studies. The determined failure rate to intubate on the first attempt of over 50% in our study seems high, but retrospective analysis of our own research projects also suggests rates between 25 and 40%. The additional increase in this trial can easily be attributed to the lack of intubation experience of the performing participants. Furthermore, TTs with a diameter of 7 mm are relatively large compared to standard procedures suggested by other research groups [8, 19]. While this may have caused an increased failure rate in the CI group compared to smaller tubes, successful placement following FFI suggests a technique-related problem and not an anatomical one. Especially research protocols relying on low ventilation pressures and decreased lung stress could benefit from the possibility to use larger bore tubes. Since piglets can be easily ventilated non-invasively with a suitable mask, intubation problems rather represent a time factor than an actual hazard, delaying eventual tube placement. However, as more intensive manipulation is necessary to establish the airway during CI, increased stress and hypoxia-induced changes might affect the results of planned projects. Since no data on this cause-effect relation exist, this remains speculative. Nonetheless, our study suggests a potentially systematic benefit of a FFI approach to porcine models, which could improve scientific accuracy of experimental results. This would simultaneously decrease the animal numbers needed, thus warranting the additional economical effort of establishing the infrastructure necessary.

Conclusion

Video-enhanced flexible fibreoptic intubation is an excellent method to safely secure the airway in swine. It can be used to provide more realistic training conditions for inexperienced providers and may simultaneously prevent airway complications, negative experimental effects and unnecessary animal losses in translational research.

Supplementary information

Additional file 1. Video recorded with the Ambu aScope™ system. The video depicts laryngeal passage after epiglottis mobilisation (see Fig. 1) and endotracheal insertion of the endoscope. Note the narrow space available to pass the larynx and the anatomical angle of the trachea. Porcine tracheas tend to be longer than in humans. Additionally, the upper main bronchus usually parts above the carina (00:37). This has to be considered to prevent inadequate placement of the tracheal tube. The endoscope should not be removed until definitive visualisation of the correct tube positioning was successful.

Acknowledgements
Excerpts of this study are part of the professorial dissertation (habilitation) of RR.

Authors' contributions
RR and EKH designed and supervised the experiments. AZ, TO and DD conducted the experiments and helped analyse the data. RR wrote the article, EKH and TO revised and approved the final draft. The author(s) read and approved the final manuscript.

References
1. Peterson GN, Domino KB, Caplan RA, Posner KL, Lee LA, Cheney FW. Management of the difficult airway: a closed claims analysis. Anesthesiology. 2005;103:33–9.
2. Cook TM, Woodall N, Frerk C, Fourth National Audit P. Major complications of airway management in the UK: results of the fourth National Audit Project of the Royal College of Anaesthetists and the difficult airway society. Part 1: anaesthesia. Br J Anaesth. 2011;106:617–31.
3. Frerk C, Mitchell VS, McNarry AF, et al. Difficult airway society 2015 guidelines for management of unanticipated difficult intubation in adults. Br J Anaesth. 2015;115:827–48.
4. Schauble JC, Heidegger T. Management of the difficult airway : overview of the current guidelines. Anaesthesist. 2018;67:725–37.
5. Apfelbaum JL, Hagberg CA, Caplan RA, et al. Practice guidelines for management of the difficult airway: an updated report by the American Society of Anesthesiologists Task Force on Management of the Difficult Airway. Anesthesiology. 2013;118:251–70.
6. Piepho T, Cavus E, Noppens R, et al. S1 guidelines on airway management : guideline of the German society of anesthesiology and intensive care medicine. Anaesthesist. 2015;64(Suppl 1):27–40.
7. Law JA, Broemling N, Cooper RM, et al. The difficult airway with recommendations for management--part 2--the anticipated difficult airway. Can J Anaesth. 2013;60:1119–38.
8. Judge EP, Hughes JM, Egan JJ, Maguire M, Molloy EL, O'Dea S. Anatomy and bronchoscopy of the porcine lung. A model for translational respiratory medicine. Am J Respir Cell Mol Biol. 2014;51:334–43.
9. Dondelinger RF, Ghysels MP, Brisbois D, et al. Relevant radiological anatomy of the pig as a training model in interventional radiology. Eur Radiol. 1998;8:1254–73.
10. Duke-Novakovski T, Ambros B, Auckland CD, Harding JC. The effects of succinylcholine or low-dose rocuronium to aid endotracheal intubation of adult sows. Can J Vet Res. 2012;76:57–61.
11. Gorti GK, Birchall MA, Haverson K, Macchiarini P, Bailey M. A preclinical model for laryngeal transplantation: anatomy and mucosal immunology of the porcine larynx. Transplantation. 1999;68:1638–42.
12. Benson GJ. Anesthetic management of ruminants and swine with selected pathophysiologic alterations. Vet Clin North Am Food Anim Pract. 1986;2:677–91.
13. Bowman J, Juergens A, McClure M, Spear D. Intubation of the Right Atrium During an Attempted Modified Surgical Airway in a Pig. J Spec Oper Med. 2017;17:96–100.
14. Steinbacher R, von Ritgen S, Moens YP. Laryngeal perforation during a standard intubation procedure in a pig. Lab Anim. 2012;46:261–3.
15. KL R, Bautista A, Duan X, et al. Teaching basic fiberoptic intubation skills in a simulator: initial learning and skills decay. J Anesth. 2016;30:12–9.
16. Boulton AJ, Balla SR, Nowicka A, Loka TM, Mendonca C. Advanced airway training in the UK: A national survey of senior anesthetic trainees. J Anaesthesiol Clin Pharmacol. 2019;35:326–34.
17. Forbes RB, Murray DJ, Albanese MA. Evaluation of an animal model for teaching fibreoptic tracheal intubation. Can J Anaesth. 1989;36:141–4.
18. Ruemmler R, Ziebart A, Moellmann C, et al. Ultra-low tidal volume ventilation—A novel and effective ventilation strategy during experimental cardiopulmonary resuscitation. Resuscitation. 2018;132:56–62.
19. Pehbock D, Dietrich H, Klima G, Paal P, Lindner KH, Wenzel V. Anesthesia in swine : optimizing a laboratory model to optimize translational research. Anaesthesist. 2015;64:65–70.
20. Collins SR, Blank RS. Fiberoptic intubation: an overview and update. Respir Care. 2014;59:865–78 discussion 78-80.
21. Schaefer HG, Marsch SC, Keller HL, Strebel S, Anselmi L, Drewe J. Teaching fibreoptic intubation in anaesthetised patients. Anaesthesia. 1994;49:331–4.

22. Johnson C, Roberts JT. Clinical competence in the performance of fiberoptic laryngoscopy and endotracheal intubation: a study of resident instruction. J Clin Anesth. 1989;1:344–9.
23. Da Conceicao M, Genco G, Favier JC, Bidallier I, Pitti R. Fiberoptic bronchoscopy during noninvasive positive-pressure ventilation in patients with chronic obstructive lung disease with hypoxemia and hypercapnia. Ann Fr Anesth Reanim. 2000;19:231–6.
24. Boet S, Bould MD, Schaeffer R, et al. Learning fibreoptic intubation with a virtual computer program transfers to 'hands on' improvement. Eur J Anaesthesiol. 2010;27:31–5.
25. El-Boghdadly K, Onwochei DN, Cuddihy J, Ahmad I. A prospective cohort study of awake fibreoptic intubation practice at a tertiary Centre. Anaesthesia. 2017;72:694–703.
26. Costa DL, Lehmann JR, Harold WM, Drew RT. Transoral tracheal intubation of rodents using a fiberoptic laryngoscope. Lab Anim Sci. 1986;36:256–61.
27. Paladino L, DuCanto J, Manoach S. Development of a rapid, safe, fiber-optic guided, single-incision cricothyrotomy using a large ovine model: a pilot study. Resuscitation. 2009;80:1066–9.
28. Johnson DH. Endoscopic intubation of exotic companion mammals. Vet Clin North Am Exot Anim Pract. 2010;13:273–89.
29. Yokoyama T, Tomiguchi S, Nishi J, et al. Hyperoxia-induced acute lung injury using a pig model: correlation between MR imaging and histologic results. Radiat Med. 2001;19:131–43.
30. Wang HM, Bodenstein M, Duenges B, et al. Ventilator-associated lung injury superposed to oleic acid infusion or surfactant depletion: histopathological characteristics of two porcine models of acute lung injury. Eur Surg Res. 2010;45:121–33.
31. Steffey EP. Some characteristics of ruminants and swine that complicate management of general anesthesia. Vet Clin North Am Food Anim Pract. 1986;2:507–16.
32. Kurita T, Morita K, Kazama T, Sato S. Comparison of isoflurane and propofol-fentanyl anaesthesia in a swine model of asphyxia. Br J Anaesth. 2003;91:871–7.
33. Takala RS, Soukka HR, Salo MS, et al. Pulmonary inflammatory mediators after sevoflurane and thiopentone anaesthesia in pigs. Acta Anaesthesiol Scand. 2004;48:40–5.
34. Goldmann K, Kalinowski M, Dieterich J, Wulf H. Use of the LMA-ProSeal in an experimental pig model -- a potential animal model for laryngeal mask airway research: results of a pilot study. Anasthesiol Intensivmed Notfallmed Schmerzther. 2006;41:223–7.
35. Goldmann K, Kalinowski M, Kraft S. Airway management under general anaesthesia in pigs using the LMA-ProSeal: a pilot study. Vet Anaesth Analg. 2005;32:308–13.

14

Dislocation rates of postoperative airway exchange catheters: A prospective case series of 200 patients

Fredy-Michel Roten[1][*][†][iD], Richard Steffen[1][†], Maren Kleine-Brueggeney[1,2], Robert Greif[1], Marius Wipfli[3], Andreas Arnold[4], Henrik Fischer[5] and Lorenz Theiler[1]

Abstract

Background: The dislocation rate of oral versus nasal airway exchange catheters (AEC) in the postoperative care unit (PACU) are unknown. Our aim was to establish dislocation rates and to assess the usefulness of waveform capnography to detect dislocation.

Methods: In this non-randomized, prospective observational trial at the University Hospital Bern, Switzerland, we included 200 patients admitted to PACU after extubation via AEC, having provided written informed consent. The study was approved by the local ethical committee. AEC position was assessed by nasal fiberoptic endoscopy at beginning of PACU stay and before removal of the AEC. Capnography was continuously recorded via the AEC. Additional measurements included retching and coughing of the patient, and re-intubation, if necessary.

Results: Data from 182 patients could be evaluated regarding dislocation. Overall dislocation rate was not different between oral and nasal catheters (7.2% vs. 2.7%, $p = 0.16$). Retching was more often noted in oral catheters (26% vs. 8%, $p < 0.01$). Waveform capnography was unreliable in predicting dislocation (negative predictive value 17%). Re-intubation was successful in all five of the nine re-intubations where an AEC was still in situ. In four patients, the AEC was already removed when re-intubation became necessary, and re-intubation failed once, with a front of neck access as a rescue maneuver.

Conclusions: We found no difference in dislocation rate between nasal and oral position of an airway exchange catheter. However, nasal catheters seemed to be tolerated better. In the future, catheters like the staged extubation catheter may further increase tolerance.

Keywords: Airway, Extubation, Intubation, Airway exchange catheter, Oral, Nasal, Postoperative, Dislocation

Background

Tracheal extubation requires as much dedication and attention as tracheal intubation, but this is often neglected, and thus adverse events during extubation are frequent. The British National Audit Project 4 showed that one sixth of all reported cases of serious adverse events occurred upon emergence or during recovery from anesthesia [1]. Likewise, complications during extubation are potentially harmful, with a reported mortality rate of 5% and a 13% rate of severe adverse outcomes with extubation failure related to general anesthesia [1]. Hence, the use of a staged extubation plan is recommended, which may include an airway exchange catheter (AEC) [2, 3]. The AEC was initially designed as an airway exchange catheter, not as an extubation catheter, hence its name. The AEC is a device, designed to maintain access to the airway after extubation to facilitate reintubation. As such, the rate of reported complications during exchange of a tracheal tube is quite high. A retrospective report in 2013 reported a

* Correspondence: fredy-michel.roten@insel.ch
†Roten F.M. and Richard S. are contributed equally to this work and share the first authorship.
[1]Department of Anesthesiology and Pain Therapy, Bern University Hospital and University of Bern, CH-3010 Bern, Switzerland

failure rate of 9.3% (39.3% when exchanging to a double lumen tube) and the airway injury rate was 7.8% with a 1.5% rate of pneumothorax [4]. In that study, difficult tube exchange was encountered in 6 of 8 patients with pneumothorax.

When used as a back-up device for extubation, the AEC were successful in 7 of the 9 cases (78%) when patient had to be re-intubated postoperatively [4]. In a study in ICU, the AEC showed an overall success rate of 92% (47 of 51) and a first-pass success rate of 87% [5]. Three out of 51 (6%) patients could not be intubated even after multiple attempts, and dislocation of the AEC may have been a reason for this. The report does not indicate whether these patients had oral or nasal AECs, which might have made a difference.

Based on these studies, it is unclear whether a nasally or orally placed AEC would show a lower dislocation rate and which position would be better tolerated by the patient.

We therefore prospectively evaluated the position of the AEC in patients admitted to the PACU who were extubated via an AEC. We expected the dislocation rate of the AEC to be different, depending on nasal versus oral position.

Methods

The local ethics committee approved this prospective observational study (Kantonale Ethikkommission KEK, Bern, Switzerland, reference number 060/10) and the study was registered in a clinical study registry (ISRCTN 96726807). For this observational, nonrandomized quality control study, we prospectively included two hundred adult patients (> 18 years old) admitted to the PACU who were extubated via an AEC (Cook Airway Exchange Catheter, Cook Medical Inc., Bloomington, IN, USA) and who gave written informed consent to use their data obtained during the PACU stay. There were no other exclusion criteria defined. As the decision for an AEC was made by the attending anesthesia team in the OR, obtaining informed consent while the patient was still awake prior to surgery was not possible. Therefore, informed consent was obtained at the time of discharge from the PACU when the patient was awake, fully oriented, free of pain and with stable vital signs. If this was not the case, the patients were consented on the day after surgery on the ward or, if the patients had already left the hospital, by telephone and postal letter. The decision to place an AEC was based on clinical judgment of the attending anesthesiologist and the surgeon in the operating room who were not part of the study group and not involved in PACU care, as was the choice of nasal vs. oral placement and the size of the AEC.

At admission to the PACU, the following AEC parameters were obtained: location, size, depth from either the corner of the mouth or the nares, and indication of the AEC. Coughing and retching as part of the patient's tolerance of the AEC were also noted throughout the PACU stay. Other recorded parameters included demographic parameters, the real and the planned period the AEC remained in situ, as well as side effects.

End-tidal carbon dioxide was measured and recorded continuously as waveform capnography until removal of the AEC using a Philips Sidestream™ system (Philips Medizin Systeme, Böblingen GmbH, Germany) by connecting the CO_2 sample line (Straight Sample Line H, Philips) to the adapter on the AEC. We assumed that the ability to measure CO_2 would reflect correct position.

The position of the AEC was verified by the attending anesthesiologist of the PACU with a flexible 2.8 mm nasopharyngoscope (Karl Storz GmbH & Co. KG, Tuttlingen, Germany) on arrival to the PACU and before removal of the AEC. Finally, the incidence of re-intubation was recorded along with the success of re-intubation.

Statistical analysis

Our primary outcome parameter was overall dislocation rate. Secondary outcomes were patients' characteristics, size of AEC, depth of AEC and position on arrival at PACU, length of stay of AEC and side effects (coughing and retching) and reintubation rate.

We hypothesized that nasally placed AECs remain significantly more often in the correct position in the trachea up until the time of removal, and that the difference of correct position compared to oral AECs would be at least 10%. H_0 = Dislocation rate oral − Dislocation rate nasal < 10%.

The sample size was based on a pilot observation which showed 3 of 30 (10%) dislocated AEC in the oral group vs. 0 of 30 (0%) dislocated AEC in the nasal group. To reach a power of 80% with a one-sided alpha of $p = 0.05$, a total of 158 patients are necessary. To compensate for missing data and drop-outs, we decided to include 200 patients.

Binary data were analyzed by Chi square test, or by Fisher's exact test if more than 20% of expected values were below 5. Ordinal data were evaluated using Kruskal-Wallis test. Continuous data were checked for normality by Q-Q plots and Shapiro-Wilk test. Normally distributed data were analyzed by Student's t-test, otherwise Mann-Whitney u-test was used.

Binary data are presented as numbers (%), continuous data as mean ± standard deviation (SD) if normally distributed, and otherwise as median with interquartile range (25th to 75th percentile). A probability of $p < 0.05$ was considered statistically significant. Data were analyzed using stata V.15.1 (StataCorp™, College Station, TX, USA).

Results

We prospectively included 200 patients who were admitted to the PACU after tracheal extubation via an oral or nasal AEC between December 2009 and May 2011. Two datasheets had to be dismissed because of an excess of missing data, leaving 198 patients for analysis. All patients provided written informed consent to use their data.

Seventy-four patients presented with an oral AEC in place after extubation, and 124 patients had a nasal AEC. Patients were treated predominantly in ENT, followed by orthopedics (Table 1). There was no difference in demographics between the two groups regarding sex, American Society of Anesthesiologists (ASA) class, weight, or body mass index. Patients with an oral catheter were slightly older. Most often, an 11 French catheter was used (71%, Table 2).

Dislocation rate and side effects

At the time of entering PACU, 4% of oral catheters and 2% of nasal catheters were already displaced as determined by nasal endoscopy. When analyzing dislocation rate, 16 datasets (5 oral AEC, 11 nasal AEC) had to be excluded because of insufficient data regarding AEC position at the time of removal. These 8% missing data represented catheters being removed without prior checking by the attending anesthesiologist (Table 2). Regarding the primary outcome parameter, overall dislocation rate, there was no significant difference between the oral and the nasal position of the catheter and thus, the null hypothesis could not be rejected (7.2% vs. 2.7%, $p = 0.16$). The odds ratio of dislocation of oral AECs vs. nasal AEC was 2.86 (95% CI: 0.66–12.39).

Interestingly, significantly more patients were retching when an oral catheter was in place compared with a nasal catheter (26% vs. 8%, $p < 0.01$). In the group with oral catheters, 41% were coughing, compared to 28% in the nasal group ($p = 0.06$). The size of the AEC did not influence retching ($p = 0.53$). Following anatomical differences between the nasal and the oral position, nasal catheters were introduced deeper compared to oral catheters (26 cm vs. 29 cm, Table 1). No serious side effects such as pneumothorax were encountered.

Capnography as indicator of correct position

CO_2 data from 20 catheters were incomplete and had to be excluded. In both groups, oral and nasal, there was one catheter dislodged as verified by nasal endoscopy even though CO_2 could always be measured (oral AECs: 1 of 59 vs. nasal AECs 1 of 96). Six of 8 oral AEC and 13 of 15 nasal AEC did not show CO_2, even though the intratracheal position was confirmed by nasal endoscopy. As a test of correct tracheal position, the presence of CO_2 showed an overall sensitivity of 89% and a specificity of 67%. The overall positive predictive value (PPV) was 98.7% (indicating that a correct tracheal position was likely if CO_2 present), the negative predictive value (NPV) was only 17% (waveform capnography often did not show CO_2 even in correctly positioned catheters).

Removal of AEC and re-intubation

Oral catheters were removed earlier compared to nasal catheters, reflecting the plan for earlier removal of these catheters. Nevertheless, a marked drop in numbers of oral AECs in the first hour after PACU admission was noted (Fig. 1). Additionally, 3 oral catheters remained in place longer than 6 h (maximum of 11), whereas 16 nasal catheters remained in place longer than 6 h, 6 of them longer than 12 h (maximum of 19).

Of the 198 studied patients, re-intubation due to respiratory insufficiency was necessary in 9 patients (Table 2). In only 5 of these patients the AEC was still in situ: one patient in the oral group and four patients in the nasal group. All re-intubations were successful via the AEC. In four patients, re-intubation became necessary

Table 1 Demographics

$n = 198$	Oral AEC $n = 74$	Nasal AEC $n = 124$	p-value
Female; n (%)	25 (34)	34 (27)	0.34
Surgical intervention ENT/Orthopedics/Maxillofacial/ General/missing data n (%)	46/16/1/8/3 (62/22/1/11/4)	65/26/14/1/18 (52/21/11/1/15)	0.001
Age in years (mean ± SD)	63.2 ± 14.2	58.1 ± 16.1	0.03
Weight in kg (mean ± SD)	77.1 ± 17.5	74.8 ± 17.0	0.37
Height in cm (mean ± SD)	170.3 ± 8.2	172.4 ± 10.3	0.15
BMI kg m^{-2} (mean ± SD)	26.6 ± 5.8	25.1 ± 4.8	0.05
ASA class I/ II/ III/ IV/ missing data; n (%)	5/31/33/2/3 (7/42/45/3/4)	10/41/64/4/5 (8/33/52/3/4)	0.81

Data are mean and standard deviation (SD), or numbers and percent
AEC Airway Exchange Catheter, ENT ears, nose, and throat

Table 2 Main Outcome Parameters

n = 198	Oral AEC n = 74	Nasal AEC n = 124	p-value
Size of AEC in French 8/ 11/ 14/ 19, n (%) *missing: 3 nasal*	0/48/22/4 (0/65/30/5)	1/71/47/2 (1/59/39/2)	0.23
Depth of AEC in cm (mean ± SD)	26.2 ± 3.3	29.3 ± 2.5	<0.001
AEC was correctly positioned on arrival PACU, yes (%)	68 (96%)	118 (98%)	0.67
95% confidence interval of correct position *missing: 3 in each group*	88.1 – 99.1%	92.9 – 99.5%	
AEC was correctly positioned until removal yes/no, n (%)	64/ 5 (93/ 7)	110/ 3 (97/ 3)	0.16
95% confidence interval of correct position *missing: 5 oral, 11 nasal*	83.9 – 97.6%	92.4 – 99.4%	
Length of stay of AEC in hours, median (IQR) min. – max.	2.5 (1.25, 4.5) 0 – 11	4 (3, 6) 0 – 19	<0.001
Patients coughing in PACU, yes n (%) *missing: 6 oral, 15 nasal*	28 (41%)	30 (28%)	0.06
Patients retching in PACU, yes n (%) *missing: 6 oral, 9 nasal*	18 (26%)	8 (8%)	0.001
Re-intubation necessary	1 (via AEC)	4 (via AEC), 4 (AEC already removed)	0.56

Data are numbers and percent, mean and standard deviation (SD) or median and interquartile range (IQR)
AEC Airway Exchange Catheter

after the AEC was removed (1 to over 12 h after removal). This was successful in three patients. In one patient a surgical airway was necessary, with good outcome.

Discussion

This prospective observational study showed that orally placed AEC tended to have a higher dislocation rate compared to nasally placed AEC (odds ratio 2.86). However, and contrary to our expectations, this finding was not statistically significant (95% confidence interval of the odds ratio was 0.66–12.39).

The non-invasive capnography proofed to be a double-edged sword and not highly reliable to verify the position of the AEC. On the one hand, presence of CO_2

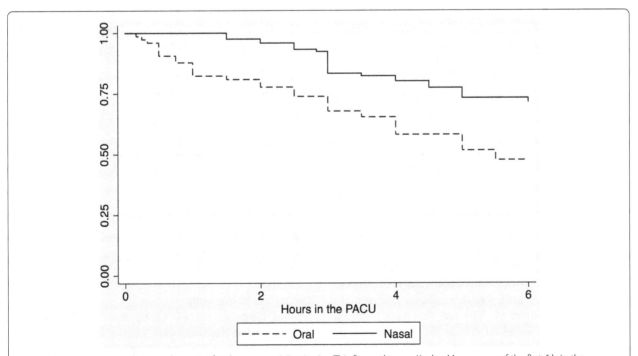

Fig. 1 Kaplan-Meyer curve showing the ratio of catheters remaining in situ. This figure shows a Kaplan-Meyer curve of the first 6 h in the post-anesthesia care unit (PACU) showing the ratio of catheters (oral and nasal) remaining in situ

was highly suggestive of correct intratracheal position, as was reflected by the high positive predictive value of 99%. On the other hand, obstruction of the AEC lumen was frequent, which led to loss of CO_2 reading and required additional care. Apparently, the only reliable option is to check AEC position via (nasal) flexible scope.

Based on our results of a relatively high overall dislocation rate of 4.4%, and our findings that dislocation cannot be ruled out by non-invasive means, we argue that the insertion of an AEC is not a reliable back-up for re-intubation in case of a known difficult airway. Furthermore, the chance of an esophageal dislocation should be a strong argument against the application of oxygen via the AEC, as has been pointed out by others [6–8]. Our dislocation rate of 4.4% was even smaller than reported before: A small audit in 18 patients revealed a dislocation rate of 11%, a further 11% did not tolerate the AEC [9].

Of note, the catheters were often inserted too deeply, compared to current guidelines: the mean insertion depth of oral catheters was 26.6 cm compared to a recommended maximum of 25 cm [10, 11]. Inserting AEC beyond recommended limits may lead to airway trauma and potentially death because of a (tension) pneumothorax, especially when additional oxygen is applied via the AEC [12]. Fortunately, we never encountered this complication in our study, but we also did not apply additional oxygen via the AEC. Catheters that feature a soft tip may have the potential to reduce the incidence of barotrauma and airway injury, but this has not been studied so far [13]. Either way, it is crucial to carefully avoid deep insertion of the AEC, and given the fact that others have reported complications from too deeply inserted AECs one must assume that this remains one of the main complications of AECs. A safer way may be to provide nasal oxygen during the re-intubation attempt, either low-flow [14] or high-flow nasal oxygen [15].

Oral catheters were removed earlier compared to nasal catheters, although this was frequently due to planned removal. However, the drop in AEC numbers over the first hour was more dominant in the oral group, perhaps reflecting frequent patient discomfort caused by coughing and retching with an oral AEC in place. In fact, the only statistically significant difference we could find was a higher incidence of postoperative retching in the oral group compared to nasally placed catheters ($p < 0.01$).

When looking at the re-intubation rate, a surprisingly high number of patients was re-intubated after removal of the AEC (4 out of 9). The fact that only 5 of 198 AECs were used for re-intubation also means that the use of 97.4% of the AECs (193 of 198) was unnecessary, which led to unnecessary patient discomfort, costs and potential adverse events. However, it is extremely difficult to predict which patients will require re-intubation, and for those patients who do require re-intubation a (correctly positioned) AEC can potentially be life-saving or at least avoid an emergency front of neck access. The overall re-intubation rate (9 of 198, 5%) was lower than the 8% reported earlier [16], although our data regarding re-intubation comprise only patients who were re-intubated in the PACU, not patients who were re-intubated in the operating room or patients who did not receive an AEC at all.

The use of an AEC for re-intubation in expected difficult extubation is recommended by many experts and guidelines [2, 6]. In our study, the success rate of re-intubation via AEC was 100% (5 out of 5), similar to the overall success rate of 92% (47 of 51) reported by Mort [5]. In that study, in addition to the benefit of high re-intubation success rates, the use of an AEC was associated with fewer episodes of severe hypoxemia (6% vs. 19%), of multiple intubation attempts (10% vs. 77%) and of esophageal intubation (0% vs. 18%), as pointed out in the accompanying editorial by Biro and Priebe [17]. To further increase the re-intubation success rate there is also the possibility to use an Aintree Intubation Catheter (Cook Medical Inc., Bloomington, IN, USA) in order to reduce the gap between a small AEC and the tracheal tube [18].

Our study also confirms the necessity of the presence of an adequate anesthesia service for high risk patients, even many hours postoperatively. As was described before, re-intubation can become necessary many hours postoperatively [5, 16]. Almost half of all re-intubations in our study occurred after removal of the AEC, between 1 and over 12 h after removal. To further improve the tolerance to the AEC, a wire-based AEC is available (Cook Staged Extubation Catheter™, Cook Medical Inc., Bloomington, IN, USA). A small preliminary study suggested high tolerance, as 17 of 23 patients (73%) tolerated the wire for 4 h, although "tolerated" was not further quantified [19]. Success rate and dislocation rate have not been proven to be different from the conventional AEC: Nasal endoscopy was performed in 11 of these patients and revealed one wire dislocated to the esophagus, which would correspond to a dislocation rate of 9%. In another recent small study, Furyk et al. reported an 8% failure rate in 23 low-risk patients when oral intubation was performed via the wire-based catheter [20].

Limitations of the study

Several limitations need to be mentioned. Foremost, several patient data sets were tainted with missing data. For example, 16 (8%, Table 2) of all catheters were removed by the patients themselves without giving us the possibility to check fiberoptically for correct position.

Finally, the power of the study was too low, as the null hypothesis could not be rejected. To find a difference between the dislocation rates of 7.2% vs. 2.6%, inclusion of over 600 patients would have been necessary, almost four times more than was anticipated. Furthermore, patients were not randomized, instead the attending anesthesiologist or the requirements of the surgical procedure decided about the placement of either an oral or a nasal AEC.

On the other hand, the combined assessment of waveform capnography and fiberoptic visualization of the correct or incorrect tube position in the PACU was never reported before. This allowed to calculate positive and negative predicted values for the use of capnography to verify correct tracheal position of the exchange catheters.

Conclusions

As a conclusion, this prospective evaluation of airway exchange catheters in the PACU revealed no statistically significant difference in dislocation rates between nasal and oral placement, but patients with nasal catheters were less prone to retching. In the difficult airway setting, it seems unjustified to exchange oral catheters to a nasal position in order to avoid dislocation. Waveform capnography is insufficient to correctly predict dislocation.

Acknowledgements
We thank Christine Riggenbach, R.N., Inselspital Bern, for her support with data collection.

Authors' contributions
FMR: contribution to conception and design; acquisition, analysis and interpretation of data; drafting and critically revising the article and giving final approval; RS: contribution to conception and design; acquisition, analysis and interpretation of data; drafting and critically revising the article and giving final approval; MKB: analysis and interpretation of data; drafting and critically revising the article and giving final approval; RG: contribution to conception and design; acquisition, analysis and interpretation of data; drafting and critically revising the article and giving final approval; MW: contribution to conception and design; acquisition, analysis and interpretation of data; critically revising the article and giving final approval; AA: contribution to conception and design; acquisition of data; critically revising the article and giving final approval; HF: contribution to conception and design; critically revising the article and giving final approval; LT: contribution to conception and design; acquisition, analysis and interpretation of data; critically revising the article and giving final approval.

Author details
[1]Department of Anesthesiology and Pain Therapy, Bern University Hospital and University of Bern, CH-3010 Bern, Switzerland. [2]Department of Anaesthesia, Evelina London Children's Hospital, Guys and St. Thomas' NHS Foundation Trust, London SE1 7EH, UK. [3]Department of Anaesthesiology and Pain Therapy, Lindenhofspital, CH-3011 Bern, Switzerland. [4]Department of Otorhinolaryngology, Head and Neck Surgery, Bern University Hospital and University of Bern, CH-3010 Bern, Switzerland. [5]Medical School, Sigmund Freud University, Kelsenstraße 2, A -1030 Vienna, Austria.

References
1. Cook TM, Woodall N, Harper J, Benger J, Fourth National Audit P. Major complications of airway management in the UK: results of the Fourth National Audit Project of the Royal College of Anaesthetists and the difficult airway society. Part 2: intensive care and emergency departments. Br J Anaesth. 2011;106(5):632–42.
2. Difficult Airway Society Extubation Guidelines G, Popat M, Mitchell V, Dravid R, Patel A, Swampillai C, et al. Difficult airway society guidelines for the management of tracheal extubation. Anaesthesia. 2012;67(3):318–40.
3. Cavallone LF, Vannucci A. Review article: Extubation of the difficult airway and extubation failure. Anesth Analg. 2013;116(2):368–83.
4. McLean S, Lanam CR, Benedict W, Kirkpatrick N, Kheterpal S, Ramachandran SK. Airway exchange failure and complications with the use of the cook airway exchange catheter(R): a single center cohort study of 1177 patients. Anesth Analg. 2013;117(6):1325–7.
5. Mort TC. Continuous airway access for the difficult extubation: the efficacy of the airway exchange catheter. Anesth Analg. 2007;105(5):1357–62.
6. Artime CA, Hagberg CA. Tracheal extubation. Respir Care. 2014;59(6):991–1002.
7. LeDez KM. Airway exchange catheters: appropriate use and gas embolism. Can J Anaesth. 2011;58(12):1142–3.
8. Duggan LV, Law JA, Murphy MF. Brief review: supplementing oxygen through an airway exchange catheter: efficacy, complications, and recommendations. Can J Anaesth. 2011;58(6):560–8.
9. Smith T, Vaughan D. Extubation over a bougie in difficult airways: are we missing a trick? Anaesthesia. 2013;68(9):974–5.
10. Frerk C, Mitchell VS, McNarry AF, Mendonca C, Bhagrath R, Patel A, et al. Difficult airway society 2015 guidelines for management of unanticipated difficult intubation in adults. Br J Anaesth. 2015;115(6):827–48.
11. Toki K, Yamaguchi Y, Miyashita T, Takaki S, Yamaguchi O, Goto T. Insertion length of airway exchange catheter during exchange of tracheal tube: a simulation study. Acta Anaesthesiol Scand. 2016;60(6):832–3.
12. Axe R, Middleditch A, Kelly FE, Batchelor TJ, Cook TM. Macroscopic barotrauma caused by stiff and soft-tipped airway exchange catheters: an in vitro case series. Anesth Analg. 2015;120(2):355–61.
13. Ramachandran SK. In response. Anesth Analg. 2014 Jul;119(1):216.
14. Weingart SD, Levitan RM. Preoxygenation and prevention of desaturation during emergency airway management. Ann Emerg Med. 2012;59(3):165–75.
15. Mir F, Patel A, Iqbal R, Cecconi M, Nouraei SA. A randomised controlled trial comparing transnasal humidified rapid insufflation ventilatory exchange (THRIVE) pre-oxygenation with facemask pre-oxygenation in patients undergoing rapid sequence induction of anaesthesia. Anaesthesia. 2017; 72(4):439–43.
16. Loudermilk EP, Hartmannsgruber M, Stoltzfus DP, Langevin PB. A prospective study of the safety of tracheal extubation using a pediatric airway exchange catheter for patients with a known difficult airway. Chest. 1997;111(6):1660–5.
17. Biro P, Priebe HJ. Staged extubation strategy: is an airway exchange catheter the answer? Anesth Analg. 2007;105(5):1182–5.
18. Law J, Duggan L. Extubation guidelines: use of airway exchange catheters. Anaesthesia. 2012;67(8):918–9 author reply 21-2.
19. McManus S, Jones L, Anstey C, Senthuran S. An assessment of the tolerability of the Cook staged extubation wire in patients with known or suspected difficult airways extubated in intensive care. Anaesthesia. 2018; 73(5):587–93.
20. Furyk C, Walsh ML, Kaliaperumal I, Bentley S, Hattingh C. Assessment of the reliability of intubation and ease of use of the cook staged extubation set- an observational study. Anaesth Intensive Care. 2017;45(6):695–9.

15

Usefulness of airway scope for intubation of infants with cleft lip and palate–comparison with macintosh laryngoscope

Yoko Okumura[*] iD, Masahiro Okuda, Aiji Sato Boku, Naoko Tachi, Mayumi Hashimoto, Tomio Yamada and Masahiro Yamada

Abstract

Background: Airway Scope (AWS) with its plastic blade does not require a head-tilt or separate laryngoscopy to guide intubations. Therefore, we hypothesized that its use would reduce the intubation time (IT) and the frequency of airway complication events when compared with the use of Macintosh Laryngoscope (ML) for infants with cleft lip and palate (CLP).

Methods: The parents of all patients provided written consents; we enrolled 40 infants with CLP (ASA-PS 1). After inducing general anesthesia using sevoflurane and rocuronium, we performed orotracheal intubations using either AWS ($n = 20$) or ML ($n = 20$), randomly. We define the duration between manual manipulation using cross finger for maximum mouth opening and the first raising motion of the chest following intubation by artificial ventilation as "IT;" further, the measured IT as primary outcomes. Airway complications were considered secondary outcomes. Moreover, we looked for associations between IT and the patient's characteristics: extensive clefts, age, height, and weight. We used the Mann–Whitney test and Fisher's exact probability test for statistical analysis; $p < 0.05$ was considered as statistically significant.

Results: The mean IT was 31.5 ± 8.3 s in AWS group and 26.4 ± 8.9 s in ML group. Statistical significant difference was not found in IT between the two groups. The IT of AWS group was statistically related to extensive clefts. Airway complications were detected in ML group.

Conclusion: AWS could be useful for intubation of infants with CLP; it required IT similar to that required using ML, with a lower rate of airway complications.

Keywords: Airway scope, Macintosh laryngoscope, Infant, Intubation time

* Correspondence: nabeko@dpc.agu.ac.jp
Department of Anesthesiology, Aichi Gakuin University School of Dentistry,
2-11 Suemori-dori, Chikusaku, Nagoya 464-8651, Japan

Background

It is recognized that intubation of infants is more difficult than that of adults [1] because infants have characteristics of macroglossia, i.e., both tongue and the epiglottis near the palate, a long and narrow epiglottis, and the large angle formed by trachea and vocal cords. Furthermore, intubation becomes difficult with craniofacial deformities or micrognathia [1]. Based on these factors, tracheal intubation is more difficult in the infants with cleft lip and palate (CLP) than in those without CLP [2, 3].

Ali et al [4] had compared intubation time for pediatric patients between pediatric Airtraq® and conventional Macintosh laryngoscope. They calculated the sample size on the bases of the mean outcome of intubation time required 30 s of the former and 40 s with a standard deviation of 8 s of the latter keeping α error 5% and power as 95% (1-β errors); therefore, the calculated sample size was 34 (17 in each group). Consequently, they concluded that Pediatric Airtaq® takes shorter time to intubate with less frequent complication than conventional laryngoscope in children.

In our hospital, Macintosh laryngoscope (ML) is the first alternative device for conventional intubation of infants with CLP. Alternatively, the blade of the Airway Scope (AWS) conforms to the upper airway and creates a groove for conducting a tracheal tube through the vocal cords, obviating the need for retroflexion of the head and spreading of the larynx. Therefore, AWS can potentially shorten intubation time (IT) compared to ML. Furthermore, AWS is unlikely to cause side effects as the blade is made of polycarbonate resin. However, it remains unclear as to which device is more useful for intubation of infants with CLP. We hypothesized that AWS would shorten IT and result in fewer side effects than ML.

Methods

Ethics approval and consent to participate

This study was approved by the Ethical Review Board of the Aichi Gakuin University School of Dentistry and was registered as a clinical trial with UMIN-CTR (No.000024763). The patients scheduled for cheiloplasty were hospitalized 2 days before the day of surgery based on specified rules of our hospital and received preanesthetic medical examination on that day. The patients were examined, and no systemic diseases or airway abnormalities were observed; therefore the anesthesiologist informed this research program, and written informed consent was obtained from the parents of the infant patients who agreed to participation in this study.

Subjects

The inclusion criteria were patients scheduled for cheiloplasty between 9 November 2016 and 31 October 2017, aged 3–11 months, and American Society of Anesthesiologists physical status I. The exclusion criteria were patients whose

parents declined to participate in this study, patients with medical history of airway abnormalities that needed tracheal intubation, or patients with cardiovascular complications.

We defined the duration between manual manipulation using cross finger for maximum mouth opening and the first raising motion of the chest following intubation by artificial ventilation as "IT;" further, we measured IT as the primary outcome. Based on the mean outcome of our pilot study including seven individuals for each group taken as 21 s in ML group and as 31 s in AWS group, we calculated effect size 1.00 using Cohen's d first and subsequently the sample size keeping α error as 5%, and power of the study as 80% (1-β errors). the minimum sample size thus calculated was 34 (17 in each group) using G*Power 3.1.9.2. (http://www.gpower.hhu.de/). We allocated the patients to one of the two groups using the sealed envelope technique. The envelopes were opaque and stapled with the allocation card inside stored in one opaque storage box, which were prepared before the start of this study by our hospital clerk who was not related to this study. Finally, 40 cases of ASA-PS 1 CLP infants were finally included in this study because we prepared 40 envelopes to avoid numerical lack for this study. The investigating anesthesiologists included four expert anesthesiologists with experience of ML technique of more than 5 years and of using AWS few times in both adults and infants. They intubated the patients according to the allocation card which was handed by our hospital clerk on the morning of the operation. A Φ3.5 mm tracheal tube of Halyard micro cuff® was used in all patients as a first choice; the ML group patients were then intubated with No. 1 blade; the AWS group patients were intubated with AWS with NK PBLADE ITL-PL®. We recorded and analyzed the research data (Fig. 1).

Evaluation parameters

We measured IT as primary outcomes. We also studied the visibility of the vocal cords, blade insertion, and tracheal tube insertion. Visibility of the vocal cords was evaluated by Cormack and Lehane grade and "quality of visual recognition of vocal cords," which is a point system of evaluation of subjects on a scale of 0–100 according to the anesthesiologist. Difficulty in blade insertion was evaluated by the presence of backward or forward movement of the blade at the pharynx, number of blade insertions, and "blade insertion difficulty," a point system of blade insertion operability evaluation on a scale of 0–100 according to the anesthesiologist. Difficulty of tracheal tube insertion was evaluated by the presence of changing head presentation, external compression of larynx, resizing of the tracheal tube if the Φ3.5 tube could not pass the glottis, and "difficulty of tracheal tube insertion," which was a point system of evaluation of subjects from 0 to 100 according to the anesthesiologist. We also assessed the correlation

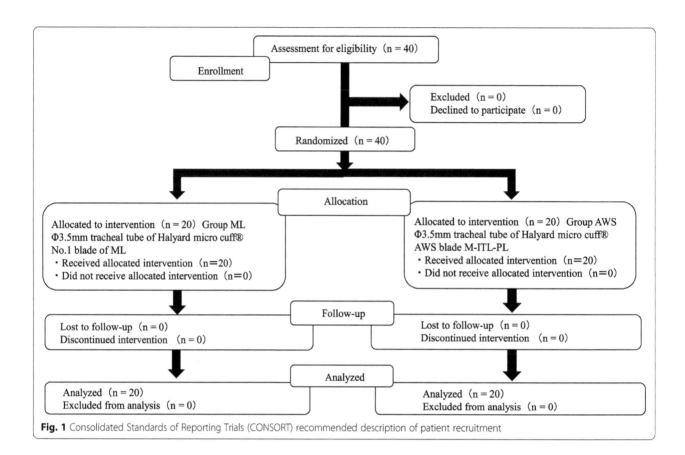

Fig. 1 Consolidated Standards of Reporting Trials (CONSORT) recommended description of patient recruitment

between patient background and IT. Moreover, we recorded complications regarding intubation maneuver as secondary outcomes, which included desaturation (< 94%), bleeding from oral or pharyngeal tissue, esophageal intubation, and hoarseness after extubation.

Statistical analysis
Characteristic of the patients, IT, numbers of attempts of intubation, visibility of vocal cords, and difficulty of blade insertion, and tracheal tube insertion were examined using the Student's t-test or Mann–Whitney test. The items

Table 1 Preoperative patient characteristics and observation of difficulty in securing the respiratory tract

	ML				AWS				p value
Degree of cleft and Region of fissure (n)	CL		CLP		CL		CLP		0.53
	unilateral	bilateral	unilateral	bilateral	unilateral	bilateral	unilateral	bilateral	
	4	2	10	4	8	1	6	5	
Sex: Male or Female (n)	male		female		male		female		0.25
	12		8		15		5		
Age (month)	5.8 ± 1.7				5.1 ± 1.2				0.22
Height (cm)	65.1 ± 3.0				64.8 ± 2.8				0.71
Weight (kg)	7.2 ± 0.8				7.1 ± 0.6				0.73
Megaloglossia or hyperplasia of palatine tonsil (n)	0				0				1
Interincisor Distance (mm)	31.0 ± 3.9				29.2 ± 7.3				0.34
limitation of cervical spine mobility (< 90°) (n)	0				0				1
Difficulty of mask ventilation (n)	0				0				1

CL cleft lip, *CLP* cleft lip and palate
The suspicious observation of difficulty in securing the respiratory tract or spreading the larynx, defined as megaloglossia, hyperplasia of palatine tonsil, trismus, limitation of cervical spine mobility, or difficulty of mask ventilation were not detected preoperatively

Table 2 IT and the factors affecting IT

		ML	AWS	P value
	Intubation time (sec)	26.4 ± 8.9	31.5 ± 8.3	0.07
Visibility of vocal cords	Cormack and Lehane grade median (IQR25%; IQR75%)	1(1; 1.5)	1(1; 1)	0.04
	Quality of visual recognition of vocal cords: good 0, bad 100 median (IQR25%; IQR75%)	0(0;10)	0(0; 20)	0.90
Difficulty of blade insertion	Number of cases with presence of backward or forward movement (n)	6	11	0.15
	Number of blade insertion: 1/2/3/4 (mean ± SD)	1	1.3 ± 0.5	0.04
	Difficulty of blade insertion: easy 0, dificult 100 median (IQR25%; IQR75%)	0(0; 10)	0(0; 20)	0.35
Difficulty of tracheal tube insertion	Number of cases with changing head presentation (n)	3	2	0.64
	Number of cases with external compression of larynx (n)	0	2	0.11
	Number of cases with resizing the tracheal tube (n)	0	1	0.32
	Difficulty of tracheal tube insertion: easy 0, dificult 100 median (IQR25%; IQR75%)	0(0; 22.5)	25(0; 40)	0.14

*:$p < 0.05$ (vs ML group)

difficulty of tracheal tube insertion and frequency of occurrence of complications were examined using Fisher's exact probability test. The correlation between patient background and IT was examined using Peason's correlation coefficient test.

Results

A total of 40 patients assessed for eligibility. All the patients were randomized for this study (Fig. 1). None of them excluded to follow up due to impossibility to intubate with the allocated method or postponement of the planned operation.

Characteristic of the patients

There were no differences in the degree and region of the cleft, sex, age, height, or weight between the two treatment groups (Table 1).

It

The average value of IT of the AWS group was 6 s greater than that of the ML group; however, significant difference was not detected in IT between the two groups (Table 2).

Visibility of vocal cords was higher in the AWS group than in the ML group. The number of blade insertion attempts in the AWS group was greater than the ML group. There was no statistical difference in the number of cases with change in head presentation, need for external laryngeal pressure, or resizing the tracheal tube between both the groups (Table 2).

Correlation between patient characteristics and IT

There was a significant correlation between IT and degree of cleft in the AWS group; however, no correlation was found between IT and patient characteristics in the ML group (Table 3).

Occurrence of complications

One case of bleeding from lip and three cases of bleeding from pharynx were observed in the ML group; however, none of these complications were detected in the AWS group. There was no correlation between occurrence of complications and IT in either group (Table 4).

Table 3 Correlation between patient characteristics and IT in AWS group

	ML						AWS					
	correlation	t value	p value	t (0.975)	95% lower limit	95% upper limit	correlation	t value	p value	t (0.975)	95% lower limit	95% upper limit
Degree of cleft:	0.11	0.47	0.644	2.10	− 0.35	0.53	0.51	2.51	0.022	2.10	0.09	0.78
Region of fissure	−0.17	− 0.72	0.483	2.10	−0.57	0.30	0.40	1.87	0.077	2.10	−0.05	0.72
Age (month)	−0.17	−0.73	0.472	2.10	−0.57	0.29	−0.18	−0.77	0.452	2.10	−0.58	0.29
Height (cm)	0.04	0.18	0.862	2.10	−0.41	0.48	−0.04	− 0.18	0.858	2.10	−0.48	0.41
Weight(kg)	0.40	1.88	0.077	2.10	−0.047	0.72	−0.14	−0.59	0.563	2.10	−0.55	0.32

*:$p < 0.05$ (vs intubation time)

Table 4 Occurrence of complications

	ML	AWS	p value
Desaturation (<94%) (n)	0	0	1
Bleeding from lips (n)	1	0	0.32
Bleeding from pharynx (n)	3	0	0.08
Bleeding from tongue (n)	0	0	1
Bleeding from palate (n)	0	0	1
Esophageal intubation (n)	0	0	1
Hoarseness after extubation (n)	1	1	1

Discussion

Yu et al [5] conducted a meta-analysis of 14 clinical studies of infant intubations, and concluded that video laryngoscope improved visibility of vocal cords but increased IT and incidence of intubation failure compared with direct viewing laryngoscope using ML. In the current study, no significant difference was observed in IT between the AWS and ML groups. Therefore, these data indicate that AWS may be a viable substitution to ML for intubation of infants with CLP.

Factors affecting IT
Visibility of vocal cords
Previous studies have attributed the difficulty of laryngoscopy in infants with CLP to young age [2], degree of cleft, and micrognathia [3]. In the current study, the Cormack and Lehane class of the ML group was statistically greater than that of the AWS group. However,

quality of view was not statistically different between the groups. This result may be obtained when the Cormack and Lehane grade is less than III, which is an index of difficult intubation; this was not observed in any of the groups. Accordingly, the quality of view was appropriate for intubation in both AWS and ML; hence, the quality of view was not related to IT.

Difficulty of blade insertion
It has previously been reported that the tip of AWS blade may inadvertently access the esophagus rather than the trachea when inserted in the infant airway [6]. In the current study, the esophagus was seen first on screen following insertion into the pharynx in the AWS cases; therefore, the number of cases in which the blade was moved backward or forward was greater in the AWS group than in the ML group. Because of this, re-insertion was favorable to moving forward and backward to avoid injuring the pharynx in the AWS group; hence, the number of attempts of blade insertions was greater than that in the ML group. Moreover, the length of the AWS blade is 65 mm, which is longer than that of infant upper airway; therefore, it may have necessitated the increased instances of moving forward and backward in this group. Conversely, the attached documents for the Halyard micro cuff® recommends a Φ3.0 mm tracheal tube for infants aged < 8 months whose weight is > 3 kg, and thus the size of blade for neonates may be suitable for most of the patients in this study. In our hospital, a Φ3.5 mm tracheal tube of Halyard micro cuff® is generally the first choice for infants with CLP.

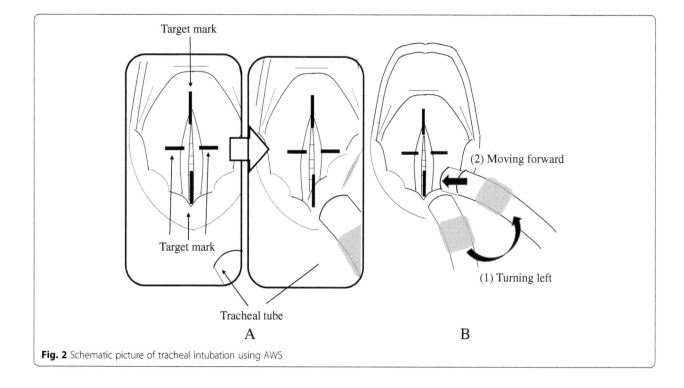

Fig. 2 Schematic picture of tracheal intubation using AWS

Therefore, we chose the blade for pediatrics that was fit for the Φ3.5 mm tracheal tube. IT might be shortened using a Φ3.0 mm tracheal tube of Halyard micro cuff® and neonate blade of AWS (length is 12 mm shorter than that for pediatrics) because of reduction in the time required to determine the location of the esophagus and detect the vocal cord by moving backward.

Difficulty of tracheal tube insertion

Unless the AWS target mark coincides with the vocal cords at the monitor screen before progression of the tube, it is easy for the tip of the tube to inadvertently hit the right Rima glottides as it is progressed to the vocal cords after removing from the blade groove in infants [6] (Fig. 2a). Therefore, the tube needs to be turned left following removal of the tube from the blade groove prior to progressing to the vocal cords (Fig. 2b). "Difficulty of tracheal tube insertion" was not statistically different between the two groups in this study; however, this maneuver might be administered as needed with the progression of the tube; hence, average of IT of AWS may be longer than that of ML.

Correlation between patient characteristics and IT

In bilateral CLP, the premaxilla and cleft palate edge protrude to the oral cavity and narrow the space. This formation may limit controllability of the AWS blade, explaining the correlation of degree of cleft and IT in the AWS group.

Complications

The AWS method has an increased risk of pharynx damage owing to the limited space between the blade and pharynx wall [7]. However, bleeding from upper airway was observed only in the ML group. The bleeding observed in the ML group was detected after fixing the tracheal tube with tapes on the lip. Nevertheless, anesthesiologists could watch the blade directly from the beginning of insertion to complete intubation when using ML. Therefore, the upper airway damage by ML may have been caused when the blade was removed from the pharynx or oral cavity. The number of cases with bleeding was not statistically different between the two groups; however, upper airway damage should be avoided, particularly in CLP surgery. More attention to upper airway mucosa is required not only at blade insertion but also at blade removal in ML even if an expert user of ML intubates, which might increase the IT time.

Conclusion

AWS could be useful for the intubation of infants with CLP; it required IT similar to that required using ML with lower rate of airway complications.

Abbreviations

AWS: Airway scope; CL: Cleft lip; CLP: Cleft lip and palate; IT: Intubation time; ML: Macintosh laryngoscope

Acknowledgements

The authors would like to thank the Department of Anesthesiology at Aichi Gakuin University Dental Hospital for their help in recruiting patients for this study.

Authors' contributions

As wrote this manuscript under supervision of AS and MO. YO designed the study. YO, NT and MH performed the investigation and analyzed the date. TY and MY made substantial contribution to the interpretation of the data. MO was responsible for the study design, writing of the manuscript, analysis and interpretation of the date. All authors have read and approved the final manuscript.

References

1. Aoyama K. Basic knowledge and skills, abnormal airway of child. LiSA. 2015; 22(7):662–7.
2. Gunawardana RH. Difficult laryngoscopy in cleft lip and palate surgery. Br J Anaesth. 1996;76:757–9.
3. Xue FS, Zang GH, Li P, Sun HT, Li CW, Liu KP, Tong SY, Liao X. The clinical observation of difficult laryngoscopy and difficult intubation in infants with cleft lip and palate. Pediatr Anesth. 2006;16:283–9.
4. Ali QE, Amir SH, Firdaus U, Siddiqui OA, Azhar AZ. A comparative study of the efficacy with conventional laryngoscope in children. Minerva Anesthesiol. 2013;79:1366–70.
5. Sun Y, Lu Y, Huang Y, Jiang H. Pediatric videolaryngoscope versus direct laryngoscope: a meta-analysis of randomized controlled trials. Pediatr Anesth. 2014;24:1056–65.
6. Kasuya S, Suzuki Y. Abnormal airway of child, approach to difficult airway. LiSA. 2015;22(7):668–73 Jananese.
7. Ueshima H. Video laryngoscope, variety and characteristic of video laryngoscope, explore the standing position at airway management in present day, Journal of clinical anesthesia. LiSA. 2016;23(12):1136–7 Japanese.

16

Comparison of disinfection effect between benzalkonium chloride and povidone iodine in nasotracheal intubation

Aiji Sato-Boku[1]* , Keiji Nagano[2], Yoshiaki Hasegawa[3], Yuji Kamimura[4], Yoshiki Sento[4], MinHye So[4], Eisuke Kako[4], Masahiro Okuda[1], Naoko Tachi[1], Hidekazu Ito[5], Yushi Adachi[6] and Kazuya Sobue[4]

Abstract

Background: Nasotracheal intubation can potentially result in microbial contamination from the upper respiratory tract to the lower respiratory tracts. However, an ideal nasotracheal disinfection method is yet to be determined. Therefore, we compared the disinfection effects between benzalkonium chloride and povidone iodine in nasotracheal intubation.

Methods: Overall, this study enrolled 53 patients aged 20–70 years who were classified into classes 1 and 2 as per American Society of Anesthesiologists-physical status and were scheduled to undergo general anesthesia with NTI. Patients who did not give consent ($n = 2$) and who has an allergy for BZK or PVI were excluded from the study. The patients were randomly divided into two groups on the basis of the disinfection method: BZK ($n = 26$, one patient was discontinued intervention) and PVI ($n = 25$). 50 patients were assessed finally.
The subjects' nasal cavities were swabbed both before (A) and after disinfection (B), and the internal surface of the endotracheal tube was swabbed after extubation (C). The swabs were cultured on Brain heart infusion agar and Mannitol salt agar. The number of bacteria per swab was determined and the rates of change in bacterial count (B/A, C/B) were calculated. The growth inhibitory activity of the disinfectants on *Staphylococcus aureus* were also investigated in vitro.

Results: Although the initial disinfection effects (B/A) were inferior for benzalkonium chloride compared with those for povidone iodine, the effects were sustained for benzalkonium chloride (C/B). In the in vitro growth inhibitory assay against *S. aureus*, benzalkonium chloride showed higher inhibitory activity than povidone iodine.

Conclusion: Although both disinfectants were inactivated or diffused/diluted over time, benzalkonium chloride maintained the threshold concentration and displayed antimicrobial effects longer than povidone iodine; therefore, benzalkonium chloride appeared to show a better sustained effect. Benzalkonium chloride can be used for creating a hygienic nasotracheal intubation environment with sustained sterilizing effects.

Keywords: Nasotracheal intubation, Benzalkonium chloride, Povidone iodine, Bacteremia

* Correspondence: bokuaiji@dpc.agu.ac.jp
[1]Department of Anesthesiology, Aichi Gakuin University School of Dentistry,
2-11 Suemori-dori, Chikusa-ku, Nagoya 464-8651, Japan

Background

Nasotracheal intubation (hereafter referred to as "NTI") is frequently necessary during dental, maxillofacial, and oropharyngeal surgeries. This method is also useful while operating on patients with respiratory insufficiency, patients who require long-term maintenance of the airway in the intensive care unit and patients in whom orotracheal intubation is difficult because of trismus. However, some complications associated with NTI include epistaxis [1, 2], bacteremia [3], retropharyngeal perforation [4], and partial or complete obstruction of the tube [5, 6]. NTI complications are some of the many causes of anesthesia-related mortality [7].

Although several effective preventive measures against epistaxis and retropharyngeal perforation have been reported [8–10], an effective disinfection method during NTI is yet to be determined. In fact, dental procedures under general anesthesia with NTI demonstrate a higher incidence of bacteremia compared with those conducted under local anesthesia [3]; moreover, patients with prosthetic heart valves, immunodeficient patients, diabetic patients, and patients taking steroids are at an increased risk of bacteremia, and such patients require antibiotic prophylaxis [11]. Reports describing the presence of NTI-related bacteremia also exist [11, 12]. Bacteremia is likely caused by transferring intranasal bacteria into the respiratory tract. Therefore, the disinfection of the nasal mucosa before nasal intubation is crucial for avoiding the contamination of respiratory organs by nasal microorganisms.

In Japan, benzalkonium chloride (hereafter referred to as "BZK") and povidone iodine (hereafter referred to as "PVI") are generally used as NTI disinfectants. A comprehensive literature search was performed using PubMed, the Cochrane Central Register of Controlled Trials and EMBASE. However, to the best of our knowledge, the authors were unable to identify any previous reports comparing the outcomes of disinfection effects between these two disinfectants. Therefore, we investigated the disinfection effects of BZK and PVI when used for disinfection in NTI.

Methods

Ethics approval and consent to participate

This study was approved by the Ethics Committee at the School of Dentistry, Aichi Gakuin University (Approval No. 495) and was registered prospectively in the UMIN-CTR as a clinical trial on 21 Oct 2017. (Registration No. UMIN000029645). Our study adhered to CONSORT guidelines. The first patient was recruited and registered on 23 Oct 2017 (https://upload.umin.ac.jp/cgi-bin/ctr/ctr_view_reg.cgi?recptno=R000033873). We obtained written informed consent from all patients after providing them with adequate explanation regarding the research aims.

Subjects

Overall, this study enrolled 53 patients aged 20–70 years who were classified into classes 1 and 2 as per American Society of Anesthesiologists-physical status (hereafter referred to as "ASA-PS") and were scheduled to undergo general anesthesia with NTI. Patients who did not give consent ($n = 2$) and who has an allergy for BZK or PVI were excluded from the study. The patients were randomly divided into two groups on the basis of the disinfection method: BZK ($n = 26$, one patient was discontinued intervention) and PVI ($n = 25$). 50 patients were assessed finally (Fig. 1).

Anesthesia, sample collection, and microbial count

The same method of anesthesia was employed for all patients. No premedication was administered. After a patient walked independently to the operating theater, the standard vital monitors (electrocardiogram, blood pressure and oxygen saturation) were monitored. Anesthesia was induced using propofol (1–2 mg/kg), remifentanil (0.2 μg/kg/min.), and fentanyl (100 μg), with rocuronium (0.6 mg/kg) used as a neuromuscular blocking agent. Until the effects of the neuromuscular blocking agent became apparent, mask ventilation was implemented for all patients using 100% oxygen. While mask ventilation was being performed, the subjects' inferior nasal passage was swabbed with a sterile cotton swab before disinfection (A). The subjects' nasal cavities and inferior nasal passages were adequately disinfected twice each using a sterile cotton swab with BZK (ZALKONIN® SOLUTION 0.025, Kenei Phamaceutical Co., Ltd., Osaka) or PVI (POVIDONE-IDOINE SOLUTION 10% 「MEIJI」 Nitto Medic Co., Ltd., Toyama). BZK and PVI were applied at normal clinical concentrations of 0.025 and 5%, respectively. Next, the patients' inferior nasal passages were swabbed again with sterile cotton swabs after disinfection (B). Then, tramazoline nasal drops were administered to the nasal cavity and NTI was conducted after the muscle relaxant was observed to take effect. In all cases, we maintained general anesthesia using Total Intra Venous Anesthesia. After the surgery, the internal surface of the endotracheal tube (inner surface 1 cm from the tip of the tube) was swabbed immediately after extubation (C). We focused on how much bacteria that invaded from the upper airway to the lower airway during intubation was suppressed by long-term disinfection effect. If we swabbed the outer surface of the endotracheal tube, we could not avoid contamination by nasal bacteria during extubation. Therefore, we swabbed the the internal surface of the endotracheal tube.

After collecting the specimens, only the swab head was cut off. The samples from (A) and (C) were placed in 10 ml of sterile physiological saline and the samples from (B) were placed in 40 ml of sterile physiological

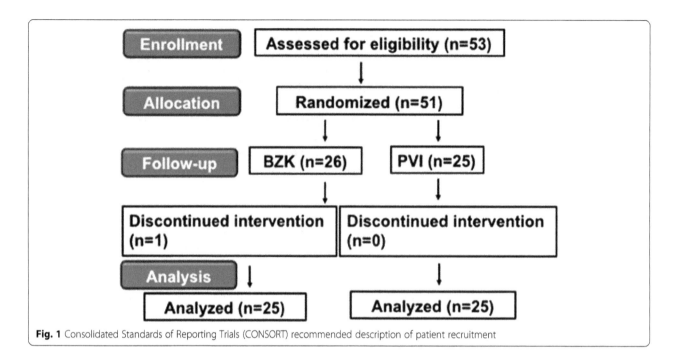

Fig. 1 Consolidated Standards of Reporting Trials (CONSORT) recommended description of patient recruitment

saline to dilute the disinfectants (BZK or PVI) that were absorbed by the swab. The samples were refrigerated and submitted for examination within six hours as described in the following sections.

Viable microbes in the swab samples were measured using a culture method. The samples were vigorously vortexed at maximum speed for 30 s to extract the microbes from the swab head in saline. After the swab heads were removed, the samples were centrifuged at 4000×*g* for 15 min at 4 °C to concentrate the extracted microbes, and then the precipitates were suspended in 1 ml of saline. The precipitates were serially diluted, and 50 μl of the dilutions was spread on agar plate medium. Brain heart infusion agar (hereafter referred to as "BHI", Becton, Dickinson and Company, Franklin Lakes, NJ, USA) was used for assessing the total number of microbes. Mannitol Salt Agar (hereafter referred to as "MTS", Nissui Pharmaceutical Co., Ltd., Tokyo, Japan) was used for detecting *Staphylococcus*. After culturing at 37 °C for 24 h under aerobic conditions, the colonies were counted and were expressed as colony-forming units (hereafter referred to as "CFU").

Assay for minimum inhibitory concentration (hereafter referred to as "MIC")

The MICs of the gram-positive bacterium *S. aureus* strain FDA 209P JC-1 against BZK and PVI were examined using both BHI agar and broth media. Approximately 10^6 CFU of bacterial cells were inoculated in the media and cultivated at 37 °C for 24 h under aerobic conditions. The MICs were visually determined.

The evaluation of parameters

The preoperative patient attributes of sex, age, anesthesia time, and patient distribution after extubation were evaluated. The numbers of bacteria (in CFU) in the samples from (A), (B), and (C) per cotton swab were assessed, and the rates of change in bacterial count (B/A, C/B) were calculated. The MICs were also visually determined.

Statistical analysis

We calculated the required minimum number of samples ($n = 46$ cases; BZK group, 23 cases; PVI group, 23 cases; effect size, 0.47; α-error, 0.05; power, 0.95). The effect size was calculated on the basis of the statistical results of a pilot study in which the patient distribution for the change in the number of bacteria after disinfection was used as a standard [BZK group, 10 cases; PVI group, 10 cases]. As application of statistical tests in the absence of reliable sample size calculation decrease its weightage, we calculated our final sample size as follows. The dropout rate in a preliminary study was 0.05. If an R dropout rate is expected, a simple but adequate adjustment is provided by $N_d = N/(1-R)^2$ where N is sample size calculated assuming no dropout and N_d that required with dropouts [13]. Therefor our adjustment was 50.9 and 50 patients were assessed finally. Student's t test was used for assessing the effects of age and anesthesia time. Chi-square independence test m × n contingency table was used for assessing sex and patient distributions. Based on the results of QQ plot from the sample (A), (B) and (C), Mann–Whitney U test was used for the number of bacteria found in the samples from

(A), (B), (C) and the rates of change in bacterial count (B/A, C/B). The level of statistical significance was set at $p < 0.05$.

Results

From October 2017 to December 2017, 53 patients were selected as subjects for this study. Figure 1 shows the consort flow diagram. Fifty-one subjects were randomly assigned into two groups on the basis of the disinfection method used: BZK and PVI. One subject dropped out during the trial.

Table 1 shows patient sex, age, and anesthesia time. No statistical differences in any parameters were observed between the two groups.

For examining the total number of bacteria, we used BHI for the general bacterial culture (Table 2). The number of nasal bacteria before disinfection (A) was equivalent in the BZK and PVI groups (30,000 and 50,000 CFU/swab, respectively) and no statistically significant differences were noted. However, individual patient differences were large and ranged from 1900 to 400,000 CFU/swab. After disinfection (B), the bacterial numbers of 1300 CFU/swab for BZK and 20 CFU/swab for PVI were reported, which correspond to a difference of 65 times ($p = 0.00005$). The rate of change (B/A) was also significantly lower for PVI than for BZK. Conversely, postoperatively (C), both groups reported a median of 1900 CFU/swab. Compared with the samples from (B), there was barely any change in the number of bacteria in the samples from (C) after BZK treatment, whereas after PVI treatment, an approximately 100-fold proliferation was observed: The rate change (C/B) for BZK and PVI was 100 and 9867, respectively ($p = 0.002$).

Table 3 shows the number of bacteria in the samples from (A), (B), and (C) in MTS and the rates of change for B/A and C/B. The number of nasal bacteria before disinfection (A) was equivalent in patients in the BZK and PVI groups (10,000 and 7000 CFU/swab, respectively) and there was no statistically significant difference noted. However, the individual differences were large and ranged from 900 to 30,000 CFU/swab. After disinfection (B), bacterial numbers of 200 CFU/swab for BZK

and 20 CFU/swab for PVI were reported, and a difference of 100 times was confirmed ($p = 0.002$). The rate of change (B/A) was significantly lower after PVI disinfection than after BZK disinfection. Conversely, postoperatively (C), both groups reported an identical median of 20 CFU/swab. Compared with the samples from (B), the number of bacteria found in the samples from (C) decreased after BZK disinfection, whereas an increase in the number of bacteria in the samples from (C) after PVI disinfection was observed, when compared between their quartiles.

Tables 4 and 5 show patient distribution regarding the change in the number of bacteria after disinfection. Compared to BZK, more patients with PVI disinfection displayed increased numbers of bacteria after extubation in both media.

The MICs of BZK and PVI against *S. aureus* were examined (Table 6). BZK inhibited *S. aureus* when diluted up to 2^9 times, but PVI only inhibited *S. aureus* when diluted up to 2^6 times.

Discussion

Previous reports have discussed the development of bacteremia due to bacterial flora associated with the upper respiratory tract (hereafter referred to as "URT") during treatment [3, 14–17]. Notably, during tracheal intubation, there is a high possibility for the bacterial flora in the nasopharyngeal region to gain access to the trachea. During intubation, host defense mechanisms that remove bacterial pathogens from URT, which would subsequently enter the lower respiratory tract, are impaired. In addition, the frequency of bacteremia after nasotracheal intubation is not related to the use of drugs for blood vessel contraction or the degree of trauma during the procedure [11].

Based on the hypothesis that *Staphylococcus* sp. is an important etiological agent associated with NTI, we used MTS, a selective medium for *Staphylococcus* sp., in this study. Although yellow colonies were frequently isolated, some white colonies were also isolated. On Gram staining of selective specimens, because the yellow and white colonies obtained appeared to be gram-positive cocci

Table 1 Characteristics of patients in this study

Characteristics of patients in this study			
	Group BZK	Group PVI	P Value
Sex Male	11	12	0.98
Sex Female	14	13	
Age (year)	37.9 ±17.1	40.3 ±13.7	0.61
Anesthesia Time(min)	175.6±85.8	154.6 ±69.7	0.36
Values are mean 1SD or number			

Table 2 The effect of BZK or PVI for General bacteria

The effect of BZK or PVI for General bacteria			
	Group BZK	Group PVI	P Value
A (CFU)	30000 (1900-100000)	50000 (6000-400000)	0.23
B (CFU)	1300 (100-9400)	20 (20-20)	0.00005
C (CFU)	1900 (320-7700)	1900 (40-2200)	0.93
B/A (%)	7.25 (2.7-18.25)	0.05 (0.01-0.31)	0.000001
C/B (%)	100 (29-1430)	9867 (200-80000)	0.002
Values are median (quartile)			

forming grape-like clusters, they were considered to be *S. aureus* and *S. epidermidis*, respectively.

In this study, the main bacterial isolates obtained from the nasal cavity were *S. aureus* and *S. epidermidis*. Because *Staphylococcus* sp. causes endocarditis [18], disinfection of the nasal cavity prior to nasotracheal intubation is extremely important to reduce the bacterial load.

Following antisepsis of the nasal cavity, the swab sampling the mucous membrane was placed in 40 ml of saline. The swab head can absorb approximately 0.135 ml of fluid. When the same volume of antiseptic (BZK or PVI) is absorbed by a swab during mucosal membrane swabbing and placed in 40 ml of saline, the sample is diluted 296-fold. Although *S. aureus* MICs of BZK and PVI were achieved after 512-fold and 64-fold dilutions, respectively, no antibacterial effect was expected theoretically because PVI was diluted below the MIC. However, the initial disinfection efficacy of PVI was higher than that of BZK, suggesting that dilution does not affect disinfection efficacy.

Because PVI has wide-spectrum disinfection properties with low levels of irritation, it is used for local applications during surgery and for infections of the oral and vaginal mucosa. Although PVI displays a rapid disinfection efficacy at low concentrations (approximately 0.1%) under experimental conditions, it can lose significant disinfection efficacy in the presence of organic matter; therefore, a 5–10% concentration is used in clinical settings. It is reported that 10 min was required for appearance of the bactericidal effect of PVI in clinical application, which organic matter was present [19]. However, we intubated immediately (1 to 2 min) after the disinfections in this study, but B/A values indicate that PVI was superior to BZK for initial disinfection. Our results suggest that reconsideration is necessary for PVI usage including an incubation time after application. Additionally, it does not seem to wait for 10 min after PVI treatment in general application. As mentioned above, PVI normally exhibits sufficient disinfection effect by waiting for 10 min after disinfection.

Table 3 The effect of BZK or PVI for Staphylococci

The effect of BZK or PVI for *Staphylococci*			
	Group BZK	Group PVI	P Value
A (CFU)	10000 (900-37500)	7000 (2000-30000)	0.93
B (CFU)	200 (20-2000)	20 (20-20)	0.002
C (CFU)	20 (20-60)	20 (20-200)	0.77
B/A (%)	4.4 (1.5-11.1)	0.3 (0.04-1.4)	0.001
C/B (%)	29 (3-100)	100 (100-1000)	0.0003
Values are median (quartile)			

Comparison of disinfection effect between benzalkonium chloride and povidone iodine in nasotracheal...

105

Table 4 Patient distribution regarding the change in the number of General bacteria after disinfection

	Patient distribution regarding the change in the number of *General bacteria* after disinfection		
	Group BZK	Group PVI	P Value
C<B	10	0	
C≑B	3	6	0.02
C>B	12	19	
Values are number			

In this study, although we intubated 1–2 min after disinfection with PVI, the initial disinfection effect was sufficient. However, if intubation was performed 10 min after disinfection, it may have been possible to suppress bacterial growth in C by exerting the original disinfection effect.

BZK continued to demonstrate a high disinfection efficacy following extubation, whereas increased bacterial levels were found after PVI disinfection. Because the clinical samples following extubation represent specimens incide the endtracheal tube, re-contamination due to bacterial flora in the nasal cavity during extubation is considered to be extremely unlikely. Therefore, the increased bacterial levels detected after extubation indicated that the growth of bacteria originally introduced into the trachea at the time of intubation develops even in a short intubation time during surgery and the disinfection effect of PVI is not sustained.

This study clearly showed that the disinfection efficacy of BZK was sustainable. In vitro, BZK inhibited the growth of *S. aureus* even at a dilution of 2^9, whereas PVI inhibited growth at a dilution of 2^6. Although both disinfectants were inactivated or diffused/diluted over time,

BZK maintained the threshold concentration and displayed antimicrobial effects longer than PVI; therefore, BZK appeared to show a better sustained effect.

There are some limitations of this study. First, with respect to bacterial counts, there were major differences in callosity among patients. There are many reasons for the variation in callosity. The level of mucosal membrane dryness in the nasal cavity can affect callosity. In the future, it may be necessary to adjust for mucosal membrane dryness prior to specimen collection. Second, multiple practitioner were participated in this study. Prior to beginning the study, disinfection methods were standardized as much as possible; however, disinfection efficacy did not account for differences among individuals. Although this study demonstrated that PVI showed immediate effects, the results may have differed if one healthcare person performed all procedures.

Third, since we only disinfect the nasal cavities and inferior nasal passages, we cannot rule out that naso- and oro-pharyngeal contamination during intubation contributed to our results. We also have not performed blood tests before and after disinfection. Therefore, we

Table 5 Patien distribution regarding the change in the number of Staphylociccu after disinfection

	Patient distribution regarding the change in the number of *Staphylococci* after disinfection		
	Group BZK	Group PVI	P Value
C<B	14	0	
C≑B	10	18	0.00006
C>B	1	7	
Values are number			

Table 6 Growth inhibition effect of *Staphylococcus aureus* (MICs)

	Growth inhibition effect on *Staphylococcus aureus* (MICs)	
	BZK	**PVI**
Dilution	2^9 **times**	2^6 **times**

may have had to discuss more solid evidence based on blood test for bacteremia.

Forth, since our research is a single-institutional research, longitudinal, multicentric, large population randomized controlled studies comparing the disinfection effects of variety of disinfectants over variety of microorganisms may be necessary to derive a valid conclusion.

Conclusion

We investigated the disinfection effects of benzalkonium chloride and povidone iodine when used for disinfection in nasotracheal intubation. Although both disinfectants were inactivated or diffused/diluted over time, benzalkonium chloride maintained the threshold concentration and displayed antimicrobial effects longer than povidone iodine. Benzalkonium chloride can be used for creating a hygienic nasotracheal intubation environment with sustained sterilizing effects.

Abbreviation
ASA-PS: American Society of Anesthesiologists-physical status; BHI: Brain heart infusion agar; BZK: Benzalkonium chloride; CFU: Colony-forming units; MICs: Minimum inhibitory concentration; MTS: Mannitol Salt Agar; NTI: Nasotracheal intubation; PVI: Povidone iodine; URT: Upper respiratory tract

Acknowledgements
The authors would like to thank the Department of Anesthesiology at Aichi Gakuin University Dental Hospital for their help in recruiting patients for this study.

Authors' contributions
AS and KN did the same contribution to this study. AS and KN wrote this manuscript under supervision of YH, MO and KS. AS, KN, YH, MO, NT, YA and YS designed the study. AS, KN, HI performed the investigation and analyzed the data. YH, YK, YS, MS, EK, MO, YA NT, HI made substantial contribution to the interruption of the data. KS was responsible for the study design, writing of the manuscript, analysis and interpretation of the data. All authors have read and approved the final manuscript.

Author details
[1]Department of Anesthesiology, Aichi Gakuin University School of Dentistry, 2-11 Suemori-dori, Chikusa-ku, Nagoya 464-8651, Japan. [2]Department of Oral microbiology, School of Dentistry Health Sciences University of Hokkaido 757 Kanazawa, Ishikari-Tobetsu, Hokkaido 061-0293, Japan. [3]Department of Microbiology, Aichi Gakuin University School of Dentistry, 1-100 Kusumotocho, Chikusa-ku, Nagoya 464-8650, Japan. [4]Department of Anesthesiology and Intensive Care Medicine, Nagoya City University Graduate School of Medical Sciences, 1 Kawasumi, Mizuho-cho, Mizuho-ku, Nagoya 467-8601, Japan. [5]Department of Anesthesiology, Aichi Developmental Disability Center Central Hospital, 713-8 Kagiya-cho, Kasugai-city, Aichi 480-0392, Japan. [6]Department of Anesthesiology, Nagoya University Graduate School of Medicine, 65 Tsurumaicho, Showaku, Nagoya 466-8550, Japan.

References
1. Lee J-H, Kim C-H, Bahk J-H, Park K-S. The influence of endotracheal tube tip design on nasal trauma during nasotracheal intubation: magill-tip versus murphy-tip. Anesth Analg. 2005;101:1226–9.
2. Chen YN, Chen JY, Hsu CS, Huanq CT, So E. Recurrent epistaxis following nasotracheal intubation: a case report. Acts Anaesthesiol Sin. 1996;34:93–6.
3. Berry FA, WI B, Ball CG. A comparison of bacteremia occurring with nasotracheal and orotracheal intubation. Anesth Analg. 1973;52:873–6.
4. Chait DH, Poulton TJ. Case report: retropharyngeal perforation, acomplication of nasotracheal intubation. Nebr Med J. 1984;69:68–9.
5. Kenney JN, Laskin DM. Nasotracheal tube obstruction from a central incisor. Oral Surg Oral Med Oral Pathol. 2005;67:266–7.
6. Tintinalli JE, Claffey J. Complications of nasotracheal intubation. Ann Emerg Med. 1981;10:142.
7. Harrison GG. Death attributable to anaesthesia: a 10 yr survey (1967–1976). Br J Anaesth. 1978;50:1041–6.
8. Boku A, Hanamoto H, Hirose Y, Kudo C, Morimoto Y, Sugimura M, Niwa H. Which nostril should be used for nasotracheal intubation: the right or left? A randomized clinical trial. J Clin Anesth. 2014;26:390–4.
9. Sanuki T, Hirokane M, Matsuda Y, Sugioka S, Kotani J. The Parker flex-tip tube for nasotracheal intubation: the influence on nasal mucosal trauma. Anaesthesia. 2010;65:8–11.
10. Morimoto Y, Sugimura M, Hirose Y, Taki K, Niwa H. Nasotracheal intubation under curve-tipped suction catheter guidance reduces epistaxis. Can J Anaesth. 2006;53:295–8.
11. Dinner M, Tjeuw M, Artusio JF. Bacteremia as a complication of nasotracheal intubation. Anesth Analg. 1987;66:460–2.
12. Berry FA, Yaubrough S, Yaubrough N. Transient bacteremia during dental manipulation in children. Pediatrics. 1973;51:476–9.
13. Lachin JM. Introduction to sample size determination and power analysis for clinical trials. Control Clin Trials. 1981;2:93–113.
14. Storm W. Transient bacteremia following endotracheal suctioning in ventilated newborns. Pediatrics. 1980;65:487–90.
15. LeFrock JL, Klainer AS, Wen-Hsien W. Transient bacteremia associated with nasotrachaal suctioning. JAMA. 1976;236:1610–1.
16. Beyt BE, King DK, Glue RH. Fatal pneumonitis and septicemia after fiberoptic bronchoscopy. Chest. 1977;72:105–7.
17. Baltch AL, Pressman HL, Hammer MC, Sutphen NC, Smith RP, Shayegani M. Bacteremia following dental extractions in patients with and without penicillin prophylaxis. Am J Med Sci. 1982;283:129–39.
18. Minegishi S, Mochida Y, Furihata S, Ichikawa S, Fukuoka M, Kanbara K, Niinami H, Umemura S. A case of vertebral osteomyelitis and native valve endocarditis caused by *Staphylococcus lugdunensis*. J Jpn Soc Intensive Care Med. 2017;24:9–13.
19. Payne DN, Babb JR, Bradley CR. An evaluation of the suitability of the European suspension test to reflect in vitro activity of antiseptics clinically siginificant organisms. Left Appl Microbiol. 1999;28:7–12.

17

A comparison between the disposcope endoscope and fibreoptic bronchoscope for nasotracheal intubation

Junma Yu[1,2*†] 🔟, Rui Hu[2†], Lining Wu[2], Peng Sun[2] and Zhi Zhang[1]

Abstract

Background: Nasotracheal intubation (NTI) is frequently performed for oral and maxillofacial surgeries. This study evaluated whether NTI is easier when guided by Disposcope endoscopy or fibreoptic bronchoscopy.

Methods: Sixty patients (30 per group) requiring NTI were randomly assigned to undergo fibreoptic bronchoscopy-guided (fibreoptic group) or Disposcope endoscope-guided (Disposcope group) NTI. The NTI time, which was defined as the time from when the fibreoptic bronchoscope or aseptic suction catheter was inserted into the nasal cavity to the time at which the tracheal tube was correctly inserted through the glottis, was recorded. Epistaxis was evaluated by direct laryngoscopy five minutes after completing NTI and was scored as one of four grades according to the following modified criteria: no epistaxis, mild epistaxis, moderate epistaxis, and severe epistaxis.

Results: The time to complete NTI was significantly longer in the fibreoptic group than in the Disposcope group (38.4 s vs 24.1 s; mean difference, 14.2 s; 95% confidence interval (CI), 10.4 to 18.1). Mild epistaxis was observed in 8 patients in the fibreoptic group and in 7 patients in the Disposcope group (26.7% vs 23.3%, respectively; relative risk, 1.2; 95% CI, 0.4 to 3.9), though no moderate or severe epistaxis occurred in either group. Furthermore, no obvious nasal pain was reported by any of the patients at any time point after extubation ($P = 0.74$).

Conclusion: NTI can be completed successfully using either fibreoptic bronchoscopy or Disposcope endoscope as a guide without any severe complications. However, compared to fibreoptic bronchoscopy, Disposcope endoscope requires less execution time (the NTI time).

Keywords: Disposcope endoscope, Nasotracheal intubation, Fibreoptic, Video stylet, Endotracheal tube

Background

Nasotracheal intubation (NTI) is frequently used during oral and maxillofacial surgeries [1], and possible complications, especially epistaxis and trauma to the airway, can occur [2]. Fibreoptic bronchoscopy-guided NTI is associated with less epistaxis and better navigability and has a lower redirection rate [3]. In other studies, compared with the Macintosh laryngoscope, fibreoptic bronchoscopy-guide NTI resulted in a lower rate of sore throat and significantly shortened the total intubation time, and improved field of view during intubation and shortened intubation time were reported for the McGrath MAC laryngoscope [4, 5].

The Disposcope endoscope (Dexscope™, Yangzhou Dex Medical Device Co., Ltd., Yangzhou, China, produced in 2014) is a video stylet used for endotracheal intubation. Its wire tube body is composed of rigid metal, but it can easily be bent during surgery, enabling doctors

* Correspondence: majuny163@163.com
†Junma Yu and Rui Hu contributed equally to this work.
[1]Hefei National Laboratory for Physical Sciences at the Microscale, Department of Biophysics and Neurobiology, University of Science and Technology of China, Hefei 230027, People's Republic of China
[2]Department of Anesthesiology, The First People's Hospital of Hefei, Anhui Medical University, Hefei, Anhui 230061, People's Republic of China

to adjust it to the optimum angle for each patient and situation (Fig. 1, a and b). Compared to the Macintosh laryngoscope, the Disposcope endoscope yields a higher success rate for endotracheal intubation and provides a better view of the glottis; it is also associated with a shorter intubation time and causes fewer dental injuries when used to imitate intubation on a manikin wearing a semi-rigid neck collar [6]. Moreover, the Disposcope endoscope demonstrated a promising ability to guide successful endotracheal intubation in trauma patients wearing a semi-rigid neck collar [6]. Another study showed that the Disposcope endoscope can also be applied successfully in double-lumen tube placement [7].

We hypothesized that Disposcope endoscope would be as effective as fibreoptic bronchoscopy in guiding NTI.

Methods

In a pilot study (5 patients in each group intubated by a trained anaesthesiologist who was familiar with both techniques) prior to this research, the NTI time, which was defined as the time from when the fibreoptic bronchoscope or aseptic suction catheter was inserted into the nasal cavity to the time at which the tracheal tube was correctly inserted through the glottis, was significantly longer in the fibreoptic group than in the Disposcope group (43.0 ± 13.4 s vs 24.0 ± 3.2 s). For this study, the total sample size to achieve 95% power and an α-

error of 5% was 8 patients per group according to G*Power 3.1.9.4 software. Sixty adult patients rated American Society of Anaesthesiologists (ASA) I and II who were scheduled to undergo elective oral and maxillofacial surgery requiring NTI under general anaesthesia were selected. We excluded patients from our study if they fell into any of the following categories: (1) age younger than 18 years or older than 80 years; (2) a body mass index (BMI) ≥ 30 kg/m^2; (3) a preoperative Mallampati score of III or higher; (4) a history of nasal abnormality (e.g., nasal trauma, surgery, obstruction, and polyps); (5) current anticoagulation therapy; (6) the presence of an oral malignant tumour or difficulty anticipated in airway management; (7) a mental disorder diagnosis; and (8) cervical vertebra instability, trauma or rheumatoid arthritis. None of the patients were premedicated, and standard monitoring equipment was used in the operating room. All study subjects were randomized by a researcher blinded to the study, and envelopes containing randomization numbers were used to allocate the patients to the following two groups (n = 30 per group) according to the airway device that would be used to guide NTI: the fibreoptic bronchoscopy-guided group (fibreoptic group) and the Disposcope endoscope-guided group (Disposcope group).

General anaesthesia was induced with 1.5–2 mg/kg intravenous propofol and 0.3 µg/kg sufentanil, and

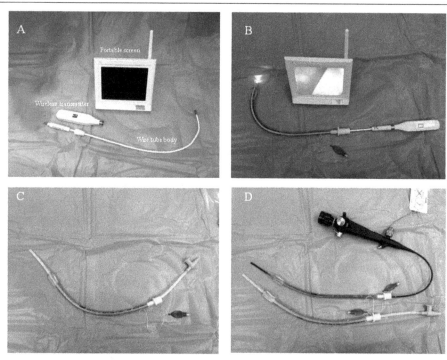

Fig. 1 The Disposcope endoscope (Dexscope™, Yangzhou Dex Medical Device Co., Ltd., Yangzhou, China, **a**). The depth of wire transfer was premeasured to ensure that the wire tip did not exceed the tube before NTI. (**b**) An aseptic suction catheter (OD, 5.33 mm, TUORen Medical Equipment Co., Henan, China, **c** and **d**) was inserted through the tracheal tube (TUORen Medical Equipment Co., Henan, China) and fibreoptic bronchoscope (Pentax FI-10BS, Pentax Corporation, Tokyo, Japan, **d**)

muscle relaxation was achieved by intravenous adminis- tration of 0.15 mg/kg cisatracurium. Airway size and pa- tency were estimated by fibreoptic bronchoscopy (Pentax FI-10BS, Pentax Corporation, Tokyo, Japan) in each nostril. Before intubation, manual ventilation was performed with 100% oxygen through a facemask for 3 min. Five drops of 1% ephedrine solution were instilled into larger nasal cavities to prevent bleeding. Males and females were intubated with 6.5-mm and 6.0-mm wire- reinforced tracheal tubes, respectively (TUORen Medical Equipment Co., Henan, China) with high-volume, low- pressure cuffs. Anaesthesia was maintained with propo- fol and remifentanil at rates of 0.1–0.15 mg/kg/min and 0.1–0.2 μg/kg/min, respectively.

In the fibreoptic group, intubation was performed with the one-hand manoeuvre by putting the little finger below the mandible angle, the ring finger below the mandible body, and the middle finger under the mental region; this gesture mimics the one-handed facemask ventilation technique. By applying this manoeuvre, the operator can simultaneously insert the fibreoptic bron- choscope and lift the chin [8]. In the Disposcope group, the depth of the wire body that was lubricated with aseptic liquid paraffin for insertion was pre-measured to ensure that the wire tip did not protrude from the tube before NTI, and the shape of the wire transfer was curved by the operator before NTI. An aseptic suction catheter (OD, 5.33 mm, TUORen Medical Equipment Co., Henan, China) lubricated with aseptic liquid paraf- fin was then inserted through the tracheal tube (Fig. 1, c and d). The tip of the catheter was directed ventrally with the tip of the catheter protruding from the distal end of the tube by approximately 10 cm [9], and the tra- cheal tube was then advanced through the nasopharynx. The suction catheter was withdrawn after the above steps were completed. The operator then used the thumb and index finger of one hand to lift the mandible during intubation [6]. The entire intubation process is shown in Fig. 2 (a-f). All intubations were performed by an anaesthesiologist who was familiar with both tech- niques and had 15 years of experience and a trained as- sistant. Minute adjustments to ventilation were performed to maintain end-tidal CO_2 pressures at 35– 45 mmHg after intubation.

The NTI time was recorded. Epistaxis was assessed by an investigator blinded to the group assignments using direct laryngoscopy at five minutes after completing NTI and was scored as one of four grades according to the following modified criteria: no epistaxis (no blood ob- served on either the surface of the tube or the posterior pharyngeal wall); mild epistaxis (blood apparent on the surface of the tube or posterior pharyngeal wall);

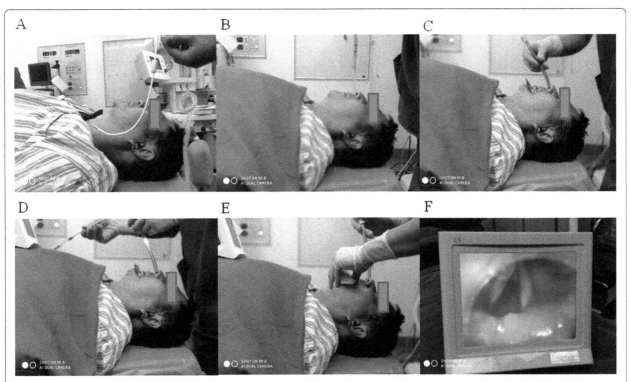

Fig. 2 The entire process for nasotracheal intubation using the Disposcope endoscope (**a-f**). (**a**) The wire tube body was bent along the radian of the nasal cavity. (**b** and **c**) The tracheal tube was inserted through the nasopharynx under suction catheter guidance until the placement depth reached 15 cm. (**d-f**) The suction catheter was withdrawn, and NTI was then performed under the guidance of the Disposcope endoscope

moderate epistaxis (pooling of blood on the posterior pharyngeal wall); and severe epistaxis (a large amount of blood in the pharynx impeding NTI and necessitating urgent orotracheal intubation) [10].

Each patient received 0.1 µg/kg sufentanil intravenously for postoperative analgaesia upon completion of the operation. Neuromuscular blockade was reversed using neostigmine (1 mg) and atropine (0.5 mg), and the trachea was extubated when the patient was awake. At 15 min, 1 h and 24 h after extubation, the patients were asked to rate their nasal pain on a visual analogue scale (VAS) according to a 10-cm vertical score ranging from 0 = no pain to 10 = worst pain imaginable by an independent anaesthetist who was unaware of which method had been used for NTI.

The study protocol was reviewed and approved by the Institutional Research Ethics Committee of The First People's Hospital of Hefei (No. 2016–6) on 3 March 2016. The study was also registered in the Chinese Clinical Trial Registry (www.chictr.org.cn, ChiCTR-IPR-17011462). Informed written consent was obtained from all patients in this study, and the study was conducted in accordance with the Declaration of Helsinki.

Data are expressed as the mean (SD). Parametric data were compared between the groups by analysis of variance and post hoc testing. The mean difference and the 95% confidence interval (CI) of the mean difference were calculated. Categorical data were analysed using Fisher's exact test. The relative risks of the proportion of categorical data and 95% CIs were calculated. Statistical significance was considered at P values < 0.05. All statistical analyses were performed with Statistical Package for Social Sciences (SPSS) software 13.0.

Results

Sixty patients consented to participate in the study. Figure 3 shows the CONSORT flow diagram for patient inclusion. No significant differences were identified between the groups with regard to patient age, height, weight, BMI, ASA score, Mallampati score, sex ratio or duration of tracheal tube indwelling time (Table 1).

The time to complete NTI (the NTI time) was significantly longer in the fibreoptic group than in the Disposcope group (38.4 s vs 24.1 s; mean difference, 14.2 s; 95% CI, 10.4 to 18.1) (Table 2).

Mild epistaxis (nasal bleeding) was observed in 8 patients in the fibreoptic group and in 7 patients in the Disposcope group (26.7% vs 23.3%, respectively; relative risk, 1.2; 95% CI, 0.4 to 3.9). No moderate or severe epistaxis occurred in either group (Table 2).

Furthermore, no obvious nasal pain was reported at any time point after extubation in the Disposcope group or the fibreoptic group, with no significant difference between the two groups ($P = 0.74$, data not shown).

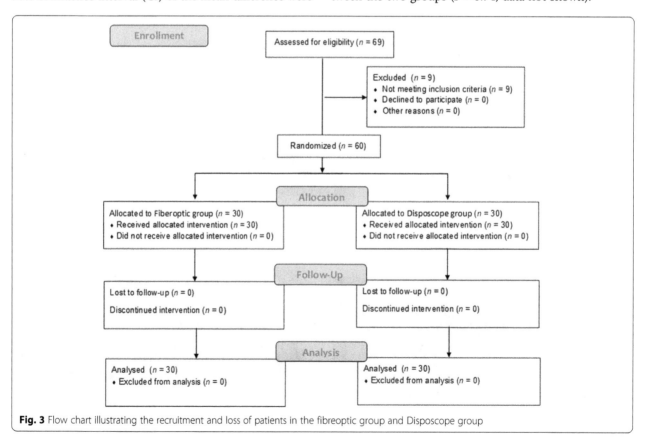

Fig. 3 Flow chart illustrating the recruitment and loss of patients in the fibreoptic group and Disposcope group

Table 1 Patient characteristics and the duration of anaesthesia

Variable	Fibreoptic group (n = 30)	Disposcope group (n = 30)	P value
Age (years)	43.4 ± 15.5	47.2 ± 15.5	0.69
Height (cm)	165.6 ± 7.6	164.1 ± 7.1	0.75
Weight (kg)	63.8 ± 7.6	64.1 ± 11.0	0.21
ASA physical status (I/II)	20/10	18/12	0.59
Sex (male:female)	14/16	12/18	0.60
BMI (kg·m^{-2})	23.3 ± 2.7	23.8 ± 3.2	0.54
Mallampati score	1.5 ± 0.5	1.4 ± 0.5	0.36
Duration of anaesthesia (min)	69.1 ± 27.0	72.1 ± 29.2	0.98

Values are expressed as a number or the mean (SD)

Discussion

Fibreoptic bronchoscopy-guided NTI is a well-established and safe technique with a high success rate and low morbidity. In this study, both fibreoptic bronchoscopy and Disposcope endoscope-guided NTI were successfully completed without any severe adverse reactions. However, less execution time was required when using the Disposcope endoscope, which is a video laryngoscope, than when using fibreoptic bronchoscopy. This is the first study in which the Disposcope endoscope was used for NTI.

Fibreoptic bronchoscopy-guided NTI is a favoured and popular procedure. For example, Shih et al. [8] reported that performing the one-hand manoeuvre not only saves time but also reduces the need for assistance in patients requiring fibreoptic bronchoscopy-guided NTI for reasons other than a difficult airway. However, these authors did suggest that the one-hand manoeuvre was not suitable for novices and that a trained assistant should always be available in cases of finger and hand fatigue or other unpredictable conditions [8]. Head tilt with chin lift techniques provides adequate airway support for patients with and without a limited mouth opening [11]. In this study, the NTI time was significantly lower in the Disposcope group than in the fibreoptic group. The main reasons were as follows. First, the wire tube body of the Disposcope endoscope is rigid but can be bent along the radian of the nasal cavity; thus, the left hand is fully available to lift the mandible to perform a chin lift. Second, in the fibreoptic group, we needed to use the left hand to facilitate insertion of the wire tube body because of its softness [8], and in most cases, we spent more time searching for the glottis.

Previous studies have discussed many strategies to reduce the risk of epistaxis during NTI in clinical practice. First, data have shown that less epistaxis occurs during NTI and that intubation is faster in the right as opposed to the left nostril, which is related to the anatomy of the structures located on the posterior nasopharyngeal wall; thus, the right nostril should be selected if patency appears to be equal on both sides of the nose [1, 12, 13]. Measurement of the nasal flow rate has also been reported to be a useful clinical strategy for selecting which nostril to use for NTI [14]. Second, using a Parker Flex-Tip tube not only helps to minimize the incidence of nasal mucosal trauma during NTI but may also increase patient safety and comfort [15]. Another study reported that using a stylet-Parker tube enhanced the ease of insertion through the nasopharynx and reduced the risk of epistaxis during NTI [16]. In contrast, Earle et al. [9] found that a Parker tube did not significantly reduce epistaxis during NTI compared to a standard tube. Therefore, stylet-Parker tubes were not used in our study. Furthermore, performing NTI under suction catheter guidance represents a simple and effective method for smoothly introducing a nasal endotracheal tube and reducing nasal bleeding during NTI [9]. In other studies, the placement of a bougie through the nasopharyngeal airway also protected the nasal mucosa, helped guide the tracheal tube and was associated with less epistaxis as well as better navigability and a lower redirection rate [3, 17]. In the present study, no moderate or severe epistaxis occurred in either group, perhaps for the following reasons: each nostril was pre-measured for size and patency by fibreoptic bronchoscopy, and five drops of 1%

Table 2 NTI time and epistaxis incidence in the groups

Variable	Fibreoptic group (n = 30)	Disposcope group (n = 30)	Difference in the means or relative risks (95% CI)	P value
NTI time (s)	38.4 ± 9.7	24.1 ± 3.9	14.2 (10.4 to 18.1)	0.01
Mild epistaxis	8/30 (26.7%)	7/30 (23.3%)	1.2 (0.4 to 3.9)	0.77
Moderate epistaxis	0	0	–	–
Severe epistaxis	0	0	–	–

Values are expressed as a number, a proportion (%) or the mean (standard deviation). Relative risks were calculated for categorical data. CI = confidence interval

ephedrine solution were instilled into larger nasal cavities to prevent bleeding. NTI was also performed under the guidance of suction catheters. Overall, the use of wire-reinforced tracheal tubes and aseptic suction catheters may also decrease the incidence of epistaxis.

In the Disposcope group, a rigid wire transfer was inserted into the tube during NTI. However, in this study, no obvious nasal pain was reported at any time point after extubation in the Disposcope group, and no significant difference was found between the groups. We hypothesized that the wire-reinforced tracheal tubes may have protected the nasal mucosa and the entire nasal passage during surgery. In previous studies, a lower rate of sore throat after NTI was observed in the fibreoptic group than when using the Macintosh laryngoscope [4]. However, we did not assess the rate of sore throat in our study because some of the surgeries were on the vocal cords.

Admittedly, several limitations to our study should be considered. First, fibreoptic bronchoscopy-guided NTI is widely known for its effectiveness in patients with difficult airways. Unfortunately, patients with preoperative Mallampati scores of III or greater were excluded from our study because we aimed to evaluate two methods of guided NTI in elective oral and maxillofacial surgeries. Therefore, an additional study, which we plan to conduct, will be needed to confirm this effect. Second, only one anaesthesiologist performed all the intubations, which may reflect a limitation and possible bias in the study. Furthermore, the NTI time is probably not clinically important when the difference is only a dozen seconds, which may not indicate clear superiority but may suggest an optimal choice. Nonetheless, we consider the NTI time to be important in emergency cases, possibly shortening the first aid time.

Conclusion

NTI can be successfully completed using fibreoptic bronchoscopy or a Disposcope endoscope as a guide without any severe complications. However, less time for NTI was required when using the Disposcope endoscope, which is a video laryngoscope, than when using fibreoptic bronchoscopy, and we consider the Disposcope necessary in emergency cases.

Abbreviations
ASA: American Society of Anaesthesiologists; BMI: Body mass index; NTI: Nasotracheal intubation; VAS: Visual analogue scale

Acknowledgments
The authors would like to thank all the staff of the Department of Anesthesiology, The First People's Hospital of Hefei, Anhui Medical University for their help in conducting and finishing this research.

Authors' contributions
JMY, RH, LNW and PS were responsible for the study design and planning. JMY and RH were responsible for the study. JMY and ZZ performed the data analysis. JMY and ZZ wrote the paper. All authors participated in revising the paper. All authors have read and approved the manuscript submitted for publication.

References
1. Sanuki T, Hirokane M, Kotani J. Epistaxis during nasotracheal intubation: a comparison of nostril sides. J Oral Maxillofac Surg. 2010;68(3):618–21.
2. Kihara S, Komatsuzaki T, Brimacombe JR, Yaguchi Y, Taguchi N, Watanabe S. A silicone-based wire-reinforced tracheal tube with a hemispherical bevel reduces nasal morbidity for nasotracheal intubation. Anesth Analg. 2003;97(5):1488–91.
3. Kwon MA, Song J, Kim S, Ji SM, Bae J. Inspection of the nasopharynx prior to fiberoptic-guided nasotracheal intubation reduces the risk epistaxis. J Clin Anesth. 2016;32:7–11.
4. Tachibana N, Niiyama Y, Yamakage M. Less postoperative sore throat after nasotracheal intubation using a fiberoptic bronchoscope than using a Macintosh laryngoscope: a double-blind, randomized, controlled study. J Clin Anesth. 2017;39:113–7.
5. Sato Boku A, Sobue K, Kako E, Tachi N, Okumura Y, Kanazawa M, Hashimoto M, Harada J. The usefulness of the McGrath MAC laryngoscope in comparison with Airwayscope and Macintosh laryngoscope during routine nasotracheal intubation: a randomaized controlled trial. BMC Anesthesiol. 2017;17(1):160.
6. Park SO, Shin DH, Lee KR, Hoog DY, Kim EJ, Baek KJ. Efficacy of the Disposcope endoscope, a new video laryngoscope, for endotracheal intubation in patients with cervical spine immobilisation by semirigid neck collar: comparison with the Macintosh laryngoscope using a simulation study on a manikin. Emerg Med J. 2013;30(4):270–4.
7. Chen PT, Ting CK, Lee MY, Cheng HW, Chan KH, Chang WK. A randomised trial comparing real-time double-lumen endobronchial tube placement with the Disposcope® with conventional blind placement. Anaesthesia. 2017;72(9):1097–106.
8. Shih CK, Wu CC, Ji TT. One-hand maneuver to facilitate flexible fiber-optic bronchoscope-guided nasotracheal intubation insedated patients. Acta Anaesthesiol Taiwanica. 2015;53(4):150–1.
9. Morimoto Y, Sugimura M, Hirose Y, Taki K, Niwa H. Nasotracheal intubation under curve-tipped suction catheter guidance reduces epistaxis. Can J Anaesth. 2006;53(3):295–8.
10. Earle R, Shanahan E, Vaghadia H, Sawka A, Tang R. Epistaxis during nasotracheal intubation: a randomized trial of the Parker flex-tip™ nasal endotracheal tube with a posterior facing bevel versus a standard nasal RAE endotracheal tube. Can J Anaesth. 2017;64(4):370–5.
11. Cheng KI, Yun MK, Chang MC, Lee KW, Huang SC, Tang CS, Chen CH. Fiberoptic bronchoscopic view change of laryngopharyngeal tissues by different airway supporting techniques: comparison of patients with and without open mouth limitation. J Clin Anesth. 2008;20(8):573–9.
12. Boku A, Hanamoto H, Hirose Y, Kudo C, Morimoto Y, Sugimura M, Niwa H. Which nostril should be used for nasotracheal intubation: the right or left? A randomized clinical trial. J Clin Anesth. 2014;26(6):390–4.
13. Takasugi Y, Futagawa K, Konishi T, Morimoto D, Okuda T. Possible association between successful intubation via the right nostril and anatomical variations of the nasopharynx during nasotracheal intubation: a multiplanar imaging study. J Anesth. 2016;30(6):987–93.
14. Lim HS, Kim D, Lee J, Son JS, Lee JR, Ko S. Reliability of assessment of nasal flow rate for nostril selection during nasotracheal intubation. J Clin Anesth. 2012;24(4):270–4.
15. Sanuki T, Hirokane M, Matsuda Y, Sugioka S, Kotani J. The Parker flex-tip™ tube for nasotracheal intubation: the influence on nasal mucosal trauma. Anaesthesia. 2010;65(1):8–11.
16. Sugiyama K, Manabe Y, Kohjitani A. A styletted tracheal tube with a posterior-facing bevel reduces epistaxis during nasal intubation: a randomized trial. Can J Anaesth. 2014;61(5):417–22.
17. Abrons RO, Vansickle RA, Ouanes JP. Seldinger technique for nasal intubation: a case series. J Clin Anesth. 2016;34:609–11.

18

Effects of benzydamine hydrochloride on postoperative sore throat after extubation in children

Hyung-Been Yhim[1] , Soo-Hyuk Yoon[1] , Young-Eun Jang[1] , Ji-Hyun Lee[1] , Eun-Hee Kim[1] , Jin-Tae Kim[1,2] and Hee-Soo Kim[1,2]*

Abstract

Background: Postoperative sore throat (POST) is a common, undesirable result of endotracheal intubation during general anaesthesia. This study aimed to evaluate the effectiveness of benzydamine hydrochloride (BH) spray in reducing the incidence of POST in paediatric patients.

Methods: This randomized, double-blind, prospective study included 142 children 6–12 years of age, who were randomly assigned to receive either BH spray or control. After induction of anaesthesia, direct laryngoscope was placed and BH spray was applied to the upper trachea and vocal cord in the BH group and intubation was performed using a cuffed tube lubricated with normal saline. Intubation in the control group was performed using a cuffed tube lubricated with normal saline without any intervention. The balloon was inflated to a pressure of 20 cmH$_2$O. Patients were extubated after fully awakened and transferred to the post-anaesthetic care unit (PACU), where they were examined for the presence of POST and any adverse events 30 min after arrival to the PACU. Postoperative pain was evaluated using a smartphone application.

Results: Seventy-one patients were allocated to each group. The incidence of POST in the BH group did not differ from that in the control group (control: BH = 35 (49.3%): 42 (59.2%); $P = 0.238$); postoperative pain was also similar between the groups. Other complications, such as breath holding, secretions, coughing, laryngospasm and desaturation events, did not differ between the groups.

Conclusions: Application of prophylactic BH spray to the vocal cords and upper trachea was not proven to reduce POST in paediatric patients.

Keywords: Benzydamine hydrochloride, Children, Postoperative sore throat

* Correspondence: dami0605@snu.ac.kr
[1]Department of Anesthesiology and Pain Medicine, Seoul National University Hospital, #101 Daehakno, Jongnogu, Seoul 03080, Korea
[2]Department of Anesthesiology and Pain Medicine, College of Medicine, Seoul National University, #101 Daehak-ro, Jongno-gu, 03080 Seoul, Republic of Korea

Background

One of the most common side effects following endotracheal intubation is postoperative sore throat (POST). The overall incidence of POST in the adult population varies from 22 to 62% [1–3], and that in paediatric population has been observed ranging from 24 to 44% [2, 4]. Some reported POST to occur at a peak incidence of 2 to 4 h after extubation in adult population whereas only limited publications regarding the incidence or peak time of POST were found among paediatric population [2, 5]. Several publications evaluated POST in children as early as 15 min since POST is worse in the early postoperative period, then decreases over time [6]. Although POST is usually alleviated over time, it lingers for 12 to 24 h, which results in significant dissatisfactions postoperatively [4].

POST is induced by direct mucosal inflammation caused by mechanical trauma with endotracheal intubation [7]. The known risk factors for POST are presence of upper respiratory tract infection, duration of anaesthesia, intubation without neuromuscular blockers, the number of intubation attempts, high cuff pressure, and the operator's experience [2]. In particular, the use of uncuffed-endotracheal tubes and higher cuff pressure of cuffed-endotracheal tube were identified as main risk factors for POST in children [3, 4].

Several systemic reviews have suggested the use of preemptive local anaesthetics or anti-inflammatory drugs, such as benzydamine hydrochloride (BH), [8] lidocaine, [5, 9] ketamine, [5, 10] aspirin, [11] and dexpanthenol [12] for the prevention of POST. BH is a topical nonsteroidal anti-inflammatory drug with additional analgesic and antipyretic properties easily applicable to children [13]. BH is available in both topical and systemic formulations; however, due to its high volume of distribution, along with its low systemic clearance, BH is preferably used topically as an oral spray, mouthwash, or vaginal administration [13]. When topically absorbed, BH demonstrated low bioavailability with 5% or less and late peak plasma concentration occurring more than 24 h after application. This temporal residence at mucosal area benefits in treating soft tissue injury and mitigating any systemic side effects such as numbness, tingling sense of oral cavity, cough, and dry mouth [13]. Especially in alleviating POST, different topical application methods have been used, such as direct spraying at the oropharyngeal cavity, gargling, spraying the endotracheal tube cuff, lubricating at the endotracheal cuff, or in combination at both the cuff and oropharyngeal cavity [14–16]. To the best of our knowledge, there have been no clinical trials comparing the effects of BH on POST in targeting a specific population of children.

In this study, we aimed to evaluate whether spraying BH along the oropharyngeal space before intubation reduced POST in children.

Methods

Patient recruitment

A prospective, randomised, comparative study was conducted between March and June 2017 at Seoul National University Hospital (SNUH, Seoul, Korea). The study was approved by the SNUH Institutional Review Board (1612–061-813) and was registered at ClinicalTrials.gov (NCT03074968, Feb 26, 2017, https://register.clinicaltrials.gov/prs/app/template/EditProtocol.vm?listmode=Edit&uid=U0000Y58&ts=5&sid=S0006WDR&cx=-hdb51u). Each participant and corresponding parent were given a verbal explanation with an opportunity to ask questions about the study. Written informed consent was obtained from participants ≥7 years of age and their parents. Verbal assent was obtained from participants < 7 years of age, in addition to written informed consent from their parents. All procedures adhered to the principles of the Declaration of Helsinki.

A total of 150 children 6–12 years of age were screened, of whom 144 were ultimately enrolled. All were classified as American Society of Anaesthesiologists (ASA) physical status I-II and scheduled for elective surgery under general anaesthesia with endotracheal tube intubation. Individuals with intellectual disabilities, history of preoperative sore throat, recent upper respiratory infection, history of difficult or expected difficult airway, were excluded. In specific, difficult airway was defined as Cormack-Lehane class 3 or 4 by laryngoscopy, and ≥ 2 intubation attempts. Those who required postoperative mechanical ventilation were also excluded. Another exclusion was made depending on the type of the surgery. Ear-Nose-Throat (ENT) surgeries were limited to those not involving the airway. ENT surgeries were included only when the surgical target was limited to ear, such as myringotomy, myringoplasty, or canal wall mastoidectomy. Any surgery that invaded oropharynx, or required gastric tube insertion was not enrolled as well.

Children were prospectively screened and randomly allocated into one of the following two groups using a randomization table (online randomization software; http://www.randomisation.com): control group, and BH group. Children were enrolled by one of the investigators, while another independent investigator generated the random allocation sequence, prepared sealed opaque envelopes, opened the envelope immediately before the start of anaesthesia, and assigned participants to their respective study group.

Anaesthetic methods

All patients arrived at the operating room without premedication and appropriately fasted according to practice guidelines from the ASA. Peripheral pulse oximetry (i.e., oxygen saturation [SpO$_2$]), non-invasive blood pressure (NIBP) at 1-min intervals, and electrocardiography were monitored. N_2O-free general anaesthesia was induced with 2–2.5 mg/kg of propofol after the 0.5 mg kg^{-1} of 1% lidocaine administration. After loss of consciousness, the patients were manually ventilated with 8% sevoflurane and 100% oxygen at a rate of 6 L/min of fresh gas flow. For facilitation of endotracheal intubation, 0.6 mg/kg of rocuronium was administered. After confirmation of full relaxation of muscles by neuromuscular monitoring, under direct laryngoscope 4 puffs of BH spray 0.15% (Tantum, Riker Canada Inc.) 15 mg/mL was applied on the vocal cords and upper trachea in the BH group (1 puff = 175 µl) by one skilled anaesthesiologist to minimize the dose differences induced by applicator. The exact dose of BH absorbed to target was unmeasureable due to the spraying administration method. An endotracheal tube (ETT, Mallinckrodt Medcial, Athlone, Ireland) with cuff was lubricated with normal saline and inserted thereafter in both groups by paediatric anaesthesiologists with expertise and more than 2 years of experience. The use of stylet was abandoned. The size was determined using the formula: [age (in years)/4] + 3.5 and the cuff was inflated to a unifying pressure of 20 cmH_2O using the same manometer (Cuff Pressure, Posey Co, USA) in all patients since to this date, cuff pressure of 20 cmH_2O is known as the standard cuff that reduce the need for tube changed without additional risk for post-extubation stridor [17]. Afterwards, auscultation was done to reassure that the cuff pressure of 20 cmH_2O leaves air-leakage presence. During the operation additional cuff pressure measurement was not planned due to the possible mucosal irritation by air leak test measurement and manometer manipulation.

Anaesthesia was maintained using 1 minimum alveolar equivalent sevoflurane at a total flow rate of 2 L/min with 0.1–0.5 µg/mg/min of remifentanil continuous infusion. The fraction of inspired oxygen (F_IO_2) of inhaled gas was maintained at 40%. Minute ventilation was adjusted to maintain a partial pressure of end-tidal carbon dioxide (E_TCO_2) between 35 and 40 mmHg with 7 ml/kg of tidal volume. An oesophageal temperature probe (Top Probe, Meditop corporation, Republic of Korea) of 9fr was inserted immediately after intubation in a blind technique. To minimize any trauma, a smaller size of oesophageal temperature probe was used, instead of the standardized size according to children's age. If any resistance was found, oesophageal temperature probe was not forced through the oesophagus, but the tip was placed at oral cavity, measuring oral temperature instead. In about 15 to 20 min before the completion of surgery, patient-controlled analgesia (PCA) with fentanyl (total 25 mcg/kg of fentanyl with loading dose of 1 mcg/kg, basal infusion dose of 2 mcg/kg/h, bolus dose of 0.5 mcg/kg per demand with lock out interval of 15 min) or

15 mg/kg of propacetamol was administered for postoperative pain control. The distinction between these two different postoperative analgesic practices was according to the customary dosing according to the type of the surgery.

After the end of surgery, sevoflurane and remifentanil were discontinued and the patients were manually ventilated using 6 L/min of fresh gas flow. Antagonism of neuromuscular blockade was made with 20 mcg/kg of atropine and 40 mcg/kg of neostigmine. The patients were extubated when they maintained adequate, non-paradoxical breathing after following signs were observed; able to generate a negative inspiratory pressure > 30 cmH_2O with spontaneous respiration; lift the head and/or limb for more than 5 s; cough forcefully after careful and gentle oral suction. During extubation, any adverse events, including breath holding for ≥20 s, coughing more than twice, excessive endotracheal secretions requiring suction, laryngospasm, or desaturation (defined as SpO_2 < 93% [18]) were recorded. All patients were assessed at 30 min after arrival to the post-anaesthesia care unit (PACU) for severity of POST by the independent investigator who was blinded to the group allocation. To minimize any confounders of residual anaesthesia, patients were evaluated only when sufficiently awake, cooperative, and able to appropriately answer question or express their needs. The POST was evaluated using a four-point scale: (0, no sore throat; 1, mild sore throat, with complaint only on prompting; 2, moderate sore throat, with complaint without prompting; 3, severe sore throat that accompanies change in voice or hoarseness [15]. And postoperative pain was evaluated with kids pain scale (application of smartphone developed by *Societa di Anestesia e Rianimazione Neonatale e Pediatrica Italiana*, Fig. 1). Additionally, postanaesthetic emergence delirium (PAED) was verified by an independent investigator who was not formerly notified of the patient's assigned group and the cut-off score of 12 or more was defined as PAED [19].

The primary outcome was the incidence of sore throat defined as grade > 1 on the POST four-point scale in the PACU. The secondary outcome variables were the postoperative pain, incidences of adverse events (breath holding ≥20 s, coughing ≥2 times, heavy secretion, laryngospasm, or desaturation < 93%), sore throat pain and PAED.

Sample size estimation and statistical analysis
A previous study reported a POST incidence of 17% with BH, and 40.8% with normal saline in adults [20]. Based on this information, and the probability of a type I error (α) being 0.05 and type II error (β) being 0.05, with a statistical power at 80%, a minimum of 54 patients in each group was required according to the R program.

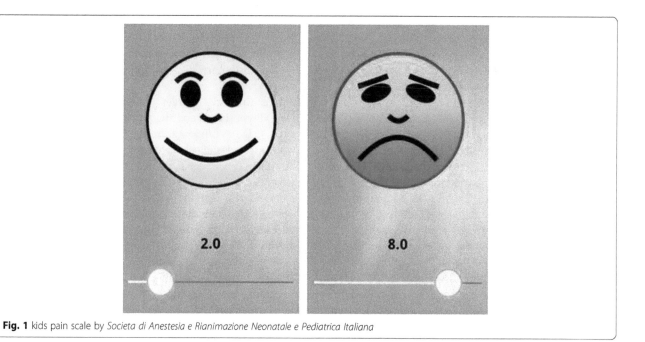

Fig. 1 kids pain scale by *Societa di Anestesia e Rianimazione Neonatale e Pediatrica Italiana*

Projecting a 20% loss in cases, 72 patients were enrolled per group.

Statistical analysis was performed using SPSS version 23.0 (IBM Corporation, Armonk, NY, USA) for Windows (Corporation, Redmond, WA, USA). The normal distribution of continuous data was evaluated using the Kolmogorov-Smirnov test, and normally distributed variables were analysed using the Student's t test for comparison of the two groups. Categorical variables, including POST and adverse events, were analysed using Pearson's chi-squared test (or Fisher's exact test if expected count < 5). The results are expressed as mean ± SD with corresponding 95% confidential interval, or median (interquartile rage [25–75%]). A *P*-value < 0.05 was considered to be statistically significant. The Kruskal-Wallis test was used to compare differences in the severity of POST.

Results
From March to June 2017, a total of 150 children were screened, of whom 144 were recruited and considered eligible for study inclusion. As in Fig. 2, two patients, one in each group, were excluded for the following reasons. One patient from the control group dropped out due to multiple attempts at intubation (i.e., > 2 attempts). One patient from the BH group was excluded due to denial of measurement reports in the PACU. Finally, the data of the 142 patients were analysed.

Patient demographics and surgery-related parameters are shown in Table 1. There were no significant differences between the control and BH groups. In Table 2. the incidence of POST scoring > 1 demonstrated no

significant difference as well. 35 (49.3%) patients in the control group experienced POST compared with 42 (59.2%) in the BH group (*P* = 0.238).

Other adverse events related to extubation and the evaluation of postoperative pain are summarized in Table 3. All adverse events including breath holding, secretions, coughing, laryngospasm, desaturation event, and PAED did not show any significant difference between two groups. And postoperative pain evaluated with smartphone application was similar between the two groups. However, interestingly, PAED was found in more than one-half of the patients in each group. A total of 56 (78.9%) patients were evaluated with PAED in the control group, with 49 (69.0%) patients in BH group (*P* = 0.18).

We reviewed the ward electric medical records for the postoperative sore throat in the recruited patients. There were no subjective significant complaints during the postoperative 24 h.

Discussion
In our study, applying BH spray, targeting the vocal cords and upper trachea before intubation in children, did not reduce the incidence of POST compared with the control group. However, previous meta-analysis involving an adult population of randomised controlled trials (RCTs) reviewed 13 studies where reduction in the incidence of POST was reported with prophylactic BH application to the oral cavity [14].

Compared with other positive-result studies, the main difference lies in the evaluation and application time. Currently, the guideline for POST evaluation time has

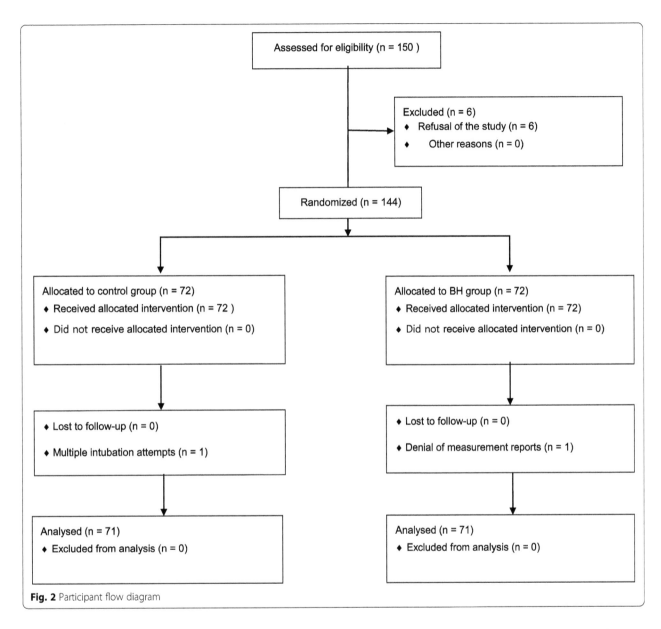

Fig. 2 Participant flow diagram

not been established yet. Previous RCTs evaluated POST for maximum 24 h at varying check points [15, 16]. However, we evaluated the patients at 30 min after entering the PACU, and only once. We focused on investigating POST in the immediate postoperative period,

Table 1 Demographic variables of each group

Characteristics	Control group	BH group	P-value
Number (M/F)	71 (31/40)	71 (29/42)	
Age (yr)	9.3 ± 2.1	9.5 ± 1.9	0.46
Height (cm)	137.7 ± 15.7	138.0 ± 12.8	0.90
Weight (kg)	35.8 ± 13.1	37.9 ± 12.4	0.34
Anesthesia time (min)	146.3 ± 60.8	159.8 ± 72.3	0.08
Operation time (min)	106.2 ± 56.6	114.1 ± 66.3	0.16

BH Benzydamine hydrochloride
Results are expressed as mean ± SD with corresponding 95% confidential interval or median with interquartile rage [25–75%]

Table 2 Incidence of postoperative sore throat

POST		Control group (n = 71)	BH group (n = 71)	P-value
No (score = 0)		36 (50.7%)	29 (40.8%)	0.238
Yes (score ≥**1**)		35 (49.3%)	42 (59.2%)	
score	1	25 (35.2%)	27 (38.0%)	
	2	7 (9.9%)	9 (12.7%)	
	3	3 (4.2%)	6 (8.5%)	

BH Benzydamine hydrochloride, *POST* Postoperative sore throat
All *P*-values are calculated by Chi-square test

Table 3 Incidences of adverse events

Adverse events	Control group (n = 71)	BH group (n = 71)	P-value
Breath holding	3 (4.2%)	2 (2.8%)	1.0
Secretion	29 (40.8%)	35 (49.3%)	0.31
Coughing	13 (18.3%)	8 (11.3%)	0.24
Laryngospasm	1 (1.4%)	0 (0.0%)	1.0
$SpO_2 < 93\%$ within 30 min since extubation	3 (4.2%)	4 (5.6%)	1.0
PAED	56 (78.9%)	49 (69.0%)	0.18
Postoperative pain	5.3 ± 3.1	5.5 ± 3.2	0.69

All P-values are calculated by Chi-square or Fischer's exact test
SpO_2 Peripheral oxygen saturation

since after transferring from PACU to ward, many children were given additional analgesics by the attending physicians which is out of anaesthesiologists' control. Moreover, unlike adult patients who are able to overtly express and verbalize their pain score after several hours, children may not be able to conceptualize or articulate the intensity of their pain after several hours. We speculated that by focusing on the early and single time period, when the postoperative pain become the new unfamiliar concern for children, assessing score through Visual Analog Scale (VAS): kids pain scale (Fig. 1) may be effective. Yet, according to common findings of previous studies regarding BH spray (rather than gargle or gel) in adults, the highest incidence of POST occurred at 4–6 h, rather than at 0–1 h [12, 15]. The single and very early time point of our evaluation may have attributed to masking or mitigating POST by postoperative pain killers, including PCA or propacetamol, and residual anaesthetic gas. Patients might not have been sufficiently awake, cooperative, and free of delirium to answer appropriately on POST questions at this time point. In addition, the application was done at least 5 min before induction in most of the previous researches. However, we applied BH spray just before the intubation because of bitter taste of BH. This 5 min might be negligible considering that the peak effect of BH was 2–4 h.

Typically divided into the oropharyngeal space versus the ETT cuff, our study focused only on targeting the vocal cords and upper trachea. Previously, one study compared oropharyngeal space with the ETT cuff and reported that spraying BH on the ETT cuff reduces incidence and severity of POST, while spraying BH on the oropharyngeal cavity showed no additional benefit, which is consistent with our results [16]. This implies that it is difficult to reach the exact cuff inflation point only through oropharyngeal spraying. Mucosal irritation occurs at the level of ETT cuff. Applying BH directly to the cuff can definitely concentrate BH at the exact mucosal irritation, thereby significantly reducing both

POST incidence and severity without further unpleasant side effects such as numbness, tingling sensation, and burning irritation, all of which children might refer to as POST [14]. While direct BH spraying easily reaches upper side of the vocal cord, it needs to overcome the vocal fold barrier to reach the cricoid level, which is the narrowest point in the paediatric airway. Thus, while BH spray may reach the trauma point in the adult airway, in paediatric patients, it may be insufficient to reach the target site.

Methodologically, differing formulations of BH, such as gel, spray or gargle, have been widely reviewed. Gel types target the tube cuff, including the endotracheal tube and supraglottic airway device tubes. Gargling covers the entire oral cavity, including the oropharynx, posterior pharyngeal wall, anterior surface of the epiglottis, and the uvula. BH gargling has demonstrated conflicting results [11, 21]. Meanwhile, spraying, as in our study, can aim both the cuff and/or oropharyngeal space, including the vocal cords and upper trachea. Spraying enables easy and fast application, with less worry about aspiration of the substances. Sprayed aerosols are smaller and widely scattered to form less tension between substances, thereby making BH widely and quickly deposited on the targeted surface area [22]. However, at the same time, this mechanism may also contribute to less convergence and lower concentration of BH to the exact airway trauma site, which is suspected to be the cricoid level in paediatric cases. Therefore, alternative aerosol delivery methods using pressurized inhalers or nebulizers may have been more effective in delivering BH to the cricoid level [22].

Additionally, the effects of normal saline as lubricant may have confounded our results, but to a low probability. In the present study, all the endotracheal tube was lubricated with normal saline immediately before intubation, and the normal saline itself may have already been sufficiently effective for the prevention of POST, thus not requiring any additional anti-inflammatory effect of BH. Normal saline can reduce the friction between ETT and airway tissues. However, the effect of such water lubrication on ETT has not been proved to significantly reduce any POST. Also, normal saline lubrication had been reported to be unrelated to diminishing POST event in diverse studies regarding adult population [2, 23, 24].

ETT cuff pressure was measured only at the time of intubation, and no measurements were taken during or at the end of surgery in our study. We found 50.7% at control group, and 40.8% at BH group reporting POST, which is higher than previously reported in the literature [1–3]. Initial ETT intubation and setting of a cuff inflation of 20 cmH_2O may have induced impairment of subglottic mucosal perfusion and oedema leading to higher incidence of POST in our study. We designed cuff target of 20 cmH_2O based on the previous report that leak at 20 to 25 cmH_2O ensures minimal mucosal pressure without definite air leak [25]. Although only ETT cuff pressure exceeding 30 cmH_2O is well-known to impair mucosal blood flow, in paediatric patients, even cuff pressure exceeding 10 cmH_2O has been reported to cause POST, recently [3]. Higher cuff pressures result in larger contact area and higher transmitted pressure exceeding the perfusion pressure of tracheal mucosae [3]. Since, children's mean arterial pressure is lower than that of adult's, cuff pressure should target inflation below 20 cmH_2O and continuous monitoring should be obligated to reduce unwanted cuff hyperinflation.

The present study has other several limitations, as well. First, the BH concentration at the target site was inaccurate owing to variable effect-site limiting factors, such as secretion, mucosal thickness, and spraying range, which could have influenced the results. Second, the estimation of POST severity encompasses a wide range of conditions, including pharyngitis, laryngitis, and trache-itis. Moreover, the grading even included cough and hoarseness on grading severity. It is particularly difficult to determine the cause of hoarseness because hoarseness commonly prevails in children due to children's emergence agitation or delirium. Restless crying was often mistaken as emergence delirium, and it was difficult to define true hoarseness from heavy crying. Therefore, the severity of POST may have been overestimated in the children with occurrence of emergence delirium. At the same time, the underestimation was also easily instigated due to easy sedation and postoperative pain management using PCA or propacetamol. To compare extra mucosal irritation, checking common BH side effects, such as burning sensation, numbness and dry mouth, may have been helpful. Lastly, postoperative analgesic choice (e.g., fentanyl in PCA or bolus of propacetamol) was not randomized between the two groups because of standard protocol of administration of analgesics in our institute. Nonetheless, PCA and propacetamol incidence was similar between the two groups and different manage of postoperative pain control or use of PCA did not affect the incidence of POST in both groups.

Conclusion

There was no benefit in using BH spray in the oropharyngeal space to reduce POST in paediatric population. However, due to the relative short period of evaluation in this study, well-designed and powered RCTs investigating the long-term effect of BH in paediatric populations must be conducted in future. Also, by comparing different application methods of BH, future studies may enable finding more accurate and practical pre-emptive local anaesthetic application within paediatric populations.

Abbreviations
ASA: American Society of Anaesthesiologists; BH: Benzydamine hydrochloride; ENT: Ear-nose-throat; E_TCO_2: End-tidal carbon dioxide; ETT: Endotracheal tube; FIO_2: Fraction of inspired oxygen; NIBP: Non-invasive blood pressure; PACU: Post-anaesthetic care unit; PAED: Postanaesthetic emergence delirium; PCA: Patient-controlled analgesia; POST: Postoperative sore throat; RCT: Rrandomised controlled trial; SpO2: Peripheral pulse oximetry; VAS: Visual analog scale

Acknowledgements
Not applicable.

Authors' contributions
Conceptualization; HBY, SHY, HSK. Data curation; YEJ, JHL. Formal analysis; EHK, JTK. Investigation; YEJ, JHL, EHK, JTK. Supervision; JTK, HSK. Writing original draft; HBY. Writing – review and editing; HSK. The authors read and approved the final manuscript.

References
1. Piriyapatsom A, Dej-Arkom S, Chinachoti T, Rakkarnngan J, Srishewachart P. Postoperative sore throat: incidence, risk factors, and outcome. J Med Assoc Thail. 2013;96(8):936–42.
2. El-Boghdadly K, Bailey CR, Wiles MD. Postoperative sore throat: a systematic review. Anaesthesia. 2016;71(6):706–17.
3. Calder A, Hegarty M, Erb TO, von Ungern-Sternberg BS. Predictors of postoperative sore throat in intubated children. Pediatr Anesth. 2012;22(3):239–43.
4. Patki A. Laryngeal mask airway vs the endotracheal tube in paediatric airway management: a meta-analysis of prospective randomised controlled trials. Indian J Anaesthesia. 2011;55(5):537–41.
5. Mostafa RH, Saleh AN, Hussein MM. A comparative study of three nebulized medications for the prevention of postoperative sore throat in the pediatric population. Open Anesthesia J. 2018;12(1):85–93.
6. Lee JY, Sim WS, Kim ES, Lee SM, Kim DK, Na YR, et al. Incidence and risk factors of postoperative sore throat after endotracheal intubation in Korean patients. J Int Med Res. 2017;45(2):744–52.
7. Chandler M. Tracheal intubation and sore throat: a mechanical explanation. Apparatus. Anaesthesia. 2002;57(2):155–61.
8. Chen CY, Kuo CJ, Lee YW, Lam F, Tam KW. Benzydamine hydrochloride on postoperative sore throat: a meta-analysis of randomized controlled trials. Can J Anaesth. 2014;61(3):220–8.
9. Tanaka Y, Nakayama T, Nishimori M, Tsujimura Y, Kawaguchi M, Sato Y. Lidocaine for preventing postoperative sore throat. Cochrane Database Syst Rev. 2015;7:CD004081.
10. Mayhood J, Cress K. Effectiveness of ketamine gargle in reducing postoperative sore throat in patients undergoing airway instrumentation: a systematic review. JBI Database Syst Rev Implementation Rep. 2015;13(9):244–78.
11. Agarwal A, Nath SS, Goswami D, Gupta D, Dhiraaj S, Singh PK. An evaluation of the efficacy of aspirin and Benzydamine hydrochloride gargle for attenuating postoperative sore throat: a prospective, randomized, single-blind study. Anesth Analg. 2006;103(4):1001–3.
12. Gulhas N, Canpolat H, Cicek M, Yologlu S, Togal T, Durmus M, et al. Dexpanthenol pastille and benzydamine hydrochloride spray for the prevention of post-operative sore throat. Acta Anaesthesiol Scand. 2007;51(2):239–43.
13. Baldock GA, Brodie RR, Chasseaud LF, Taylor T, Walmsley LM, Catanese B. Pharmacokinetics of benzydamine after intravenous, oral, and topical doses to human subjects. Biopharm Drug Dispos. 1991;12(7):481–92.
14. Kuriyama A, Aga M, Maeda H. Topical benzydamine hydrochloride for prevention of postoperative sore throat in adults undergoing tracheal intubation for elective surgery: a systematic review and meta-analysis. Anaesthesia. 2018;73(7):889–900.
15. Mekhemar NA, El-Agwany AS, Radi WK, El-Hady SM. Comparative study between benzydamine hydrochloride gel, lidocaine 5% gel and lidocaine 10% spray on endotracheal tube cuff as regards postoperative sore throat. Braz J Anesthesiol. 2016;66(3):242–8.
16. Huang Y-S, Hung N-K, Lee M-S, Kuo C-P, Yu J-C, Huang G-S, et al. The effectiveness of Benzydamine hydrochloride spraying on the endotracheal tube cuff or Oral mucosa for postoperative sore throat. Anesth Analg. 2010;111:887–91.

17. Weiss M, Dullenkopf A, Fischer JE, Keller C, Gerber AC. Prospective randomized controlled multi-Centre trial of cuffed or uncuffed endotracheal tubes in small children # #this article is accompanied by editorial I. Br J Anaesth. 2009;103(6):867–73.

18. Bodily JB, Webb HR, Weiss SJ, Braude DA. Incidence and duration of continuously measured oxygen desaturation during emergency department intubation. Ann Emerg Med. 2016;67(3):389–95.

19. Bajwa SA, Costi D, Cyna AM. A comparison of emergence delirium scales following general anesthesia in children. Pediatr Anesth. 2010;20(8):704–11.

20. Hung N-K, Wu C-T, Chan S-M, Lu C-H, Huang Y-S, Yeh C-C, et al. Effect on postoperative sore throat of spraying the endotracheal tube cuff with Benzydamine hydrochloride, 10% lidocaine, and 2% lidocaine. Anesth Analg. 2010;111(4):882–6.

21. Faiz SH, Rahimzadeh P, Poornajafian A, Nikzad N. Comparing the effect of ketamine and benzydamine gargling with placebo on post-operative sore throat: a randomized controlled trial. Adv Biomed Res. 2014;3:216.

22. Smith C, Goldman RD. Nebulizers versus pressurized metered-dose inhalers in preschool children with wheezing. Can Fam Physician. 2012;58(5):528–30.

23. Puebla I, Kim E, Yang SM, Kwak SG, Park S, Bahk J-H, et al. Tracheal tubes lubricated with water to reduce sore throat after intubation: a randomized non-inferiority trial. PLoS One. 2018;13(10):e0204846.

24. Taghavi Gilani M, Miri Soleimani I, Razavi M, Salehi M. Reducing sore throat following laryngeal mask airway insertion: comparing lidocaine gel, saline, and washing mouth with the control group. Braz J Anesthesiology. 2015; 65(6):450–4.

25. Timmerman K, Thomas JM. Endotracheal tubes in paediatric anaesthesia: the cuffed versus uncuffed debate. Southern Afr J Anaesthesia Analgesia. 2014;16(3):88–91.

19

Incidence of airway complications associated with deep extubation in adults

Jeremy Juang[1,2*†] ⓘ, Martha Cordoba[1,2†], Alex Ciaramella[1,2], Mark Xiao[1,2], Jeremy Goldfarb[1,2], Jorge Enrique Bayter[3] and Alvaro Andres Macias[1,2]

Abstract

Background: Endotracheal extubation is the most crucial step during emergence from general anesthesia and is usually carried out when patients are awake with return of airway reflexes. Alternatively, extubations can also be accomplished while patients are deeply anesthetized, a technique known as "deep extubation", in order to provide a "smooth" emergence from anesthesia. Deep extubation is seldomly performed in adults, even in appropriate circumstances, likely due to concerns for potential respiratory complications and limited research supporting its safety. It is in this context that we designed our prospective study to understand the factors that contribute to the success or failure of deep extubation in adults.

Methods: In this prospective observational study, 300 patients, age ≥ 18, American Society of Anesthesiologists Physical Status (ASA PS) Classification I - III, who underwent head-and-neck and ocular surgeries. Patients' demographic, comorbidity, airway assessment, O_2 saturation, end tidal CO_2 levels, time to exit OR, time to eye opening, and respiratory complications after deep extubation in the OR were analyzed.

Results: Forty (13%) out of 300 patients had at least one complication in the OR, as defined by persistent coughing, desaturation $SpO_2 < 90\%$ for longer than 10s, laryngospasm, stridor, bronchospasm and reintubation. When comparing the complication group to the no complication group, the patients in the complication group had significantly higher BMI (30 vs 26), lower O_2 saturation pre and post extubation, and longer time from end of surgery to out of OR ($p < 0.05$).

Conclusions: The complication rate during deep extubation in adults was relatively low compared to published reports in the literature and all easily reversible. BMI is possibly an important determinant in the success of deep extubation.

Keywords: Tracheal extubation, Deep extubation, Airway, Anesthesia, Ambulatory surgery, Emergence, Complications, Adult, Volatile anesthetics

* Correspondence: jeremy_juang@meei.harvard.edu
†Jeremy Juang and Martha Cordoba contributed equally to this work.
[1]Department of Anesthesiology, Massachusetts Eye and Ear, 243 Charles St, Boston, MA 02114, USA
[2]Harvard Medical School, Boston, MA 20114, USA

Background

Endotracheal extubation is the final and arguably the most crucial step during emergence from general anesthesia (GA). Normally, it is carried out when patients are awake with return of airway reflexes. However, extubations can also be accomplished while patients are deeply anesthetized but maintaining spontaneous breathing, a technique known as "deep extubation". Deep extubation is frequently performed in the setting of eye surgery as well as head and neck surgery. The intention is to minimize bucking and limit increase in intraocular and intracranial pressure [1–4].

When surveyed, even in appropriate clinical situations, many anesthesiologists are still reluctant to perform deep extubation in adults because of concerns for potential respiratory complications [5]. This apprehension may be unfounded as most published experiences (and reported complications) center around pediatric patients [6–9] and not adult patients. To our knowledge, there have only been a couple of adult deep extubation studies, with around 30 patients in each arm, comparing respiratory complications in patients deeply extubated after inhaled anesthetics with and without adjuvants [10, 11]. More robust data in a larger adult population are needed to inform clinical practice.

Therefore, in this prospective observational cohort study, we set out to assess the rate of respiratory complications after deep extubation in a larger sample size of 300 adult patients undergoing ocular and head and neck surgery. Our goal was to determine if there are intraoperative factors that may influence the success of deep extubations.

Methods

Study population

This single arm, unblinded, observational study was approved by the Institutional Review Board (IRB) of Massachusetts Eye and Ear Infirmary, Boston, Massachusetts (#1047249). The study was conducted in accordance with all rules and regulations laid out by the IRB and human studies committee. A waiver of written informed consent was obtained for this study. This study was registered at Clinicaltrials.gov (NCT04557683).

Patients greater than 18 years of age at the time of surgery and selected by the anesthesiologist as a candidate for deep extubation were enrolled in this study without specific exclusion criterion. All patients were evaluated by the preoperative anesthesia staff prior to surgery and a detailed preoperative note detailing vital signs, health history, and airway assessment (Mallampati score I-IV, neck ROM, TM distance, mouth opening, and artificial airway, facial hair, dental exam) was documented in the electronic medical record. Over the course of six months, 300 patients were enrolled in this observational study. Each day during this six-month period, a research coordinator would report to the main operating room and determine the possible candidates for the day based on age and anesthetic plan. Towards the end of each surgery the research coordinator would ask each anesthesiologist utilizing inhalation anesthetics about the extubation plan. If the anesthesiologist selects the patient for deep extubation, the patient would be followed from the end of surgery to Post Anesthesia Care Unit (PACU) for data collection. The deep extubation technique was the only controlled procedural variable among our patient cohort; other anesthesia procedural variables were selected at the provider's discretion.

Anesthetic management

At the end of the case, the fraction of inspired oxygen (FiO_2) was increased to 100% and the end inspired concentration of inhaled anesthetic was adjusted to be at least 1 Minimum Alveolar Concentration (MAC) or higher if needed. The depth of anesthesia was considered adequate clinically when the patient was spontaneously breathing with a regular pattern, at a MAC of 1 or higher, and if the patient did not exhibit any response to suctioning and to deflation and reinflation of the endotracheal tube cuff. Before extubation, an oral airway was placed in all the patients, and jaw thrust was applied if needed after extubation. The oral airway was removed, either in the operating room by anesthesia provider or in PACU by trained PACU nursing staff with 1-to-1 nurse to patient ratio under the supervision of an anesthesiologist, when the patient regained airway reflexes. Patients were administered oxygen at 6 L/min, via a face mask; supplemental oxygen was discontinued in PACU as per usual recovery room management.

Statistical analysis

For comparison, patients were classified into two groups: those without respiratory complications to those with respiratory complications as defined by persistent coughing, desaturation measured by saturation of peripheral oxygen (SpO_2) by pulse oximetry of less than 90% for longer than 10s, laryngospasm, stridor, bronchospasm, and reintubation. Patient demographics, baseline characteristics, procedures, intubation notes, and intraoperative variables were obtained from the electronic medical records and analyzed. Statistical analysis and graphs were performed and presented using Prism 8.4.2 (GraphPad Software Inc., La Jolla, CA). The normality of the distribution of continuous variables was assessed using the Shapiro-Wilk normality test. Mann-Whitney tests were used to compare continuous variables among groups. A 2-tailed P-value less than 0.05 was considered significant. Fisher's exact test was used to compare categorical variables among groups. Continuous variables are presented as median with interquartile ranges (q1-q3), while categorical variables are summarized using frequencies and percentages.

Results

A total of 300 adult patients were recruited for the study. Among them, 40 (13%) patients had at least one complication in the OR post deep extubation that included persistent coughing, desaturation $SpO_2 < 90\%$ for longer than 10s, sore throat, laryngospasm, stridor, bronchospasm (Fig. 1a). None of the 300 patients required re-intubation.

When comparing patient's demographic of the complications group to the no complications group, there were no differences in patient age (50.0(34.4–60.5) vs 50.0(30.3–52.0), $p = 0.9506$) (Fig. 1b) and sex (Fig. 1c). In contrast, patients in the complications group had significantly higher BMI (30.0(25.3–35.0) vs 26.0(23.0–29.0), $p < 0.0001$) when compared to the no complications group (Fig. 1d).

We observed no significant difference in patient ASA PS classification or type of surgery class (ear, eye, neck, nose, throat, thyroid) (Fig. 2 a&b). Furthermore, there were no significant differences in rates of pre-existing respiratory pathology, Mallampati Score, Cormack and Lehane's classification between complications and no-complications groups (Fig. 2c-e). Lastly, all the patienta were able to be masked.

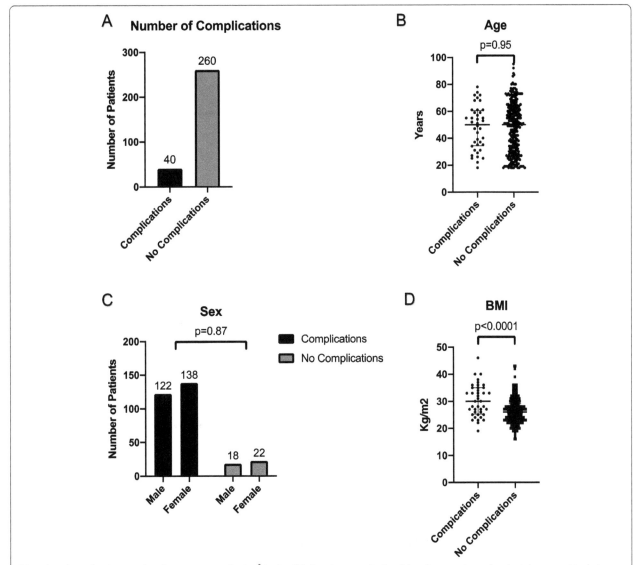

Fig. 1 Number of patients with at least one complication* in the OR after deep extubation (**a**) and comparison of patient demographics between complications and no complications group by (**b**) Age, (**c**) BMI, and (**d**) Sex. *Complications include desaturation SpO2 < 90% for longer than 10s, persistent cough, laryngospasm, stridor, bronchospasm, and reintubation

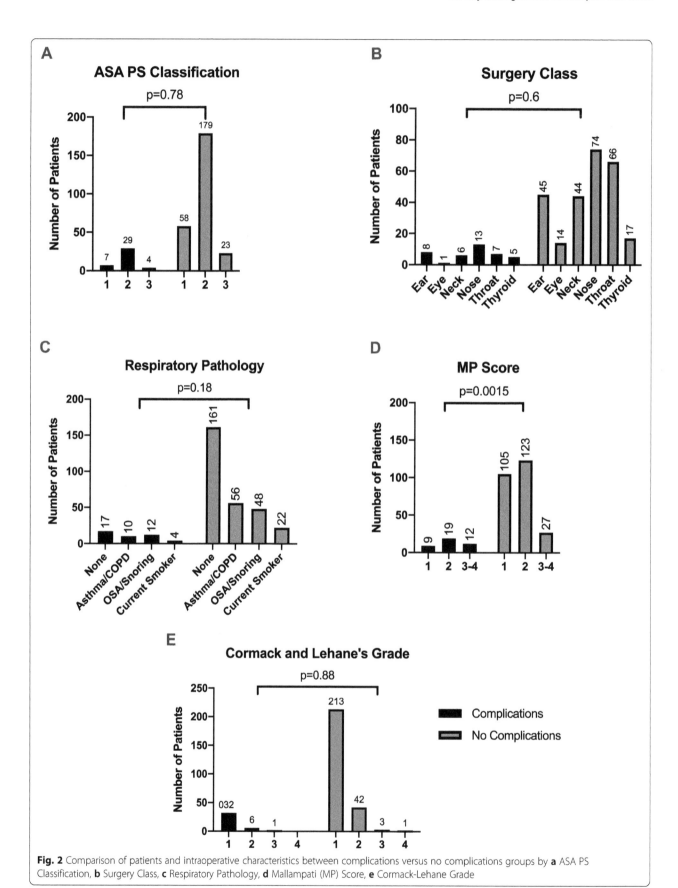

Fig. 2 Comparison of patients and intraoperative characteristics between complications versus no complications groups by **a** ASA PS Classification, **b** Surgery Class, **c** Respiratory Pathology, **d** Mallampati (MP) Score, **e** Cormack-Lehane Grade

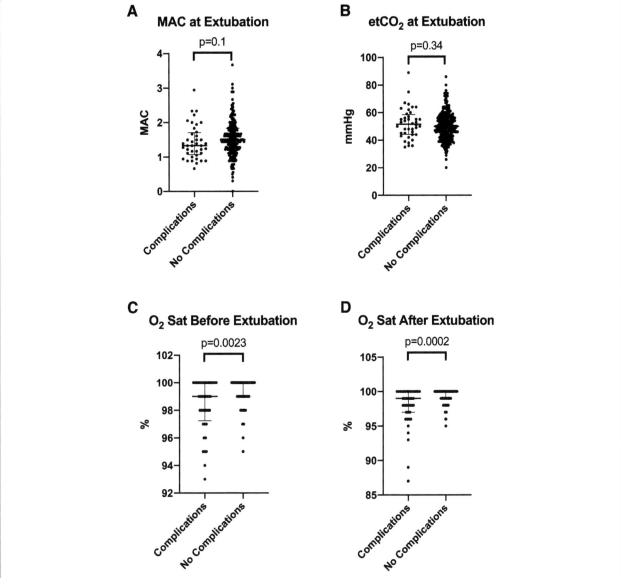

Fig. 3 Comparison of emergence conditions between complications versus no complications groups by **a** MAC, **b** end-tidal CO_2 (etCO_2), (C) O_2 Saturation (Sat) before and (D) O_2 Sat after extubation

Anesthetic depth did not appear to impact complications at the time of extubation MAC (1.33(1.07–1.71) vs 1.50(1.22–1.83, $p = 0.1002$), nor did etCO_2 (51.5(44.3–58.5) vs 50.0 (43.0–57.0), $p = 0.3352$) (Fig. 3a & b). However, patient percent O_2 saturation levels are significantly lower for the complication group compared to the no complications group at 5 mins before deep extubation (99.0(97.3–100) vs 100 (99.0–100), $p = 0.0023$) (Fig. 3c).

The time from deep extubation to leaving the OR was longer, at 12.0(9.00–14.8) mins, in the complications group compared to 9.00(7.00–13.0) mins in the no complications group ($p = 0.0098$) (Fig. 4a). The time to eye opening was also longer in the complications group than the no complications group (15.0(9.00–21.0) vs 18.0(13.3–25.0), $p = 0.0036$) (Fig. 4b). The total intraoperative opioid use and muscle relaxant and reversal use are not significantly different between the two groups (Table 1).

Discussion

In this study, 13% of adult patients (40 out of 300) had at least one or more respiratory complications with deep extubation. This is within range of a previous publication by Kim and colleagues in which one group that

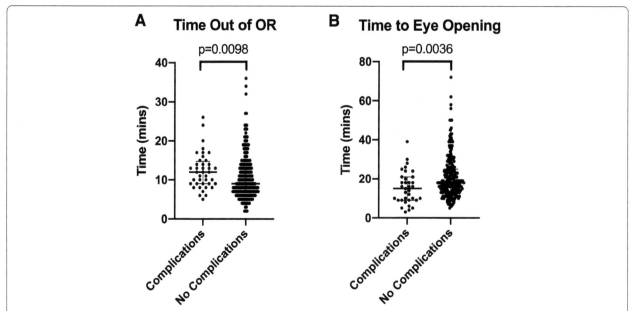

Fig. 4 Comparison of emergence times between complications versus no complications groups from end of surgery to **a** time out of OR and from extubation to **b** time to eye opening

received desflurane had a 48% complications rate (12 out of 25 patient) while the other group that received desflurane with remifentanil had a 3.4% complication rate (1 out of 29 patients) [10]. It is also consistent with Fan et al's report, where percentage of patient with airway complications ranges from 12 to 37.5% [11]. An important difference between ours and prior studies is how respiratory complications are defined. For example, whereas Kim et al's defined complications as coughing and breath holding, we expanded the criteria to capture additional complications, including significant desaturation, laryngospasm, stridor, bronchospasm and reintubation, that could also influence the success of deep extubation. It is worth noting that all of these complications were easily corrected by the anesthesia providers in our study with no need for drastic interventions such as reintubation. However, our data also showed that patients who had complications

with deep extubation tended to stay longer in the OR compared with patients who did not.

It is well understood that deep extubation can minimize adverse hemodynamic reflexes in appropriate situations [12]. Nonetheless, many anesthesiologists are reluctant to perform deep extubation in adults because of concerns for potential respiratory complications [5]. The present study indicates that deep extubations in adults is likely safer than in the pediatric population. Our airway complication rate of 13% in adult patients is significantly lower than the 40% complication rate (64 out of 159 patients) reported in a recent meta-analysis of pediatric patients [13]. While it is possible that patient selection and provider difference account for the lower rate; it is also conceivable that the pediatric airway is more irritable and sensitive to stimulation than the adult airway [14].

Table 1 Comparison of intraoperative dose of medications. Drug name (dosing unit) are listed in the left column. Data are expressed as median (q1-q3)

Drugs	Complications (n = 40)	No Complications (n = 260)	P-Value
Fentanyl (mcg)	100 (0.0–100.0)	100 (0.0–100.0)	0.3674
Remifentanil (mg)	0.580 (0.15–0.973)	0.435 (0.100–0.960)	0.3133
Morphine (mg)	0.0 (0.0–2.0)	0.0 (0.0–2.0)	> 0.9999
Hydromorphone (mg)	0.200 (0.00–0.900)	0.00 (0.00–0.500)	0.3374
Rocuronium (mg)	10.0 (0.00–10.0)	10.0 (0.00–10.0)	0.5999
Succinylcholine (mg)	100 (0.00–100)	80.0 (0.00–100)	0.6332
Neostigmine (mg)	0.00 (0.00–0.00)	0.00 (0.00–0.00)	0.5735

Present study suggests that patient selection plays an integral part in the success of endotracheal deep extubations. Our anesthesia providers selected patients for deep extubations per clinical discretion without predetermined criterion. Overwhelmingly, the patients selected had easy airway placement based on the Cormack and Lehane's Grade as only 1 patient out of 300 had a grade 4 view, which is a probable factor contributing to an overall complications rate near the lower limits of previously published ranges [10, 11]. On the flip side, our data also shows that when the provider chose to deep extubate patient with lower O_2 saturation levels 5 mins prior to extubation, these patients are more likely to have significant airway complications. Our results suggest that higher BMI patients are less likely to tolerate deep extubations. We observed a statistically significant correlation between higher BMI and likelihood of complications during deep extubation. The median BMI in the complications group was 30 while the median BMI in the no complications group was 26. Obesity has been shown to worsen oxygenation through several mechanisms, including increased intraabdominal pressure and atelectasis [15–17]. Whether an isolated elevated BMI is a causal factor for complications during deep extubations will need further investigation.

The depth of anesthesia suitable for a smooth deep extubation is primarily based on the MAC of inhaled anesthetics. Previous studies suggested that extubation could be performed at an inhaled anesthetic level as low as 1 MAC [2, 11, 18–20]. Some of the differences in MAC levels were likely due to variations in adjuvant opioid use, because opioid medications have been shown to minimize coughing and various extubation related adverse events [21, 22]. Here, we allowed the providers to freely decide the type and amount of opioid use appropriate for practice and did not observe a significant difference in the amount of opioid used in the complications versus no complications groups.

There were several limitations to this study. Firstly, this is a single-center prospective study, and the anesthesiologists were not and could not be blinded to the treatment technique. Secondly, there is also significant selection bias in the study, as no patients with history of difficult airway underwent deep extubation. Thirdly, other than the deep extubation technique, the anesthetic management was not standardized. However, this is a reality of every day anesthesia practice, irrespective of the extubation technique. Lastly, an experienced anesthesia provider remained with each patient until an adequate control of the airway was achieved, which could have contributed to the low incidence rate of complications. Moving forward, we hope our data can facilitate a more informed calculation of sample size for future studies comparing the complication rate of deep

versus awake extubation in adults. As expected, time to leaving the OR was higher in the complication group, however, the general question about differences in operating room turnover times between deep and traditional extubation techniques is beyond the scope of this study. Finally, there are probably many different ways of performing a deep extubation and further studies should be done to fine tune this technique.

Conclusions

Our findings demonstrate that deep extubation in adults is associated with a relatively low complication rate. Furthermore, high BMI and low O_2 saturation levels pre-extubation are associated with increased complications. We acknowledge that deep extubation should not be performed in patients with a known of history of difficult airway or aspiration risk and should always be performed by experienced providers after careful assessment. However, our experience does support deep extubation as a feasible and safe option in appropriate clinical circumstances.

Abbreviations

ASA PS: American Society of Anesthesiologists Physical Status; BMI: Body Mass Index; FiO2: Fraction of inspired Oxygen; GA: General Anesthesia; IRB: Institutional Review Board; MAC: Minimum Alveolar Concentration; MEEI: Massachusetts Eye and Ear Infirmary; PACU: Post Anesthesia Care Unit; SPO2: Saturation of Peripheral Oxygen

Acknowledgments

Xinling Xu, Statistician. Department of Anesthesiology, Perioperative and Pain Medicine Brigham and Women's Hospital, Harvard Medical School, 75 Francis St, Boston, MA 02115 USA.

Disclosures

None.

Authors' contributions

Author: J.J. Contribution: J.J.: supervision, project administration, validation, formal analysis, investigation, data curation, writing-original draft, writing-review & editing. Attestation: J.J. approved the final manuscript and attests to the integrity of the case report presented in this manuscript. Conflicts of Interest: none. Author: M.C. Contribution: M.C.: Conceptualization, methodology, investigation, supervision, data curation, validation, writing-original draft, and writing- review & editing. Attestation: M.C. approved the final manuscript and attests to the integrity of the study presented in this manuscript. Conflicts of Interest: None. Author: A.C. Contribution: A.C.: investigation, data curation, and validation. Attestation: A.C. approved the final manuscript and attests to the integrity of the study presented in this manuscript. Conflicts of Interest: None Author: M.X. Contribution: M.X.: data analysis, writing-original draft, and writing- review & editing. Attestation: M.X. approved the final manuscript and attests to the integrity of the study presented in this manuscript. Conflicts of Interest: None. Author: J.G. Contribution: J.G.: Supervision, investigation, data curation, validation, interpretation, writing-original draft, writing- review & editing. Attestation: J.G. approved the final manuscript and attests to the integrity the study presented in this manuscript. Conflicts of Interest: none. Author: J.E.B. Contribution: J.E.B.: Conceptualization and methodology. Attestation: J.E.B. approved the final manuscript and attests to the integrity of the study presented in this manuscript. Conflicts of Interest: None. Author: A.A.M. Contribution: A.A.M.: Conceptualization, methodology, investigation, data curation, validation, formal analysis, writing-original draft, writing- review & editing, supervision, project administration, and funding acquisition. Principal Investigator. Attestation: A.A.M. approved the final manuscript and attests to the integrity of the study presented in this manuscript.

Author details
[1]Department of Anesthesiology, Massachusetts Eye and Ear, 243 Charles St, Boston, MA 02114, USA. [2]Harvard Medical School, Boston, MA 20114, USA. [3]Clinica El Pinar, Km 2 Anillo vial Floridablanca – Girón, Ecoparque Empresarial Natura Torre 2 piso 1 y 2, Piedecuesta, Colombia.

References
1. Valley RD, Ramza JT, Calhoun P, Freid EB, Bailey AG, Kopp VJ, Georges LS. Tracheal extubation of deeply anesthetized pediatric patients: a comparison of isoflurane and sevoflurane. Anesth Analg. 1999;88(4):742–5.
2. Valley RD, Freid EB, Bailey AG, Kopp VJ, Georges LS, Fletcher J, Keifer A. Tracheal extubation of deeply anesthetized pediatric patients: a comparison of desflurane and sevoflurane. Anesth Analg. 2003;96(5):1320–4 table of contents.
3. Irwin RS. Complications of cough: ACCP evidence-based clinical practice guidelines. Chest. 2006;129(1 Suppl):54S–8S.
4. Fagan C, Frizelle HP, Laffey J, Hannon V, Carey M. The effects of intracuff lidocaine on endotracheal-tube-induced emergence phenomena after general anesthesia. Anesth Analg. 2000;91(1):201–5.
5. Daley MD, Norman PH, Coveler LA. Tracheal extubation of adult surgical patients while deeply anesthetized: a survey of United States anesthesiologists. J Clin Anesth. 1999;11(6):445–52.
6. Patel RI, Hannallah RS, Norden J, Casey WF, Verghese ST. Emergence airway complications in children: a comparison of tracheal extubation in awake and deeply anesthetized patients. Anesth Analg. 1991;73(3):266–70.
7. Pounder DR, Blackstock D, Steward DJ. Tracheal extubation in children: halothane versus isoflurane, anesthetized versus awake. Anesthesiology. 1991;74(4):653–5.
8. Koga K, Asai T, Vaughan RS, Latto IP. Respiratory complications associated with tracheal extubation. Timing of tracheal extubation and use of the laryngeal mask during emergence from anaesthesia. Anaesthesia. 1998;53(6):540–4.
9. von Ungern-Sternberg BS, Davies K, Hegarty M, Erb TO, Habre W. The effect of deep vs. awake extubation on respiratory complications in high-risk children undergoing adenotonsillectomy: a randomised controlled trial. Eur J Anaesthesiol. 2013;30(9):529–36.
10. Kim MK, Baek CW, Kang H, Choi GJ, Park YH, Yang SY, Shin HY, Jung YH, Woo YC. Comparison of emergence after deep extubation using desflurane or desflurane with remifentanil in patients undergoing general anesthesia: a randomized trial. J Clin Anesth. 2016;28:19–25.
11. Fan Q, Hu C, Ye M, Shen X. Dexmedetomidine for tracheal extubation in deeply anesthetized adult patients after otologic surgery: a comparison with remifentanil. BMC Anesthesiol. 2015;15:106.
12. Jaffe RA, Schmiesing CA, Golianu B. Anesthesiologist's manual of surgical procedures. 5th ed. Philadelphia: Lippincott Williams & Wilkins; 2014. 1 online resource.
13. Koo CH, Lee SY, Chung SH, Ryu JH. Deep vs. Awake Extubation and LMA Removal in Terms of Airway Complications in Pediatric Patients Undergoing Anesthesia: A Systemic Review and Meta-Analysis. J Clin Med. 2018;7:353. https://doi.org/10.3390/jcm7100353.
14. Peat JK, Gray EJ, Mellis CM, Leeder SR, Woolcock AJ. Differences in airway responsiveness between children and adults living in the same environment: an epidemiological study in two regions of New South Wales. Eur Respir J. 1994;7(10):1805–13.
15. Eichenberger A, Proietti S, Wicky S, Frascarolo P, Suter M, Spahn DR, Magnusson L. Morbid obesity and postoperative pulmonary atelectasis: an underestimated problem. Anesth Analg. 2002;95(6):1788–92 table of contents.
16. Pelosi P, Gregoretti C. Perioperative management of obese patients. Best Pract Res Clin Anaesthesiol. 2010;24(2):211–25.
17. Lang LH, Parekh K, Tsui BYK, Maze M. Perioperative management of the obese surgical patient. Br Med Bull. 2017;124(1):135–55.
18. Inomata S, Yaguchi Y, Taguchi M, Toyooka H. End-tidal sevoflurane concentration for tracheal extubation (MACEX) in adults: comparison with isoflurane. Br J Anaesth. 1999;82(6):852–6.
19. Shen X, Hu C, Li W. Tracheal extubation of deeply anesthetized pediatric patients: a comparison of sevoflurane and sevoflurane in combination with low-dose remifentanil. Paediatr Anaesth. 2012;22(12):1179–84.
20. Hu C, Yu H, Ye M, Shen X. Sevoflurane in combination with remifentanil for tracheal extubation after otologic surgery. Am J Health Syst Pharm. 2014;71(13):1108–011.
21. Mignat C, Wille U, Ziegler A. Affinity profiles of morphine, codeine, dihydrocodeine and their glucuronides at opioid receptor subtypes. Life Sci. 1995;56(10):793–9.
22. Yarmush J, D'Angelo R, Kirkhart B, O'Leary C, Pitts MC 2nd, Graf G, Sebel P, Watkins WD, Miguel R, Streisand J, et al. A comparison of remifentanil and morphine sulfate for acute postoperative analgesia after total intravenous anesthesia with remifentanil and propofol. Anesthesiology. 1997;87(2):235–43.

20

The midline approach for endotracheal intubation using GlideScope video laryngoscopy could provide better glottis exposure in adults

Lianxiang Jiang[1], Shulin Qiu[2], Peng Zhang[1], Weidong Yao[1], Yan Chang[1] and Zeping Dai[1]*

Abstract

Background: Previous studies have demonstrated that the common laryngoscopic approach (right-sided) and midline approach are both used for endotracheal intubation by direct laryngoscopy. Although the midline approach is commonly recommended for video laryngoscopy (VL) in the clinic, there is a lack of published evidences to support this practice. This study aimed to evaluate the effects of different video laryngoscopic approaches on intubation.

Methods: Two hundred sixty-two patients aged 18 years who underwent elective surgery under general anaesthesia and required endotracheal intubation were included in the present prospective, randomized, controlled study. The participants were randomly and equally allocated to the right approach (Group R) or midline approach (Group M). All the intubations were conducted by experienced anaesthetists using GlideScope video laryngoscopy. The primary outcomes were Cormack-Lehane laryngoscopic views (CLVs) and first-pass success (FPS) rates. The secondary outcomes were the time to glottis exposure, time to tracheal intubation, haemodynamic responses and other adverse events. Comparative analysis was performed between the groups.

Results: Finally, 262 patients completed the study, and all the tracheas were successfully intubated. No significant differences were observed in the patient characteristics and airway assessments ($P > 0.05$). Compared with Group R, Group M had a better CLV ($\chi2 = 14.706$, $P = 0.001$) and shorter times to glottis exposure (8.82 ± 2.04 vs 12.38 ± 1.81; $t = 14.94$; $P < 0.001$) and tracheal intubation (37.19 ± 5.01 vs 45.23 ± 4.81; $t = 13.25$; $P < 0.001$), but no difference was found in the FPS rate (70.2% vs 71.8%; $\chi2 = 0.074$; $P = 0.446$) and intubation procedure time (29.86 ± 2.56 vs 30.46 ± 2.97, $t = 1.75$, $P = 0.081$). Between the groups, the rates of hoarseness or sore throat, minor injury, hypoxemia and changes in SBP and HR showed no significant difference ($P > 0.05$).

Conclusion: Although the FPS rate did not differ based on the laryngoscopic approach, the midline approach could provide better glottis exposure and shorter times to glottis exposure and intubation. The midline approach should be recommended for teaching in VL-assisted endotracheal intubation.

Keywords: Endotracheal intubation, Video laryngosc, Laryngoscopic approach

* Correspondence: zpdai@wnmc.edu.cn
[1]Department of Anaesthesia, Yijishan Hospital of Wannan Medical College, No. 2, Zheshan West Road, Wuhu City, Anhui Province, China

Background

In the past decade, video laryngoscopy-assisted tracheal intubation has been extensively applied in airway management because of better visualization of the laryngeal structures on a high-resolution video screen [1–3]. Common teaching in direct laryngoscopy advocates that the device is inserted into the right side of the mouth, the tongue is moved to the left by the blade flange, the blade tip is advanced into the epiglottic vallecula, and then the device is raised to obtain the laryngeal view (right-sided approach) [4]. Until now, this method has been considered the gold standard in tracheal intubation, even for teaching undergraduates. However, we found that the right-sided approach may not be appropriate for intubation using video laryngoscopy (VL) in the clinic. The midline approach without sweep of the tongue is commonly recommended to achieve an unobstructed view of the larynx by VL, but there is a lack of published supporting evidence. Israel and colleagues conducted a retrospective cohort study of children who had undergone endotracheal intubation using VL and found no difference in successful intubation on the first attempt based on the laryngoscopic approach type [5]. However, many factors, including glottis visualization, pre-shaped angulation of the tube, level of trainee and presence of difficult airway predictors, are all correlated with first-pass success (FPS) [6–8]. Other studies have also demonstrated that VL helps to decrease intubation failure but did not improve the FPS in intensive care unit patients requiring intubation or in anaesthesiology practice [9–11]. Therefore, the FPS rate may not be adequate to evaluate the performance of different laryngoscopic approaches for intubation. Urgent evidence is needed to support which approach makes a greater contribution to glottic opening.

In this study, we aimed to compare the right-sided versus midline laryngoscopic blade approach in adult patients who had undergone video laryngoscopy-assisted tracheal intubation using the following outcomes: 1) Cormack-Lehane laryngoscopic views (CLV); 2) first-pass success (FPS) rate; 3) time to glottis exposure and intubation; 4) adverse events and haemodynamic changes during intubation.

Methods

Study design

Ethical approval for this study (Ethical Committee NO.4–2019) was provided by the Ethical Issues Committee, Yiji Shan Hospital of Wannan Medical College, Anhui, China (Chairperson Prof Wu P) on March 6, 2019. Written informed consent was obtained from all the patients prior to participation. This study is an interventional, randomized controlled trial and was registered in the Chinese Clinical Trial Registry (ChiCTR1900023252). Our study was adhered to the applicable Consolidated Standards of Reporting Trials (CONSORT) guidelines. The participants were randomly and equally allocated to two groups: right-sided approach group (Group R) and midline approach group (Group M). The randomized sequence was generated by computer, and all allocations were included in sealed opaque envelopes. For randomization, the envelopes will be opened only after transporting the patient to the operating room, and only one envelope can be opened per patient. Because of the nature of the study, the outcome observer could not be blinded to the patients' group allocation. This was a single-blind clinical trial—that is, patients were blinded to interventions.

Patients older than 18 years, with American Society of Anesthesiology (ASA) physical status I-III, and scheduled to undergo elective surgical procedure under general endotracheal anaesthesia, were all included. Patients were excluded due to the following criteria: 1) patients with a predictable difficult airway: Mallampati score $\geq$ IV, an interincisor gap less than 3.5 cm, a thyromental distance less than 6.5 cm, a sternomental distance less than 12.5 cm; 2) patients with reduced neck extension and flexion, airway obstruction (infectious, traumatic, foreign body, anaphylaxis), recent airway surgery, or a history of a difficult airway; 3) patients with the need for a rapid sequence induction, an alternative intubation method or known or suspected oral, pharyngeal or laryngeal masses; 4) patients with poor dentition, symptomatic gastro-oesophageal reflux, cervical spine instability, unstable hypertension, coronary artery disease, cerebral disease or patients for whom the resources were not available to conduct the procedure on the scheduled date of surgery.

After transfer to the operative room, the patients were monitored for non-invasive blood pressure (BP), heart rate (HR), pulse oximetry (SpO_2) and end-tidal carbon dioxide partial pressure ($P_{ET}CO_2$). The demographic and clinical characteristics of the patients were collected. The patients then underwent a uniform induction technique with midazolam 0.05 mg/kg, propofol 2.0 to 2.5 mg/kg and then were adequately relaxed with cisatracurium 0.15 mg/kg as evident by the loss of all trains of four responses using a peripheral nerve stimulator. With the induction of anaesthesia, the patients could also be administered 0.5 µg/kg of sulfentanyl. All the tracheas were intubated by the oral route using a Glidescope video laryngoscope, size 3 blades (GlideScope® GVL, Verathon Inc., BAothell, WA, USA). For patients in group R, the blade flange was inserted from the right side of the mouth to obtain glottic opening. A midline approach was conducted in group M. In both groups, video laryngoscopy-assisted tracheal intubations were performed by an experienced anaesthesiologist. Intraoperative anaesthesia was intravenously maintained with propofol 4–8 mg/kg/h and remifentanil 0.1–0.2 µg/kg /min. The bispectrality index (BIS) was used to monitor the depth of anaesthesia and keep the BIS value between 45 and 60.

Outcomes

Our primary outcome was CLV and the FPS rate. The CLV was determined by the modified Cormack-Lehane view of the glottis based on the view obtained at video laryngoscopy: grade I, the glottis is completely visible; grade IIa, the glottis opening is partially visible; grade IIb, only arytenoid cartilage is visible; grade III, only the tip of the epiglottis is visible; and grade IV, no glottis structures are visible [12]. Our secondary outcomes were the times to glottis exposure, intubation procedure time and tracheal intubation time. We defined the time to glottis exposure as the time from the insertion of the blade into the mouth until exposure of the glottis, the time to intubation procedure as the time from finishing exposure of the glottis and ending at blade removal from the mouth and the time to tracheal intubation as the time from starting at blade insertion and ending at blade removal from the mouth. Other outcomes, including hypoxemia (SpO$_2$ < 90%), haemodynamic changes [systolic blood pressure (SBP) and heart rate were recorded before intubation, and 1 min, 2 min and 5 min post-intubation], minor injury (oropharyngeal mucosal injury), hoarseness or sore throat on the first postoperative day assessed by a blinded anaesthetist, were also recorded.

Sample size

We conducted a pilot study of 60 patients for sample size assessment. In this pilot study, the number of CVL grade I-II was 30 (100%) in Group M and 28 (93.3%) in Group R. A sample size of 218 (109 in each group) allowed the detection of a 20% difference between the groups, with an α of 0.05 (two tailed), a β of 0.20, and a power of 0.8. To account for 20% attrition, a total sample size of 262 (131 in each group) was selected.

Statistical analysis

Continuous variables, such as the height, weight, body mass index (BMI) of the patients and metrics of airway assessments are presented as the mean ± SD. The categorical data are presented as percentages. Ninety-five percent confidence intervals (CIs) for all counts and proportions were also calculated. The primary efficacy variable of the laryngoscopic views, FPS rate and adverse events in different groups were analysed using chi squared test ($\chi 2$) or Fisher's exact test. The Mann-Whitney U test or Student's t test was used to compare both groups with respect to basic characteristics and other outcomes including the time to glottis exposure, SBP and HR. All the statistical tests were two-sided tests (test level α = 0.05). A P value< 0.05 was considered statistically significant.

Results

Two hundred ninety-five patients were approached: 14 did not meet the inclusion criteria, 8 declined to participate, and 11 were excluded for other reasons. Finally, 262 patients completed the study, with 131 in each group (Fig. 1). Among them, 133 (50.8%; 95% CI: 44.7 to 56.9%) patients were male and 129 (49.2%; 95% CI: 43.1 to 55.3%) patients were female. The basic characteristics and metrics of airway assessment in both groups are shown in Table 1. No significant differences were observed in the age, gender, weight, height, body mass index, Mallampati score, sternomental distance, interincisor distance, thyromental distance and ASA physical status ($P > 0.05$).

In Group M, 122 (93.1%; 95% CI: 88.7 to 97.5%) patients were grade I, 9 (6.9%; 95% CI: 2.5 to 11.3%) were grade IIa and no patient was above grade IIb. In Group R, 100 (76.3%; 95% CI: 69.0 to 83.7%) patients were grade I, 29 (22.2%; 95% CI: 14.9 to 29.3%) were grade IIa, 2 (1.5%; 95% CI: 0.6 to 3.7%) were grade IIb and no patient was above grade III. Compared with Group R, Group M had a better CLV ($\chi 2$ = 14.706; P = 0.001). All the patients' tracheas were successfully intubated, and the total success rate was comparable in the two groups (P = 1.00). Ninety-two (70.2%; 95% CI: 62.3 to 78.2%) patients were successfully intubated on the first attempt in Group M, 94 (71.8%; 95% CI: 63.9 to 79.6%) were successfully intubated on the first attempt in Group R, and the FPS rate showed no difference between the groups ($\chi 2$ = 0.074; P = 0.446). Additionally, compared with Group R, Group M had a shorter time to glottis exposure (8.82 ± 2.04 vs 12.38 ± 1.81, t = 14.94, $P <$ 0.001) and tracheal intubation (37.19 ± 5.01 vs 45.23 ± 4.81, t = 13.25, $P <$ 0.001), but no difference was found in the intubation procedure time (29.86 ± 2.56 vs 30.46 ± 2.97, t = 1.75, P = 0.081) (Table 2).

During intubation, hoarseness or sore throat were the most common adverse events, although the rates of these were not different between the groups (74.8% in Group M vs 77.9% in Group R; $\chi 2$ = 0.338, P = 0.331). Seven (5.3%; 95% CI: 1.4 to 9.2%) patients had hypoxemia and 8 (6.1%; 95% CI: 2.0 to 10.3%) had minor injuries in Group M, 6 (4.6%; 95% CI: 1.0 to 8.2%) patients had hypoxemia and 9 (6.9%; 95% CI: 2.5 to 11.3%) had minor injuries in Group R. Additionally, no difference were found in the rates between the groups (hypoxemia: 5.3% vs 4.6%, $\chi 2$ = 0.081, P = 0.500; minor injury: 6.1% vs 6.9%, $\chi 2$ = 0.063, P = 0.500) (Table 2).

Regarding the haemodynamic response to intubation stress, the baseline, SBP and HR before intubation, and at 1 min, 2 min and 5 min post-intubation in the two groups were recorded. No significant difference was found in the changes of SBP and HR between the groups ($P > 0.05$) (Fig. 2 and Fig. 3).

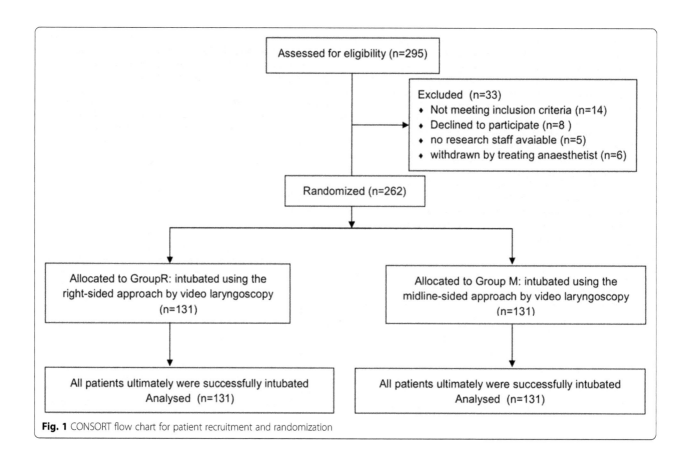

Fig. 1 CONSORT flow chart for patient recruitment and randomization

Table 1 Patient characteristics and airway assessments

	Group R (n = 131)	95%CI	Group M (n = 131)	95%CI	p value
Age;year	54.60 ± 11.16	52.67–56.53	56.87 ± 12.60	54.69–59.05	0.124
Gender; %(n)					0.388
Male; %(n)	53.4(70)	44.8–62.1	48.1(63)	39.4–56.8	
Female; %(n)	46.6(61)	37.9–55.2	51.9(68)	43.2–60.6	
Height;cm	165.67 ± 7.11	164.45–166.88	166.27 ± 8.52	164.81–167.73	0.537
Weight;kg	61.46 ± 7.81	60.11–62.81	60.00 ± 8.22	58.58–61.42	0.142
ASA physical status; %(n)					0.455
1	21.4(28)	14.3–28.5	24.4(32)	17.0–31.9	
2	74.0(97)	66.4–81.7	72.5(95)	64.8–80.3	
3	4.6(6)	1.0–8.2	3.1(4)	0.1–6.0	
Body mass index; kg.m^{-2}	22.57 ± 3.81	21.91–23.23	21.77 ± 4.01	21.08–22.46	0.119
Sternomental distance;cm	16.52 ± 0.91	16.36–16.68	16.41 ± 1.05	16.23–16.59	0.367
Interincisor distance;cm	3.95 ± 0.56	3.85–4.05	4.05 ± 0.60	3.95–4.15	0.164
Thyromental distance;cm	7.58 ± 0.61	7.48–7.69	7.62 ± 0.58	7.52–7.72	0.587
Mallampati score;%(n)					0.777
1	55.7(73)	47.1–64.3	57.3(75)	48.7–65.8	
2	38.2(50)	29.7–46.6	37.4(49)	29.0–45.8	
3	6.1(8)	2.0–10.3	5.3(7)	1.4–9.2	

Values are Number (proportion) or Mean ± SD. *Group R* right-sided approach group, *Group M* midline approach group, *95% CI* 95% confidence interval

Table 2 Details of intubation

	Group R (n = 131)	Group M (n = 131)	p value
Glottic view; %(n)			< 0.001
1	76.3(100)	93.1(122)	
2a	22.2(29)	6.9(9)	
2b	1.5(2)	0	
3	0	0	
FPS rate; %(n)	71.8(94)	70.2(92)	0.446
Total success rate; %(n)	100(131)	100(131)	1.0
Intubation procedure time;s	30.46 ± 2.97	29.86 ± 2.56	0.081
Exposure time;s	12.38 ± 1.81	8.82 ± 2.04	< 0.001
Intubation time;s	45.23 ± 4.81	37.19 ± 5.01	< 0.001
Adverse events; %(n)			
Hypoxemia	4.6(6)	5.3(7)	0.500
Minor injury	6.9(9)	6.1(8)	0.500
Hoarseness or Sore throat	77.9(102)	74.8(98)	0.331

Values are Number (proportion) or Mean ± SD. *Group R* right-sided approach group, *Group M* midline approach group

Discussion

As an available tool for difficult airway management, video laryngoscopy has been demonstrated to improve the success rate and decrease iatrogenic airway trauma [2, 3, 6]. However, the better method of video laryngoscopy-assisted tracheal intubation has not been verified. The performance of intubation using the right-sided approach versus midline approach was compared. We found that the midline approach had better Cormack-Lehane laryngoscopic views and shorter times to glottis exposure and tracheal intubation. The differences in the FPS rate, hypoxemia, haemodynamic response and other adverse events between the groups were not observed.

To obtain adequate direct visualization during intubation, the tongue is commonly swept to the left according to guidance [4, 13]. Although the midline approach

has been proposed for intubation by some experts in the early twentieth century, they point to direct laryngoscopy not video laryngoscopy [5, 13–15]. Additionally, no clear evidence exists to support the clinical experience until now. In 2015, Israel and colleagues first explored the effects of both approaches on FPS rate at a paediatric emergency department using the C-MAC video laryngoscope [5]. They found that the PFS rates did not differ based on the laryngoscopic approach type. However, this finding did not illustrate that both approaches were identical because many factors mentioned above contribute to the first-pass success. Similar to their result, the FPS rate was also comparable between the groups in our study. Thus, the success rate of endotracheal intubation was not recognized as our only main outcome. Instead, we believe it was more persuasive to add laryngoscopic

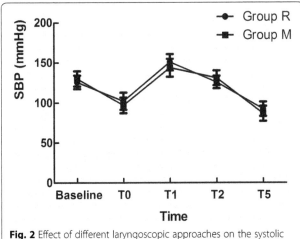

Fig. 2 Effect of different laryngoscopic approaches on the systolic blood pressure (SBP)

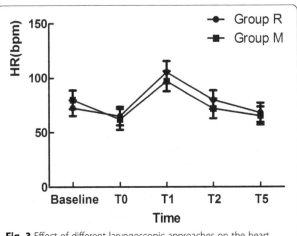

Fig. 3 Effect of different laryngoscopic approaches on the heart rate (HR)

views as an indicator to compare the effect of different approaches on intubation. Finally, we demonstrated that glottis exposure in the midline approach was better than the right approach. Additionally, different from both approaches, the left-molar approach requires that the tongue be displaced to the right. It was reported that the left molar approach can also provide a better laryngeal view in cases of unexpected difficult intubation and mitigate difficult intubation when performed by direct laryngoscopy [16, 17]. Nevertheless, whether VL provides a better laryngeal view than the conventional approach requires advanced research.

Because it is difficult to recognize key anatomic landmarks using a right-sided approach, a longer time may be needed to reach an optimal view [5, 6]. Our finding further supports this statement: the midline approach requires a shorter time to glottis exposure than the right-sided approach during tracheal intubation using VL. In the right-sided approach, the tongue was moved to the left and deviated from the median line of the mouth, resulting in angulation between the tongue and blade. Much more force was needed to expose the glottis due to the dispersion of forces. By contrast, in the midline approach, the laryngoscope blade is straight to expose the glottis, avoiding more forces. Adverse events such as oedema, tooth trauma, and soft tissue lesions can be caused by excessive forces transmitted through the laryngoscope during an intubation [18]. Thus, the rate of minor injury in the midline approach was lower than that in the right approach in theory. Increasing evidence has indicated that the video laryngoscope has an established role in tracheal intubation, decreasing the forces applied to the soft tissues of the upper airway and incidence of complications, compared with the Macintosh laryngoscope [18–20]. However, we found no difference in the rates of adverse events between the approaches in contrast to these studies and Israel's results. Two explanations are possible. First, patients with predictable difficult airways were not included in our study. All the endotracheal intubations in both groups were conducted by VL with a lower applied force. Second, the participants were children in Israel's study while they were adults in the present study. Compared with the adults, the children may be more likely to suffer from tissue damage. For the haemodynamic response to intubation, the patients did not significantly differ in SBP and HR after stress between the groups.

Our study possessed limitations. First, video laryngoscopy was originally designed as a device to manage difficult intubation with direct laryngoscopy, but the patients with predicable difficult airways were all excluded in our trial. Whether the midline approach would be effective in this population needs further study. Second, investigators were not blinded to the outcome measures. Third,

several video laryngoscopes with different designs are commercially available and have been investigated in various settings [21, 22]. All the intubation procedures were performed using a Glidescope video laryngoscope in the present study. Whether the results were applied to other video laryngoscopes may be worth discussing.

Conclusions

We observed that the midline approach was associated with a better glottis exposure and a shorter time to intubation than the right-sided approach. The midline approach should be recommended for teaching in video laryngoscopy-assisted endotracheal intubation.

Abbreviations
ASA: American Society of Anesthesiology; BIS: bispectral index; BMI: Body mass index; BP: Non-invasive blood pressure; CLV: Cormack-Lehane laryngoscopic views; FPS: First-pass success; HR: Heart rate; $P_{ET}CO_2$: End-tidal carbon dioxide partial pressure; SBP: Systolic blood pressure; SpO_2: Pulse oximetry; VL: Video laryngoscopy

Acknowledgements
Not applicable.

Authors' contributions
QSL and ZP conducted the study and collected the data. CY and JLX supervised the research and analysed the data. JLX and DZP wrote and revised the manuscript. YWD and DZP designed and conducted the study. All of the authors read and approved the final manuscript.

Author details
[1]Department of Anaesthesia, Yijishan Hospital of Wannan Medical College, No. 2, Zheshan West Road, Wuhu City, Anhui Province, China. [2]Department of Anaesthesia, Beijing Tiantan Hospital of Capital Medical University, Beijing, China.

References
1. Mcnarry AF, Patel A. The evolution of airway management-new concepts and conflicts with traditional practice. Br J Anaesth. 2017;119:154–66.
2. Mort TC, Braffett BH. Conventional versus video laryngoscopy for tracheal tube exchange: Glottic visualization, success rates, complications, and rescue alternatives in the high-risk difficult airway patient. Anesth Analg. 2015;121:440–8.
3. Lewis SR, Butler AR, Parker J, Cook TM, Schofield-Robinson OJ, Smith AF. Videolaryngoscopy versus direct laryngoscopy for adult patients requiring tracheal intubation: a Cochrane systematic review. Br J Anaesth. 2017;119:369–83.
4. Wang JK. Endotracheal intubation and endobronchial intubation. In: Guo QL, Yao SL, editors. Clinical anesthesiology. Beijing: People's Medical Publishing House; 2017. p. 41–70.
5. Green-Hopkins I, Werner H, Monuteaux MC, Nagler J. Using Video-recorded Laryngoscopy to Evaluate Laryngoscopic Blade Approach and Adverse Events in Children. Acad Emerg Med. 2015;22:1283–9.
6. Kerrey BT, Rinderknecht AS, Geis GL, Nigrovic LE, Mittiga MR. Rapid sequence intubation for pediatric emergency patients: higher frequency of failed attempts and adverse effects found by video review. Ann Emerg Med. 2012;60:259–1.
7. Sakles JC, Chiu S, Mosier J, Walker C, Stolz U. The importance of first pass success when performing orotracheal intubation in the emergency department. Acad Emerg Med. 2013;20:71–8.
8. Goto T, Gibo K, Hagiwara Y, Okubo M, Brown DF, Brown CA 3rd, Hasegawa K. Factors Associated with First-Pass Success in Pediatric Intubation in the Emergency Department. West J Emerg Med. 2016;17:129–34.
9. Lascarrou JB, Boisrame-Helms J, Bailly A. Video laryngoscopy vs direct laryngoscopy on successful first-pass Orotracheal intubation among ICU patients: a randomized clinical trial. JAMA. 2017;317:483–93.

10. Gao YX, Song YB, Gu ZJ, Zhang JS, Chen CF, Sun H, Lu Z. Video versus direct laryngoscopy on successful firstpass endotracheal intubation in ICU patients. World J Emerg Med. 2018;9:99–104.
11. Sulser S, Ubmann D, Schlaepfer M, Brueesch M, Goliasch G, Seifert B, Spahn DR, Ruetzler K. C-MAC videolaryngoscope compared with direct laryngoscopy for rapid sequence intubation in an emergency department: a randomised clinical trial. Eur J Anaesthesiol. 2016;33:943–8.
12. Yentis SM, Lee DJH. Evaluation of an improved scoring system for the grading of direct laryngoscopy. Anaesthesia. 1998;53:1041–6.
13. Xue FS, Li HX, Liu YY, Yang GZ. Current evidence for the use of C-MAC videolaryngoscope in adult airway management: a review of the literature. Ther Clin Risk Manag. 2017;3:831–41.
14. Aziz M, Brambrink A. The Storz C-MAC video laryngoscope: description of a new device, case report, and brief case series. J Clin Anesth. 2011;23:149–52.
15. Magill I. Technique in endotracheal anaesthesia. Br Med J. 1930;2:817–9.
16. Bozdogan N, Sener M, Bilen A, Turkoz A, Donmez A, Arslan G. Does left molar approach to laryngoscopy make difficult intubation easier than the conventional midline approach? Eur J Anaesthesiol. 2008;25:681–4.
17. Cuvas O, Basar H, Gursoy N, Culhaoglu S, Demir A. Left-molar approach for direct laryngoscopy: is it easy? J Anesth. 2009;23:36–40.
18. Carassiti M, Zanzonico R, Cecchini S, Silvestri S, Cataldo R, Agrò FE. Force and pressure distribution using Macintosh and GlideScope laryngoscopes in normal and difficult airways: a manikin study. Br J Anaesth. 2012;108:146–51.
19. Cordovani D, Russell T, Wee W, Suen A, Cooper RM. Measurement of forces applied using a Macintosh direct laryngoscope compared with a Glidescope video laryngoscope in patients with predictors of difficult laryngoscopy: a randomised controlled trial. Eur J Anaesthesiol. 2018;35:1–6.
20. Russell T, Khan S, Elman J, Katznelson R, Cooper RM. Measurement of forces applied during Macintosh direct laryngoscopy compared with GlideScope (R) videolaryngoscopy. Anaesthesia. 2012;67:626–31.
21. Wetsch WA, Spelten O, Hellmich M, Carlitscheck M, Padosch SA, Lier H, Böttiger BW, Hinkelbein J. Comparison of different video laryngoscopes for emergency intubation in a standardized airway manikin with immobilized cervical spine by experienced anaesthetists: a randomized, controlled crossover trial. Resuscitation. 2012;83:740–5.
22. Ruetzler K, Imach S, Weiss M, Haas T, Schmidt AR. Comparison of five video laryngoscopes and conventional direct laryngoscopy. Anaesthesist. 2015;64:513–9.

21

LMA® Gastro™ Airway for endoscopic retrograde cholangiopancreatography

Andre Tran[1] , Venkatesan Thiruvenkatarajan[2*] , Medhat Wahba[2] , John Currie[2] , Anand Rajbhoj[2] ,
Roelof van Wijk[2] , Edward Teo[3] , Mark Lorenzetti[3] and Guy Ludbrook[4]

Abstract

Background: Various airway techniques have been employed for endoscopic procedures, with an aim to optimise patient outcomes by improving airway control and preventing hypoxia whilst avoiding the need for intubation. The LMA® Gastro™ Airway, a novel dual channel supraglottic airway technique, has been described as such a device. Its utility alongside sedation with low flow nasal cannula and general anaesthesia (GA) with intubation for endoscopic retrograde cholangiopancreatography (ERCP) procedures was evaluated.

Methods: Details of all the ERCPs performed in our institution from March 2017 to June 2018 were carefully recorded in the patients' electronic case records. Data on the successful completion of ERCP through LMA® Gastro™ Airway; any difficulty encountered by the gastroenterologists; and adverse events were recorded. Episodes of hypoxia ($SpO_2 < 92\%$) and haemodynamic parameters were compared across the three groups: LMA® Gastro™ vs. sedation with low flow nasal cannula vs. GA with an endotracheal tube (ETT).

Results: One hundred seventy-seven ERCP procedures were performed during the study period. The LMA® Gastro™ Airway was employed in 64 procedures (36%) on 59 patients. Of these 64 procedures, ERCP was successfully completed with LMA® Gastro™ Airway in 63 (98%) instances, with only one case requiring conversion to an endotracheal tube. This instance followed difficulty in negotiating the endoscope through LMA® Gastro™ Airway. No episodes of hypoxia or hypercapnia were documented in both LMA® Gastro™ and GA with ETT groups. One sedation case with nasal cannula was noted to have hypoxia. Adverse intraoperative events were recognised in 2 cases of LMA® Gastro™: one had minimal blood stained secretions from the oral cavity that resolved with suctioning; the other developed mild laryngospasm which resolved spontaneously within a few minutes.

(Continued on next page)

* Correspondence: Venkatesan.Thiruvenkatarajan@sa.gov.au
This study was performed in accordance with the Strengthening the Reporting of Observational Studies in Epidemiology [STROBE] recommendations.
[2]Department of Anaesthesia, The Queen Elizabeth Hospital, 28 Woodville Rd, Adelaide, South Australia 5011, Australia

(Continued from previous page)

Conclusion: In patients undergoing ERCP, the LMA® Gastro™ airway demonstrated a high success rate for ERCP completion. Ventilation was well maintained with minimal intraoperative and postoperative adverse events. This technique may have a role in higher risk groups such as high ASA (American Society of Anesthesiologists) status, or those with potential airway difficulties such as high body mass index and those with known or suspected sleep apnoea.

Keywords: LMA® GASTRO™ airway, Endoscopic retrograde cholangiopancreatography, Airway management, Endoscopy

Core tip

The aim of this retrospective observational analysis was to evaluate the utility of the LMA® Gastro™ Airway as an airway technique for endoscopic retrograde cholangiopancreatography (ERCP) procedures, in order to improve airway control, prevent hypoxia and avoid the need for intubation. Out of 177 ERCP procedures performed during the study period, the LMA® Gastro™ Airway was employed in 64 procedures (36%) on 59 patients. Of these 64 procedures, the LMA® Gastro™ airway demonstrated a high success rate (98%) for ERCP completion, with only one case requiring conversion to an endotracheal tube. Ventilation was well maintained with minimal intraoperative and postoperative adverse events. This technique may have a role in higher risk groups such as high ASA (American Society of Anesthesiologists) status, or those with potential airway difficulties such as high body mass index and those with known or suspected sleep apnoea.

Tran A, Thiruvenkatarajan V. LMA® Gastro™ Airway for endoscopic retrograde cholangiopancreatography: a retrospective observational analysis.

Background

Endoscopic retrograde cholangiopancreatography (ERCP) is a commonly performed intervention in the management of pancreatico-biliary disorders. The patients presenting for this procedure are usually elderly with significant comorbidities, and there has been a steady increase in the demand for these procedures. Moderate to deep sedation is a commonly employed technique for ERCPs, with general anaesthesia utilising an endotracheal intubation being reserved for selected cases. Reported rates of hypoxemia during all endoscopic procedures range from 11 to 50% [1–3], and this may be as high as 60% with ERCP [4]. (Definitions of hypoxia vary between the studies.) Sustained hypoxia is a major risk factor for peri procedural cardiac arrhythmias and myocardial ischaemia [5–7]. Some of the anaesthetic challenges of ERCP are the requirement of a semi-prone position, a shared airway, the semi-urgent nature of some of the presentations, and often being required to perform these procedures in a non-operating room environment.

Various airway techniques have been employed for endoscopic procedures, aiming to avoid hypoxia, and obtain better airway control. These include the standard laryngeal mask airway (LMA), gastro-laryngeal tube (GLT), endoscopy mask, a specialised bite block and nasal positive pressure delivery devices [4, 8–15].

The LMA® Gastro™ Airway (Teleflex® Medical, Ireland), is a new device developed specifically for endoscopy procedures. A recent large, prospective observational trial on 292 patients undergoing gastrointestinal endoscopy has shown a 99% success rate for LMA® Gastro™ Airway insertion [16]. Two small case series (< 14 patients) have described their utility for ERCP procedures [17, 18].

The purpose of this observational study was to evaluate the utility of LMA® Gastro™ Airway as an advanced airway technique for ERCP procedures. The specific data assessed on the use of LMA® Gastro™ Airway were: Success rate of completion of ERCPs through LMA® Gastro™ Airway, ventilation and oxygenation parameters, airway related adverse events, and immediate postoperative complications.

Methods

This study was performed in accordance with the Strengthening the Reporting of Observational Studies in Epidemiology [STROBE] recommendations. This work was considered as a quality assurance study and exempted from ethical approval (Central Adelaide Local Health Network Reference number: Q20190607).

Electronic medical records allowed us to keep track of all patients who underwent ERCP with LMA® Gastro™ Airway from March 2017 to June 2018. This period followed a practice change at our institution when LMA® Gastro™ Airway had just been introduced and some uptake of this device was noted. Selection of the airway technique as moderate to deep sedation assisted by low flow oxygen supplementation, LMA® Gastro™ Airway and general anaesthesia with an endotracheal tube was based on clinical judgement at the discretion of the attending anaesthetist.

Perioperative medical records and discharge summaries were analysed. Data on demographic profile, disease characteristics, preoperative airway assessment, information on airway management including size of LMA® Gastro™ Airway used, any airway manipulations (jaw thrust, chin lift, realigning the device), complications such as bronchospasm, laryngospasm, regurgitation/aspiration of gastric contents, conversion to a different size of the device or endotracheal intubation, data on haemodynamics, oxygenation and ventilation during the procedure and anaesthesia management were collected. Data on the successful completion of ERCP through LMA® Gastro™ Airway and any difficulty encountered by the gastroenterologists were recorded. Any adverse events and adjuvant administered in PACU (post anaesthesia care unit) and reported immediate postoperative pharyngolaryngeal events such as sore throat, dysphagia, dysphonia, and dysarthria were also collected. Hypoxia during ERCP was defined as any documented episode of $SpO_2 < 92\%$ and hypercapnia as an average ETCO2 (end tidal carbon-dioxide) > 45 mmHg. Additionally, the duration of anaesthesia and time spent in PACU were also noted.

An extension to this retrospective study included comparison between three groups: LMA® GASTRO™ vs. sedation with low flow nasal cannula vs. general anaesthesia (GA) with an endotracheal tube (ETT) from March 2017 to June 2018, focusing on demographics, outcomes of hypoxia defined as any incidence of $SpO_2 < 92\%$, requirement of conversion to endotracheal tube, blood pressure control with vasopressors/inotropes/vagolytics, incidence of adverse intraoperative and postoperative (PACU) events and ERCP failure.

The data were entered in an Excel database and analysed using Microsoft Excel 2017.

Results

Of the 177 ERCP procedures performed at our institution from 1st March 2017 to the 25th June 2018, LMA® Gastro™™ Airway was employed in a total of 64 procedures (36%), 85 (48%) procedures were done with sedation and 28 (15%) procedures required general anaesthesia with an endotracheal tube. It is likely that the choice of sedation and general anaesthesia with an endotracheal tube would have been based on the clinical profile. Data on the 64 ERCPs utilising the LMA® Gastro™ Airway intervention is presented. Patient demographics, clinical characteristics and the periprocedural data are presented in Tables 1 and 2. Notably, 4 LMA Gastro ERCP cases had a BMI over 40, maximum being 44. All of them tolerated the procedure well. A majority of the cases in this LMA Gastro group were ASA 3 or 4 (59.7%, 37 out of 62).

In the LMA® Gastro™ group, the patients were anaesthetised by 14 different consultant anaesthetists. The 64 ERCPs were performed by two gastroenterologists. One particular consultant provided anaesthesia for 26 ERCPs, with the second most common provider anaesthetising 6

Table 1 Baseline patient clinical characteristics. Results are presented as number (%) or median (range) for continuous data

Characteristics	n
Demographics	
Male/Female	28/36
Age (years)	66 (27–91)
Average BMI kg/m^2	29 (18–44)
Nature of ERCP	
Elective	37
Emergency	26
ASA Status 1/2/3/4	3/22/32/5
Anticipated difficult airway[a]	
Yes	10
No	49
Unknown	5
Relevant comorbidity	
Suspected/Known OSA	10
Chronic Obstructive Pulmonary Disease	1
Gastro-oesophageal reflux disease	24
Bronchial asthma	2
Active/Ex- regular tobacco smoking	21
Hypertension	13
Congestive Cardiac Failure (CCF)	5
Ischaemic Heart Disease (IHD)	9

'Unknown' pertains to mean there was a lack of documentation for that many patients

ERCPs. The 2 gastroenterologists contributed 43 (66%) and 21 (33%) cases each.

Out of the 64 ERCPs reviewed, LMA® Gastro™ Airway was used as the primary airway device in 63, and in one instance it was used as a rescue airway intervention for a failed sedation technique. Of the 64 procedures, ERCP was successfully completed with LMA® Gastro™ Airway in 63 (98%) instances, with only one requiring conversion to an endotracheal tube. This instance followed difficulty in negotiating the endoscope through LMA® Gastro™ Airway. There were no documented instances of chin lift, jaw thrust, head and neck manipulations, repositioning the airway, or changing the size of the device. No episodes of hypoxia or hypercapnia were documented. Adverse intraoperative events were recognised in 2 cases. One patient had minimal blood stained secretions in the oral cavity that resolved with suctioning; and the other patient had mild laryngospasm which resolved on its own within a few minutes. Two patients were noted to have adverse events in PACU. Laryngospasm resolving within a few minutes was noted in one, whilst another patient developed significant abdominal pain treated with a proton-pump inhibitor and an anti-emetic. No major airway interventions were noted in PACU.

Table 2 ERCP Procedural characteristics. Total $n = 64$. Results are presented as number or mean (range) for continuous data

Procedural characteristics	n
ERCP Position[a]	
Lateral	42
Semi prone	11
Supine	1
LMA® GASTRO™ Airway Size[b]	
3/4/5	20/36/3
Anaesthetic agents and adjuvants	
Propofol infusion + Fentanyl	24
Propofol/Alfentanil infusion	39
Muscle relaxant use	1
Hyoscine butyl bromide	12
Vasopressor use	15
Patient Parameters	
Pre-procedural heart rate	76 (48–115)
Lowest heart rate during ERCP	72 (45–115)
Highest heart rate during ERCP	88 (55–144)
Pre-procedural SpO$_2$	97 (94–100)
Lowest SpO$_2$ during ERCP	98 (92–100)
Highest SpO$_2$ during ERCP	99 (95–100)
Lowest EtCO$_2$ during ERCP	41 (31–55)
Highest EtCO$_2$ during ERCP	44 (33–60)
Lowest BIS value	41 (31–55)
Highest BIS value	44 (33–60)
Mean Duration of Anaesthesia (in minutes)	57 (30–115)
PACU lowest SpO$_2$	97 (92–100)
PACU medications	
Nebulisation	32
Opioid analgesia	11
Anti-emetic usage	10
Time spent in PACU (minutes)	56 (9–225)

a- data available in 54 procedures
b- size not mentioned in 3, one conversion to endotracheal tube

Comparative data between sedation with low flow Nasal Cannula vs. LMA® Gastro™ Airway vs. Intubation ERCP cases

The distribution of cases between these three airway approaches represented "selected" populations according to anaesthesiologist discretion taking into account the level of patient complexity, risk of aspiration and desaturation, haemodynamic stability, surgical position, user experience and last but not least, patient preference.

Table 3 demonstrates the selectivity of these populations well. None of the patients in the LMA® Gastro™ group and GA with ETT group experienced intraoperative

hypoxia. In the sedation group, one case experienced intraoperative hypoxia.

It is unsurprising a majority of ETT cases were emergency procedures needing rapid sequence intubation, maximum BMI was the greatest at 77 and significantly higher in terms of mean duration of anaesthesia time. A large number of the 28 ETT cases were flagged as extremely high risk procedures pre-operatively relating to aspiration risk and airway difficulty, poor oxygen saturation below 95% at baseline, likely extended duration of anaesthesia and prolonged ventilation or airway protection postoperatively, and one case of severe autism requiring general anaesthesia. Of note in PACU, 1 ETT case had a minor desaturation to 94%, another case required ongoing intubation and extended inotropic support, and another demonstrated multiple apnoeic episodes in recovery.

Conversely, a majority of the low flow cannula cases were ASA 1–2, tolerated well with minimal cases needing blood pressure alterations and showed the lowest mean duration of anaesthesia. Similar to LMA® Gastro™, one case required airway conversion to ETT in the context of apnoeic episodes on nasal specs. There was a high incidence of intraoperative events in the sedation group in the setting of bronchospasm, epistaxis, desaturation and bradycardia HR 30–35. Like the LMA® Gastro™ group, the 2 ERCP failures in the low flow cannula group also related to procedural difficulty.

Discussion

Our observations confirm that the LMA® Gastro™ Airway can be successfully employed as a primary airway technique for ERCP procedures in some patients. The case that required conversion from LMA® Gastro™ Airway to an endotracheal tube was due to the gastroenterologist being unable to get the gastroscope pass through the endoscope channel of LMA® Gastro™ Airway. This happened to be the third case since this technique was adapted by us, possibly noting a difficulty during the early learning phase.

Gastroenterologists are unlikely to adopt the LMA® Gastro™ Airway for complex endoscopic intervention, unless success is demonstrated in both emergency and elective cases across a diverse group of patients. Our study group had a mixture of low and high risk cases giving rise to anaesthetic as well as procedural challenges. Although formal interviews were not conducted, it was evident that the gastroenterologists were satisfied with the device.

A medicolegal analysis of malpractice claims involving anesthesiologists, has shown that gastrointestinal endoscopy procedures comprised the largest portion of "outside operating suite" malpractice claims in the US [19]. Of these, ERCPs represented the maximum likelihood of

Table 3 Comparative Data between all 177 ERCP cases. Results are presented as number (%) or median (range) for continuous data

Characteristics	LMA® Gastro™	Low Flow Nasal cannula	Endotracheal Tube (ETT)
Number of cases (n)	64	85	28
Demographics			
Male/Female	28/36	37/48	10/18
Age (years)	66 (27–91)	73 (19–95)	78 (18–94)
Average BMI kg/m^2	29 (18–44)	28 (17–44)	29 (18–77)
Nature of ERCP			
Elective	37	52	8
Emergency	26	35	20
ASA Status 1/2/3/4/5	3/22/32/5/0	17/26/35/7/0	1/3/18/6/1
Airway conversion to ETT	1	1	N/A
Intraoperative $SpO_2 < 92\%$	0	1	0
Lowest Intraoperative SpO_2	98 (92–100)	98 (89–100)	98 (92–100)
Vasopressor/inotropic/vagolytic use			
Atropine	1	0	1
Adrenaline	1	0	1
Ephedrine	0	1	1
Metaraminol	15	5	9
Noradrenaline	1	0	3
Mean Duration of Anaesthesia (in minutes)	57	51	71
ERCP Failure	6	2	0
Adverse Intraoperative Events[a]	2	3	0
Adverse 24 h Postoperative (PACU) events[b]	2	1	3

a – adverse events included broncho/laryngospasm, epistaxis, blood-stained secretions and bradycardia
b – adverse events included episodes of laryngospasm, apnoea, minor desaturation ($SpO_2 < 94\%$) and abdominal pain

payout (91% compared with 37.5% of colonoscopies, and 25% of combined endoscopy/colonoscopy procedures). In view of the morbidity associated with endoscopy interventions, there has been an increased interest recently looking for devices that can facilitate better oxygenation and airway control. General anaesthesia with an endotracheal tube may be considered in some ways a "safe option" in the prone position in terms of having a secured airway and a lower ERCP failure rate [20], and there may be a reduction in some complication rates. However, intubation has drawbacks. In addition to the well-known problems associated with insertion of the tube, managing a paralysed intubated patient in a semi-prone position creates additional challenges. Furthermore, there may be a prolongation of anaesthetic time due to the use of muscle relaxants.

Although the first generation laryngeal mask airways have been used successfully for ERCPs, the absence of a dedicated endoscopic channel and a gastric aspiration port are obvious limitations [8–10]. The GLT is perhaps the most widely evaluated supraglottic airway device for endoscopies [4, 11, 12]. Some of the drawbacks of this device include: loss of position of the device after

insertion when turning the patient prone, only one size, and it can be used only in patients over 155 cm tall. The design is unfamiliar to many anaesthetists, and its method of use is slightly different compared to other commonly used supraglottic airways.

Difficulty introducing duodenoscope into the oesophagus may be encountered due to a tight/thick crico-pharyngeus muscle and/or significant anterior cervical osteophytes. This can occur especially in the elderly population, either during sedation without airway adjuncts or even under general anaesthesia with endotracheal intubation. Our gastroenterologists believe that this problem was not encountered during their intubation with the duodenoscope in our patient population. It may be attributed to the alignment of the endoscope channel running parallel to the airway lumen communicating distally with the upper oesophageal sphincter where the endoscope exits. This may indicate another potential benefit using LMA® Gastro™ Airway.

The LMA® Gastro™ Airway has dedicated independent channels for both endoscope insertion (16 mm internal diameter) and oxygenation. It also has an integrated bite block, and an adjustable holder to secure the device (Fig. 1). Some of the advantages that are claimed are:

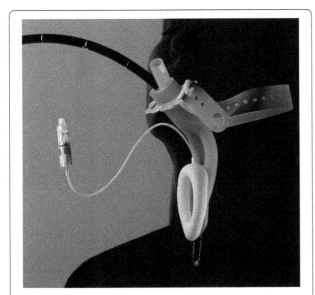

Fig. 1 LMA® Gastro™ Airway. Image obtained and adapted from Teleflex, Australia with written permission

improved airway patency, it is available in three sizes: 3, 4 and 5; familiarity and ease of insertion - it is designed similar to other LMAs; insertion possible in lateral or prone position; dynamic flexibility allowing the device to remain in place with head movement; inbuilt cuff pressure monitoring pilot balloon; and allows endoscopes up to 14 mm in size as compared to 13.8 mm with GLT [11].

The 2 cases associated with intraoperative airway events were semi-urgent presentations. Self-resolving mild oropharyngeal bleeding was noted in one. The other emergency case involved an anticipated difficult airway in the context of Down's syndrome and central obesity (BMI 31). Mild laryngospasm was noted both intraoperatively and in PACU. This was attributed to induction using a volatile anaesthetic in view of needle phobia and the patient's airway characteristics. Although the procedure was completed with LMA® Gastro™ Airway, the anaesthetic team recommended the use of an endotracheal tube for similar procedures in the future.

Interestingly, LMA® Gastro™ Airway was employed as a rescue technique in one instance where there the SpO_2 dropped to 86% despite the application of dual nasopharyngeal airways and high flow nasal oxygen therapy. The ease of insertion in a non-supine position and enabling successful ventilation is one of the notable features of this device. Although not formally evaluated, our patients positioned themselves in either lateral or prone position prior to preoxygenation. Unlike other endoscopy airway adjuvants, the LMA® Gastro™ Airway offers reliable CO_2 monitoring. Oxygenation and ventilation were well maintained in all our cases.

ERCP outcome failure was reported in 5 occasions. While failed cannulation of the bile duct was attributed

in three, inability to cannulate ampulla and failed stone extraction were identified in one each. It was evident that the failures were not due to the choice of LMA® Gastro™ Airway as an airway intervention. There is an argument that the endoscope manipulation may be difficult from the extra-oral end of a supraglottic device, rather than a more proximal oropharyngeal entry offered by other airway adjuvants [21]. Nonetheless, the success rate shown in our study diminishes this concern.

It is a contentious issue as to whether non-anaesthesia providers could deliver deep sedation with propofol for a complex intervention such as ERCP [22]. The practice varies globally. Monitoring brain function, some sources have shown that 96% of patients consenting for moderate to deep sedation for endoscopy (including ERCP) were indeed under deep general anaesthesia [23]. The sedation practice (deep propofol based) for endoscopy in Australia is predominantly driven by anaesthetists [24]. A survey on ERCP practice across gastroenterology practitioners in Australia performing the intervention revealed that 97.5% of their cases were assisted by anaesthetists [25]. It has been shown that higher ASA category (> 3) patients would require frequent airway manoeuvres during sedation for ERCPs (1). Hence, LMA Gastro may have a greater role in complex interventions attempted on sicker patients.

Limitations and strengths

This observational study did not allow for formal matched comparison of efficacy and safety with other conventional airway options such as moderate to deep sedation or other airway adjuvants including GA with ETT and sedation with low flow nasal cannula. Choice of the airway technique was at the discretion of the anaesthetist. Hence, confounding factors in patient selection for the LMA® Gastro™ Airway technique could be a further limitation. Nonetheless, this is the largest series analysing LMA® Gastro™ Airway for ERCPs. Over half of the LMA® Gastro™ cases (37 out of 64) were of the ASA III and IV category and difficult airway was anticipated in 10, implying that the technique was employed on a complex case mix. Future large trials are warranted to analyse the safety and cost implications of this technique in specific population groups such as those with known or suspected sleep apnoea, high BMI and diverse co-morbidities.

Conclusion

In patients undergoing ERCP, the LMA® Gastro™ Airway demonstrated a high success rate of ERCP completion. Ventilation was well maintained with minimal intraoperative and postoperative adverse events. While the technique may not be required for low risk patients, it may have a role in high risk groups such as high ASA (American Society of Anesthesiologists) status, high body mass index and those with known or suspected sleep apnoea.

Abbreviations
ASA: American society of anesthesiologists; BIS: Bispectral index; BMI: Body mass index; CO_2: Carbon dioxide; ERCP: Endoscopic retrograde cholangiopancreatography; $ETCO_2$: End tidal carbon dioxide; ETT: Endotracheal tube; GA: General anaesthesia; GLT: Gastro-laryngeal tube; LMA: Laryngeal mask airway; OSA: Obstructive sleep apnoea; PACU: Post anaesthesia care unit; SpO_2: Peripheral oxygen saturation; STROBE: Strengthening the Reporting of Observational Studies in Epidemiology

Acknowledgements
Not applicable.

Authors' contributions
AT and VT contributed equally to the work and should be regarded as co-first authors. VT designed the study, formatted the data collection, performed some of the cases, analysed the data and wrote the paper; AT collected and analysed the data, drafted the manuscript; MW and AR managed the cases and reviewed the manuscript; JC and RVW revised the manuscript; ET and ML performed the procedures and reviewed the manuscript; GL critically reviewed the manuscript and study design. The author(s) read and approved the final manuscript.

Author details
[1]Discipline of Medicine, The University of Adelaide, Adelaide, South Australia, Australia. [2]Department of Anaesthesia, The Queen Elizabeth Hospital, 28 Woodville Rd, Adelaide, South Australia 5011, Australia. [3]Department of Gastroenterology, The Queen Elizabeth Hospital, 28 Woodville Rd, Adelaide, South Australia, Australia. [4]Discipline of Acute Care Medicine, The University of Adelaide, Adelaide, South Australia, Australia.

References
1. Coté GA, Hovis RM, Ansstas MA, Waldbaum L, Azar RR, Early DS, Edmundowicz SA, Mullady DK, Jonnalagadda SS. Incidence of sedation-related complications with propofol use during advanced endoscopic procedures. Clin Gastroenterol Hepatol. 2000;8(2):137–42.
2. Qadeer MA, Rocio Lopez A, Dumot JA, Vargo JJ. Risk factors for hypoxemia during ambulatory gastrointestinal endoscopy in ASA I-II patients. Dig Dis Sci. 2009;54(5):1035–40.
3. De Paulo GA, Martins FP, Macedo EP, Gonçalves ME, Mourão CA, Ferrari AP. Sedation in gastrointestinal endoscopy: a prospective study comparing non anesthesiologist-administered propofol and monitored anesthesia care. Endosc Int Open. 2015;3(1):E7–E13.
4. Daskaya H, Uysal H, Çiftçi T, Baysal B, Idin K, Karaaslan K. Use of the gastro-laryngeal tube in endoscopic retrograde cholangiopancreatography cases under sedation/analgesia. Turk J Gastroenterol. 2016;27(3):246–51.
5. Bell GD, Bown S, Morden A, Coady T, Logan RF. Prevention of hypoxaemia during upper-gastrointestinal endoscopy by means of oxygen via nasal cannulae. Lancet. 1987;1:1022–4.
6. Holm C, Christensen M, Rasmussen V, Schulze S, Rosenberg J. Hypoxaemia and myocardial ischaemia during colono- scopy. Scand J Gastroenterol. 1998;33:769–72.
7. Johnston SD, McKenna A, Tham TC. Silent myocardial ischaemia during endoscopic retrograde cholangiopancrea-tography. Endoscopy. 2003;35: 1039–42.
8. Gajraj NM. Use of the laryngeal mask airway during oesophago-gastro-duodenoscopy. Anaesthesia. 1996;51(10):991.
9. Orfei P, Ferri F, Panella I, Meloncelli S, Patrizio AP, Pinto G. The use of laryngeal mask airway in esophagogastroduodenoscopy in children. Minerva Anestesiol. 2002;68(3):77–82.
10. Osborn IP, Cohen J, Soper RJ, Roth LA. Laryngeal mask airway--a novel method of airway protection during ERCP: comparison with endotracheal intubation. Gastrointest Endosc. 2002;56(1):122–8.
11. Gaitini LA, Lavi A, Stermer E, Charco Mora P, Pott LM, Vaida SJ. Gastro-laryngeal tube for endoscopic retrograde cholangiopancreatography: a preliminary report. Anaesthesia. 2010;65:1114–8.
12. Fabbri C, Luigiano C, Cennamo V, Polifemo AM, Maimone A, Jovine E, D'Imperio N, Zanello M. The gastro-laryngeal tube for interventional endoscopic biliopancreatic procedures in anesthetized patients. Endoscopy. 2012;44(11):1051–4.
13. Cai G, Huang Z, Zou T, He M, Wang S, Huang P, Yu B. Clinical application of a novel endoscopic mask: a randomized controlled trial in aged patients undergoing painless gastroscopy. Int J Med Sci. 2017;14(2):167–72.
14. Goudra BG, Chandramouli M, Singh PM, Sandur V. Goudra ventilating bite block to reduce hypoxemia during endoscopic retrograde cholangiopancreatography. Saudi J Anaesth. 2014;8(2):299–301.
15. Dimou F, Huynh S, Dakin G, Pomp A, Turnbull Z, Samuels JD, Afaneh C. Nasal positive pressure with the SuperNO(2)VA™ device decreases sedation-related hypoxemia during pre-bariatric surgery EGD. Surg Endosc. 2019. https://doi.org/10.1007/s00464-019-06721-1 [Epub ahead of print].
16. Terblanche NCS, Middleton C, Choi-Lundberg DL, Skinner M. Efficacy of a new dual channel laryngeal mask airway, the LMA®gastro™ airway, for upper gastrointestinal endoscopy: a prospective observational study. Br J Anaesth. 2018;120(2):353–60.
17. Skinner MW, Galloway PS, McGlone DJ, Middleton C. Use of the LMA® gastro™ airway, a novel dual channel laryngeal mask airway, for endoscopic retrograde cholangiopancreatography: a report of two cases. Anaesth Intensive Care. 2018;46(6):632.
18. Aiello L, Corso RM, Bellantonio D, Maitan S. LMA Gastro Airway® Cuff Pilot for endoscopic retrograde cholangiopancreatography (ERCP): a preliminary experience. Minerva Anestesiol. 2019. https://doi.org/10.23736/S0375-9393. 19.13509-2.
19. Stone AB, Brovman EY, Greenberg P, Urman RD. A medicolegal analysis of malpractice claims involving anesthesiologists in the gastrointestinal endoscopy suite (2007-2016). J Clin Anesth. 2018;24(48):15–20.
20. Raymondos K, Panning B, Bachem I, Manns MP, Piepenbrock S, Meier PN. Evaluation of endoscopic retrograde Cholangiopancreatography under conscious sedation and general anesthesia. Endoscopy. 2002;34(9):721–6.
21. Goudra B, Singh PM. Reply to "state of the art in airway management during GI endoscopy: the missing pieces". Dig Dis Sci. 2017;62(5):1388–9.
22. Garewal D, Waikar P. Propofol Sedation for ERCP Procedures: A Dilemna? Observations from an Anesthesia Perspective. Diagn Ther Endosc. 2012; 2012:639190, 5 pages. https://doi.org/10.1155/2012/639190.
23. Goudra B, Singh PM. ERCP: the unresolved question of endotracheal intubation. Dig Dis Sci. 2014;59(3):513–9.
24. Leslie K, Sgroi J. Sedation for gastrointestinal endoscopy in Australia: what is the same and what is different? Curr Opin Anaesthesiol. 2018;31(4):481–5.
25. Ting AYS, Croagh D, Alexander S, Devonshire D, Swan MP. The current practice of ERCP in Australia: 2014 survey. Gastroenterol Hepatol. 2014; 29(Suppl 2):46–67.

22

Outcomes in video laryngoscopy studies from 2007 to 2017: Systematic review and analysis of primary and secondary endpoints for a core set of outcomes in video laryngoscopy research

Jochen Hinkelbein[1*†] , Ivan Iovino[1,2†], Edoardo De Robertis[2,4] and Peter Kranke[3]

Abstract

Background: Airway management is crucial and, probably, even the most important key competence in anaesthesiology, which directly influences patient safety and outcome. However, high-quality research is rarely published and studies usually have different primary or secondary endpoints which impedes clear unbiased comparisons between studies. The aim of the present study was to gather and analyse primary and secondary endpoints in video laryngoscopy studies being published over the last ten years and to create a core set of uniform or homogeneous outcomes (COS).

Methods: Retrospective analysis. Data were identified by using MEDLINE® database and the terms "video laryngoscopy" and "video laryngoscope" limited to the years 2007 to 2017. A total of 3351 studies were identified by the applied search strategy in PubMed. Papers were screened by two anaesthesiologists independently to identify study endpoints. The DELPHI method was used for consensus finding.

Results: In the 372 studies analysed and included, 49 different outcome categories/columns were reported. The items "time to intubation" (65.86%), "laryngeal view grade" (44.89%), "successful intubation rate" (36.56%), "number of intubation attempts" (23.39%), "complications" (21.24%), and "successful first-pass intubation rate" (19.09%) were reported most frequently. A total of 19 specific parameters is recommended.

Conclusions: In recent video laryngoscopy studies, many different and inhomogeneous parameters were used as outcome descriptors/endpoints. Based on these findings, we recommend that 19 specific parameters (e.g., "time to intubation" (inserting the laryngoscope to first ventilation), "laryngeal view grade" (C&L and POGO), "successful intubation rate", etc.) should be used in coming research to facilitate future comparisons of video laryngoscopy studies.

Keywords: Airway management, Video laryngoscopy, Primary outcome, Primary endpoint

* Correspondence: Jochen.hinkelbein@uk-koeln.de
†Jochen Hinkelbein and Ivan Iovino contributed equally to this work.
[1]Department of Anaesthesiology and Intensive Care Medicine, University Hospital of Cologne, Kerpener Str. 62, 50937 Köln, Germany

Background

Airway management is at least one crucial but probably even the most important key competence in anaesthesiology, which directly influences the safety and outcome of anaesthetised patients [1, 2]. Fortunately, anaesthesia-specific mortality has been significantly decreasing over the last decades and is now estimated to be approximately 1 per 100,000 cases [3–5]. Airway-related problems were reported to cause approximately 40% of anaesthesia-related deaths [6].

Mortality rate is approximately 5.6 per million general anaesthetics or one per 180,000 patients anaesthetised [7]. Taking these numbers into account, it is not surprising that airway management is a major research focus and each year thousands of studies are published analysing many specific problems during airway management [1]. Several specific patient groups have even a higher risk of problems [2].

Endotracheal intubation by using video laryngoscopy has significantly increased over the last decade in both pre- and in-hospital airway management [8]. Today, it is considered standard for difficult airway management and specific emergencies. It is even questioned whether it should be the first choice method.

However, high-quality research is rarely published [1] and studies usually have different primary or secondary endpoints, which impedes high quality comparisons between studies and hampers the possibility to draw meaningful conclusions to significantly and systematically improve safety and quality of clinical care. Different definitions and an inconsistent outcome reporting in studies which investigate comparable clinical problems will, therefore, limit results of research [9–11].

Insufficient attention has been paid on the choice of outcomes used for clinical trials in recent years [12]. To describe and analyse the same intubation performance, some studies use different "time" definitions and intervals (e.g., time to intubation, time to visualize glottis, time to place the endotracheal tube, etc.) and others use anatomical parameters (e.g., Cormack & Lehane grade [13], POGO score [14], etc.). Hence, no standard has been established to facilitate comparisons of results among different studies.

Consensus and consistency when using appropriate outcome measures in clinical trials should enhance the interpretation of research [9]. So far, no conclusive analysis of primary and secondary endpoints being used in studies has been published.

The aim of the present study was to gather and analyse primary and secondary endpoints in video laryngoscopy studies published over the last ten years, i.e., during 2007 to 2017. This data is used to create a basis for development of a core set of outcomes items to be used to facilitate comparisons in future trials. Besides parameters found in published literature, the list would be amended by parameters considered essential in airway management studies.

Methods

Systematic PubMed search

Data gathering was performed using MEDLINE® database (http://www.ncbi.nlm.nih.gov/pubmed). To identify relevant literature, the search terms "video laryngoscopy" and "video laryngoscope" were used.

A total of 3351 studies were identified by the applied search strategy in PubMed (Fig. 1). First, a filter restricting the time period of the search (10 years range; going from 22/June/2007 to 22/June/2017) was applied. The PubMed® article categories selected were "Clinical Study", "Clinical Trial", "Comparative Study", "Controlled Clinical Trial", "Evaluation Studies", "Multicenter Study", "Observational Study" and "Randomized Controlled Trial". The final raw dataset consisted of 582 papers (the number of results is referred to a search made on 11/July/2017).

The complete list of items, including whole article names, authors and PubMed® URLs as well as the table of the results sorted by year was downloaded directly

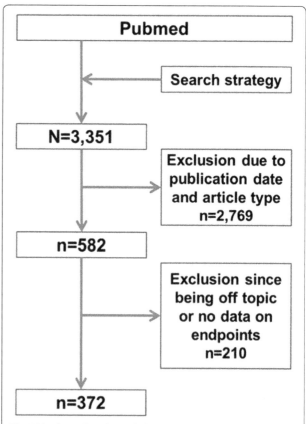

Fig. 1 Numbers of studies included and excluded for analysis. A total of $N = 211$ studies provided data on primary and secondary endpoints and were included for analysis

from PubMed® in a CSV format. Manuscripts presenting scientific data on video laryngoscopy as well as outcome parameters were included for analysis. If outcome parameters were not presented, the specific manuscript was excluded for analysis.

Data analysis

Papers were screened manually by two anaesthesiologists to identify study endpoints. For each study, "primary outcome"/"primary endpoint" or "secondary outcome"/ "secondary endpoint" were collected if clearly stated in the abstract and/or in the full text (when available in the University of Naples Federico II or University of Cologne digital libraries).

If a study did not contain parameters described as "primary outcome/endpoint" or "secondary outcome/ endpoint", alternative measurements were included in the analysis. Alternatively, the "aim/goal/objective/target/purpose/null hypothesis" information was used from the abstract. Also, all studies evaluating directly a video laryngoscopy system or evaluating how the effectiveness of these laryngoscopes could be improved by other ancillary devices (e.g., different endotracheal tubes, stylets, gum elastic boogie, etc.) were included.

A chess-like table was hence built with the several outcomes as columns and 372 papers included as rows (Fig. 2). Outcomes from different studies, having different names but concerning the same variable were fused in a single column (e.g., "dental compression" and "number of audible dental click sounds"). Outcomes concerning a group of variables, slightly different among the studies but mostly overlapping were fused, as well.

Data processing

The number of row-column matches for each column/ category was reported in a different table and the ratio between it and the total number of included articles was calculated. Derived from the percentages of each parameter, a suggestion was provided of which parameters should be reported in future video laryngoscopy studies to facilitate study comparisons.

Generation of recommendations

The chosen outcomes outcomes need to be relevant to both health care providers and healthcare users on one hand, and also to those involved in making decisions and choices about health care, on the other hand [12]. However, a lack of attention for using clinical outcomes in studies has led to avoidable losses in both the production and reporting of research. Moreover, the outcomes which have been included in studies have not always been those being most important or relevant for patients [15]. To develop a consensus between the authors

concerning use of different parameters, the Delphi system was used [16, 17].

To develop relevant recommendations for video laryngoscopy studies, the four-step Core Outcome Set (COS) process was used. First, the scope was defined, followed by checking if a set exists as a second step. Third, a procedure for the development of the COS was defined and last, it was defined what specific parameters should be measured in future studies [12].

In a COS framework, the method is used for achieving convergence of opinion from experts on the importance of different outcomes in sequential questionnaires (or rounds) sent either by post or electronically [12]. In the present study, all authors ($n = 4$) participated in the process. Three rounds were planned. The answers for each of the outcomes were summarised and fed back anonymously until a consensus was reached with at least 75%. After considering the views of others before re-rating each item, participants were able to change their initial responses based on the feedback from the previous rounds. Direct communication concerning the specific parameters was not possible. Therefore, the feedback provides a mechanism for reconciling different opinions of participants and is essential to achieving a consensus [12]. In terms of the overall validity for the final consensus, this approach has significant advantages as compared to round-table discussions [18].

Results

Number of studies

A total of 3351 studies were identified by the applied search strategy in PubMed (Fig. 1). Using the filters for date and article type, a reduction of 2769 papers was obtained. The final raw dataset consisted of 582 papers. During the detailed analysis, 210 papers were excluded because they were considered off topic or belonged to an article type different from the ones chosen during the search filters setting (e.g. meta-analysis, review, etc.). Of the $n = 210$ articles excluded, $n = 169$ (80.48% of 210) were off the topic, $n = 23$ (10.95% of 210) did not evaluate directly a video laryngoscopy system or the effectiveness of the association with ancillary devices, $n = 13$ (6.19% of 210) belonged to a category of articles not included in the search strategy and $n = 5$ (2.38% of 210) did not provide an endpoint.

After exclusion of not relevant papers, $N = 372$ were considered eligible for final analysis (Fig. 1).

Analysis

The analysis of each item, excluding the off topic articles or the not chosen article types, led to a table consisting of 49 outcome categories depicted horizontally and 372 publications depicted vertically (Fig. 2). The ratio between the number of row-column matches for each

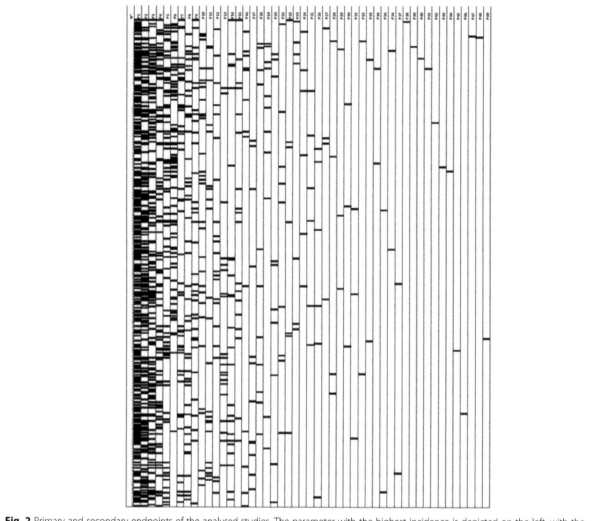

Fig. 2 Primary and secondary endpoints of the analysed studies. The parameter with the highest incidence is depicted on the left, with the lowest incidence on the right. This figure shows graphically how often parameters were used in the studies analysed. On the x-axis (columns): from P1 to P49 the different parameters analysed (for their definitions see Table 1). On the y-axis (lines): the specific studies (i.e., *n* = 372). For the percentages of each specific parameters see Table 1

outcome category (numerator) and the total number of included articles (denominator) was calculated (the total number of outcome categories was not chosen as denominator since it could be more susceptible to subjective evaluation).

Among the total of 49 collected parameters, the items *"time to intubation"* (65.86%), *"laryngeal view grade"* (44.89%), *"successful intubation rate"* (36.56%), *"number of intubation attempts"* (23.39%), *"complications"* (21.24%), *"successful first-pass intubation rate"* (19.09%) were reported most frequently in the investigated studies (Table 1). Furthermore, these items were grouped in eight parameter categories (Table 1). Besides these six parameters having the highest reporting rate in previous studies and found with the purely computationally approach, additional six parameters were identified in the Delphi round. The Delphi method was used

to find a consensus what parameters are of utmost importance. These parameters were *"time to glottis view"*, *"ease of intubation (subjective scoring)"*, *"dental compression AND number of audible dental click sounds"*, *"optimization manoeuvres AND use of airway back-up devices"*, *"haemodynamic parameters"*, and *"lowest arterial oxygen saturation"*. We, therefore, highlighted top twelve of outcomes with a prevalence range from 65.86 to 3.49% (Table 1).

Besides the previously reported parameters, seven additional parameters were identified with the Delphi round which should be reported in future airway management studies. Two of them should be reported in any study (patient and manikin study): "exact specifications of the device used" and "exact specifications of the patient group". For patient studies, the parameters "death",

Table 1 Frequency of primary and secondary endpoints used in the studies analysed. The "**Top-12**" of the used parameters are indicated in Bold-type

	Outcome Name	Number of Matches	Percent Age	Column Name
Time	**Time to intubation (#1)**	245	65,86%	P1
	Time to glottic view (#2)	36	9,68%	P9
	Endotracheal tube insertion time	18	4,84%	P15
	TTSI[a] on the first attempt	11	2,96%	P18
	Time to ventilation after intubation	7	1,88%	P23
	Total time of chest compression interruption during ETI[b]	2	0,54%	P36
	Time to supraglottic ventilation	1	0,27%	P38
Views	**Laryngeal view grade (CL AND/OR POGO[c]) (#3)**	167	44,89%	P2
Intubation Success	**Successful intubation rate (#4)**	136	36,56%	P3
	Successful first-pass intubation rate (#5)	71	19,09%	P6
	Ease of intubation (subjective scoring)[d] (#6)	48	12,90%	P7
	Failed intubation	23	6,18%	P11
	Intubation difficulty score (IDS)	22	5,91%	P12
	Factors complicating intubation[e]	11	2,96%	P19
	Proportion of difficult intubation	6	1,61%	P25
	DoubleLumenTube position	4	1,08%	P27
	Successful tracheal intubation rate after failed initial laryngoscopy	4	1,08%	P28
	Intubation success rate in patients with difficult laryngoscopy predictors	2	0,54%	P32
	Reason for intubation failure	2	0,54%	P34
	Likelihood of successful intubation	2	0,54%	P35
	Adequate ETT[f] position	1	0,27%	P41
	Factors that affect FPS[g] in trauma patients	1	0,27%	P43
	Proportion of successful to failed intubations	1	0,27%	P45
	Accuracy of correct unilateral placement	1	0,27%	P48
Number of attempts	**Number of intubation attempts (#7)**	87	23,39%	P4
	Number of tube insertions	2	0,54%	P37
Complications	**Complications[h] (#8)**	79	21,24%	P5
	Dental compression AND number of audible dental click sounds (#9)	24	6,45%	P14
	Severity of force applied to the upper airway	10	2,69%	P20
	Variables reflecting morbidity[i]	6	1,61%	P24
	Potential laryngeal trauma	2	0,54%	P33
	Gagging severity score at the time of best laryngeal visualization	1	0,27%	P44
Device use & operator variables	**Optimization manoeuvres AND use of airway back-up devices (#10)**	48	12,90%	P8
	Device difficult score	20	5,38%	P13
	Device preference	9	2,42%	P21
	Overall participant satisfaction	7	1,88%	P22
	Ergonomics[j]	3	0,81%	P29
	Postural analysis	3	0,81%	P30
	Learning process	3	0,81%	P31
	Reasons for using methods other than McGrath MAC video laryngoscope	1	0,27%	P39

Table 1 Frequency of primary and secondary endpoints used in the studies analysed. The "**Top-12**" of the used parameters are indicated in Bold-type *(Continued)*

	Outcome Name	Number of Matches	Percent Age	Column Name
	Practitioner experience	1	0,27%	P49
Monitoring	**Haemodynamic parameters (#11)**	30	8,06%	P10
	Lowest arterial oxygen saturation (#12)	13	3,49%	P16
	Cervical vertebral angle	12	3,23%	P17
	SpO2 immediately after removing the blade from the patient	1	0,27%	P40
	Bispectral index score	1	0,27%	P46
	Intraocular pressure	1	0,27%	P47
Other	Airway grade[k]	6	1,61%	P26
	Intubation conditions[l]	1	0,27%	P42

[a]Time to successful intubation
[b]Endotracheal intubation
[c]Cormack-Lehane score and Percentage Of Glottic Opening
[d]mainly a visual analogue scale score ranging from 1 (extremely easy) to 10 (extremely difficult) with several exceptions (e.g, numerical rating scale 1 = the easiest, 5 = the most difficult)
[e]e.g., visualization difficulty related to obscured view from fogging, secretions or blood in the airway; difficulty passing the tracheal tube past the vocal cords; inappropriate endotracheal tube size for the patient; or difficulty controlling the direction of the tracheal tube using the video display
[f]Endotracheal tube
[g]First-pass success
[h]Pre- and post-intubation correlated complictions (e.g., upper airway morbidity, swallowing difficulties or any dental injuries)
[i]e.g., in-hospital mortality, hospital length of stay, duration of mechanical ventilation, duration of ICU stay, ICU mortality, etc
[j]Biomechanical performance of doctors during the ETI (e.g., assessed using surface electromyography and inertial measurement units)
[k]Airway assessment predictors: Mallampati test, mouth opening, thyromental distance, cervical flexion-extension, and neck thickness, snoring, retrognathia, and other types of anomalies also considered as predictors of a difficult airway
[l]Ease of Laryngoscopy, Vocal cords position, Reaction to insertion of the tracheal tube and cuff inflation (Diaphragmatic movement/coughing), direction of the ETT by the forceps and advancement of the ETT by the forceps

Table 2 Suggested minimal endpoints categories for reporting of video laryngoscopy studies. The table consists of 12 previously reported parameters plus seven additional parameters from the Delphi round

Category	Parameter
Time	Time to intubation (taking the laryngoscope to first successful ventilation)
	Time to glottis view
View	Laryngeal view grade (CL and POGO)
Intubation Success	Successful first-pass intubation rate
	Successful intubation rate
	Ease of intubation
Number	Number of intubation attempts
Complications	Any clinically significant complication
	Dental compression AND number of audible dental click sounds
Devices	Optimization manoeuvres AND use of airway back-up devices
Monitoring	Hemodynamic parameters
Patients	Lowest arterial oxygen saturation
Additional parameters (not covered by the studies before)	
Patients outcome	Death
	ICU admission
	hospital length of stay
	dysphagia
	reduced quality of life
Patients	Exact specifications of the patient group
Devices	Exact specifications of the device used

"ICU admission", "hospital length of stay", "dysphagia", and "reduced quality of life" should be reported.

Discussion

Over the last ten years, many different and inhomogeneous parameters were used as outcome descriptors/endpoints in video laryngoscopy studies. In order to facilitate literature comparison, taking into account the percentages of items used in previous publications, we suggest that 12 parameters should be used in future video laryngoscopy studies (Table 2). Additionally, the seven patient outcome parameters not covered by the studies before should be reported.

Video laryngoscopy studies

The use of video laryngoscopes has increased significantly over the last years for many pre-hospital and in-hospital situations [8]. Today, it is considered standard for difficult airway management and emergencies and in some scenarios, it is even questioned whether it should be the method of first choice. Whereas the use of video laryngoscopes was limited to elective intubations several years ago, especially for the anticipated difficult airway, these devices are used today for a broad spectrum of indications such as anticipated difficult airway, teaching and training, or even awake intubation. As airway management is a topic of major research interest and each year thousands of studies that probe all the specific problems of airway management are published, even video laryngoscopy studies seek to compare a variety of devices, arbitrarily chosen, in a variety of settings [1].

In previous studies, a great multiplicity of measured outcomes has been subsequently used to assess the capability of video laryngoscopes to modify the intubation-related variables in comparison to the classic direct laryngoscopy or within the category itself among the different devices [1]. However, none of these outcomes are present in all studies and in some cases, like in the case of the "time to intubation" endpoint, divergence subsists in single definitions, making it difficult to perform any comparison between the outcomes obtained in different articles.

The aim of the study was, therefore, to provide a simple analysis of a part of the scientific literature on the subject so that it would be possible to derive a common basis on which future studies on video laryngoscopy can be built. Standardizing end points will also improve the validity of pooled analysis of clinical trials and assist those wanting to replicate trial results [9]. Besides parameters found in published literature, the list will be amended by parameters considered essential in airway management studies.

Set of parameters

Nearly no analysed study used the same set of parameters to quantify and qualify performance of intubation with a video laryngoscope. Furthermore, parameters used were often non-specific and not clearly defined, since so far, in this field of research, no consolidated minimal reporting dataset does exist, unlike in other fields of research [19].

This problem of definition, even for the meaning of single parameters, is well represented in the main category for prevalence, i.e. "time to intubation". Three examples could well reflect the high variability in definition since time to intubation is described as (i) the time "from the passage of the tip of the laryngoscope past the patient's teeth to the appearance of CO_2 on the capnograph trace" [20], (ii) the moment "from when the facemask was removed from the patient's face to when end-tidal CO_2 of at least 20 mm Hg was measured on

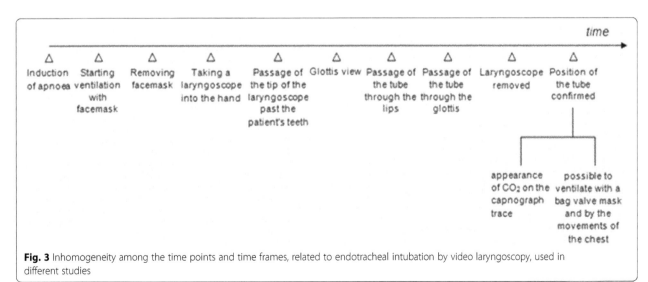

Fig. 3 Inhomogeneity among the time points and time frames, related to endotracheal intubation by video laryngoscopy, used in different studies

the end-tidal gas monitor" [21] or when (iii) "the time started to run when a participant took a laryngoscope into his/her hand and stopped when the appropriate position of the tube was confirmed by the fact that it was possible to ventilate with a bag valve mask and by the movements of the chest and the abdomen" (Fig. 3) [22].

Future aspects

From a practical point of view, several (comparable) parameters and categories should be reported in video laryngoscopy studies (Table 2). This may enhance comparisons of parameters in different studies and facilitate meta-analyses as well as systematic reviews in video laryngoscopy studies. Comparison between studies is made easier, and other investigators will have a stronger foundation on which to design future, definitive trials [9].

Usefulness of parameters

In the present study, a set of 19 parameters for video laryngoscopy studies is presented. Whereas using many different parameters increases the possibility to compare different studies, it may be cumbersome to record all parameters. Besides this practical point, the feasibility of the different parameters itself varies significantly. Whereas, e.g., "time to intubation", "number of intubation attempts", or "successful intubation rate" are quite clear and objective to assess, "ease of intubation" and "hemodynamic parameters monitoring" are far more subjective. Moreover, "laryngeal view grade" or "optimization manoeuvres AND use of airway back-up devices" clearly depends on the skills and expertise as well as anatomical factors of the patient. Therefore, it is essential to keep these limitations also in mind when comparing different studies.

Limitations

The present study provides an overview on parameters used in previous studies on video laryngoscopy. However, it has also some limitations which should be mentioned. From a total of $n = 582$ articles identified, only $n = 372$ (63.92%) could be included due to the inclusion–/exclusion-criteria mentioned.

Furthermore, not all studies provided information in which model video laryngoscopes were investigated: if in patients, in cadavers, or in manikins. Finally, the definition of video laryngoscopes is quite broad and comparison between the different available models is often impossible.

Conclusions

Over the years, many different and inhomogeneous parameters were used as outcome endpoints in video laryngoscopy studies.

The final result of parameters offers several recommendations for choosing the endpoints, but the fact remains that these endpoints are still numerous, which reflects the literature on this field although we have demanded a consensus limiting the endpoints to those most relevant and most clinical based from the experts. The example of "Laryngeal view grade" (CL and/or POGO), even if widely cited, does not reflect the difficulty of intubation in video laryngoscopy [23].

The standardization of endpoints for video laryngoscopy studies could lead to improve the effectiveness of literature review and facilitate a more valid comparison between outcomes obtained in future studies.

Abbreviations

C&L: Cormack&Lehane classification; COS: Core set of uniform or homogeneous outcomes; POGO: Portion of glottis opening score

Acknowledgements

None.

Authors' contributions

JH and PK conceived the study. JH and II performed data analysis and wrote the manuscript. PK and EDR significantly improved the manuscript and checked analyses. All authors read and approved the final manuscript.

Author details

[1]Department of Anaesthesiology and Intensive Care Medicine, University Hospital of Cologne, Kerpener Str. 62, 50937 Köln, Germany. [2]Department of Neurosciences, Reproductive and Odontostomatological Sciences, University of Naples "Federico II", Via S. Pansini, 5, 80131 Naples, Italy. [3]Department of Anaesthesia and Critical Care, University Hospital of Wuerzburg, Wuerzburg, Germany. [4]Department of Surgical and Biomedical Sciences, University of Perugia, Perugia, Italy.

References

1. Hinkelbein J, Greif R, Diemunsch P, Kranke P. Publication and innovation in airway management: quality not quantity! Eur J Anaesthesiol. 2017;34:408–10.
2. Hinkelbein J. Big data for big patients: gaining insight into risks for tracheal intubation in obese patients. Brit J Anaesth. 2018;120:901–3.
3. Bainbridge D, Martin J, Arango M, Cheng D. Perioperative and anaesthetic-related mortality in developed and developing countries: a systematic review and meta-analysis. Lancet. 2012;380:1075–81.
4. Staender S, Mahajan R. Anesthesia and patient safety: have we reached our limits? Curr Opin Anaesthesiol. 2011;24:349–53.
5. WACKER J, STAENDER S. The role of the anesthesiologist in perioperative patient safety. Curr Opin Anaesthesiol. 2014;27:649–56.
6. Schiff J, Welker A, Fohr B, et al. Major incidents and complications in otherwise healthy patients undergoing elective procedures: results based on 1.37 million anaesthetic procedures. Br J Anaesth. 2014;113:109–21.
7. Cook T, Woodall N, Frerk C, Project FNA. Major complications of airway management in the UK: results of the fourth National Audit Project of the Royal College of Anaesthetists and the difficult airway society. Part 1: anaesthesia. Br J Anaesth. 2011;106:617–31.
8. Hinkelbein J, Cirillo F, Robertis ED, Spelten O. Update on videolaryngoscopy: Most relevant publuacations of the last 12 months. Trends Anaesth Crit Care. 2015;5:188–94.
9. Myles P, Grocott M, Boney O, Moonesinghe S, Group C-S. Standardizing end points in perioperative trials: towards a core and extended outcome set. Brit J Anaesth. 2016;116:586–9.
10. Koroshetz W. A core set of trial outcomes for every medical discipline? Brit Med J. 2015;350:h85.

11. Ioannidis J. Howto make more published research true. PLoS Med. 2014;11:e1001747.
12. Williamson P, Altman D, Bagley H, et al. The COMET handbook: version 1.0. Trials. 2017;18:280.
13. Cormack R, Lehane J. Difficult tracheal intubation in obstetrics. Anaesthesia. 1984;39:1105–11.
14. Levitan R, Ochroch E, Kush S, Shofer F, Hollander J. Assessment of airway visualization: validation of the percentage of glottic opening (POGO) scale. Acad Emerg Med. 1998;5:919–23.
15. Chalmers I, Glasziou P. Avoidable waste in the production and reporting of research evidence. Lancet. 2009;374:86–9.
16. RANDCORPORATION. Delphi Method. [cited 2016 April]. Available from: http://www.rand.org/topics/delphi-method.html. Accessed 30 May 2017.
17. Diamond I, Grant R, Feldman B, et al. Defining consensus: a systematic review recommends methodologic criteria for reporting of Delphi studies. J Clin Epidemiol. 2014;67:401–9.
18. Sinha I, Smyth R, Williamson P. Using the Delphi technique to determine which outcomes to measure in clinical trials: recommendations for the future based on a systematic review of existing studies. PLoS Med. 2011;8:e1000393.
19. Apfel C, Roewer N, Korttila K. How to study postoperative nausea and vomiting. Acta Anaesthesiol Scand. 2002;46:921–8.
20. Foulds L, Mcguire B, Shippey B. A randomised cross-over trial comparing the McGrath(®) series 5 videolaryngoscope with the Macintosh laryngoscope in patients with cervical spine immobilisation. Anaesthesia. 2016;71:437–42.
21. Turkstra T, Cusano F, Fridfinnson J, Batohi P, Rachinsky M. Early endotracheal tube insertion with the GlideScope: a randomized controlled trial. Anesth Analg. 2016;122:753–7.
22. Szarpak Ł, Czyżewski Ł, Truszewski Z, Kurowski A. Pentax airway scope AWS-S200 video laryngoscope for child tracheal intubation in a manikin study with 3 airway scenarios. Am J Emerg Med. 2015;33:1171–4.
23. Gu Y, Robert J, Kovacs G, et al. A deliberately restricted laryngeal view with the GlideScope® video laryngoscope is associated with faster and easier tracheal intubation when compared with a full glottic view: a randomized clinical trial. Can J Anaesth. 2016;63:928–37.

23

Videolaryngoscopy versus direct laryngoscopy for double-lumen endotracheal tube intubation in thoracic surgery

Joachim Risse[1,2]* ⓘ, Ann-Kristin Schubert[2], Thomas Wiesmann[2], Ansgar Huelshoff[2], David Stay[2], Michael Zentgraf[2], Andreas Kirschbaum[3], Hinnerk Wulf[2], Carsten Feldmann[2] and Karl Matteo Meggiolaro[2]

Abstract

Background: Double-lumen tube (DLT) intubation is necessary for thoracic surgery and other operations with the need for lung separation. However, DLT insertion is complex and might result in airway trauma. A new videolaryngoscopy (GVL) with a thin blade might improve the intubation time and reduce complexity as well as iatrogenic airway complications compared to conventional direct laryngoscopy (DL) for DLT intubation.

Methods: A randomised, controlled trial was conducted in 70 patients undergoing elective thoracic surgery using DLT for lung separation. Primary endpoint was time to successful intubation. The secondary endpoints of this study were number of intubation attempts, the assessment of difficulty, any complications during DLT intubation and the incidence of objective trauma of the oropharynx and supraglottic space and intubation-related subjective symptoms.

Results: 65 patients were included (DL group [$n = 31$], GVL group [$n = 34$]). Median intubation time (25th–75th percentiles) in GVL group was 93 s (63–160) versus 74 (58–94) in DL group [$p = 0.044$]. GVL resulted in significantly improved visualisation of the larynx (Cormack and Lehane grade of 1 in GVL group was 97% vs. 74% in DL Group [$p = 0.008$]). Endoscopic examinations revealed significant differences in GVL group compared to DL group showing less red-blooded vocal cord [$p = 0.004$], vocal cord haematoma [$p = 0.022$] and vocal cord haemorrhage [$p = 0.002$]. No significant differences regarding the postoperative subjective symptoms of airway were found.

Conclusions: Videolaryngoscopy using the GlideScope®-Titanium shortly prolongs DLT intubation duration compared to direct laryngoscopy but improves the view. Objective intubation trauma but not subjective complaints are reduced.

Keywords: Double-lumen endotracheal tube, Intubation, Thoracic Anaesthesia, Videolaryngoscopy

* Correspondence: joachim.risse@uk-essen.de
[1]Center of Emergency Medicine, University Hospital Essen, Hufelandstrasse 55, 45122 Essen, Germany
[2]Department of Anesthesiology and Intensive Care Medicine, Philipps-University Marburg, Baldingerstraße, 35033 Marburg, Germany

Background

Lung separation is performed for thoracic surgery using several technical solutions (e.g. double-lumen intubation, bronchus blocker) [1]. Using a double-lumen tube (DLT) has become the most commonly used technique worldwide despite a more challenging procedure of tube placement compared to a conventional endotracheal tube [2–4]. Additionally, the rate of upper airway trauma including damage of pharynx, larynx (particularly vocal cords) and trachea during the insertion of a DLT using a conventional laryngoscope is significantly higher [3–5]. Reasons for this are a larger outer diameter and enhanced stiffness of a DLT compared to a conventional endotracheal tube. Due to the characteristics of a DLT, the direct view of the laryngeal structures are impaired during a DLT insertion [6, 7]. On the other hand, videolaryngoscopy has become standard for difficult airway management using conventional endotracheal tubes. In DLT intubation, the literature shows conflicting results of the benefits of videolaryngoscopy compared to direct laryngoscopy, especially intubation time as well as iatrogenic injuries [8, 9]. Moreover, meta-analysis data with moderate to low quality evidence exist, showing a higher success rate at first attempt, a higher incidence of malpositioned double-lumen tube and a lower incidence of oral, mucosal or dental injuries with videolaryngoscopy for DLT intubation [10].

A improved videolaryngoscopy device (GlideScope®-Titanium, Fa. Verathon Inc.) with a thinner blade (thickness of single use blade is 3 mm in size 3 and 2.7 mm in size 4) was introduced recently. A thinner blade design might be useful during the intubation of patients with a small oral cavity or limited mouth opening capacity. Presumably this device offers more space in the pharynx during DLT intubation than other videolaryngoscopy blades used in previous clinical trials which might result in improved intubation than previous videolaryngoscopy devices.

For GlideScope®-Titanium, single use blades are 3 mm (Size 3) and 2.7 mm (Size 4). Thus, we hypothesized that this improved GlideScope® videolaryngoscopy system (GVL) might result in a shortened intubation time and better visualisation of the anatomic structures compared with a conventional laryngoscopy approach for double lumen tube insertion. This could reduce the rate of airway trauma parameters and improve patient-centered outcome parameters.

Methods

This prospective trial adheres to CONSORT guidelines and was approved by the local ethics committee (Ethikkommission Marburg, AZ115/16; 14.09.2016; retrospectively registered at the German Clinical Trials registry DRKS [DRKS00020978]). After written informed consent, adult patients scheduled for elective thoracic surgery requiring general anaesthesia with the need of a DLT for lung separation with American Society of Anesthesiologists physical status I–IV were enrolled from 23.02.2017 until 18.09.2017. Exclusion criteria were patient age < 18 years, non-elective surgery, pregnancy, scheduled rapid-sequence induction, contraindication for DLT insertion; contraindication to one-lung ventilation as well as abnormal physical status of the Cervical spine (e.g., after C-spine trauma, Bechterew's disease).

Primary and secondary endpoints

The primary endpoint of this study was duration of endobronchial DLT intubation (s). The intubation time was defined as: blade passes mouth opening → positive capnography (visualisation of 3 expirations in the capnography). The secondary endpoints of this study were number of intubation attempts, the assessment of difficulty and any complications during DLT intubation and the incidence of intubation-related injuries in both groups. Therefore, we performed two consecutive transnasal flexible endoscopic examinations (at the end of surgery and on the first postoperative day) of the oropharynx, of the supraglottic space and of the vocal cords, a follow-up survey by questionnaire and a dental examination to detect dental trauma.

Sample size calculation

Sample size calculation was based on a previous study [7], which reported a mean (SD) time of 46 [11] s for DLT placement with videolaryngoscopy. Based on these results an a priori power analysis was performed for primary endpoint given a beta value of 0.80 and a significance level alpha of 0.05. We calculated a minimum required sample size of 29 patients per group to detect a 20% difference in the time taken for DLT intubation using non-parametric testing. Effect size of the duration of intubation used calculating sample size was 0.8 according to Cohen's D. As a drop-out rate of 20% was assumed, the sample size was increased to 35 patients per group. Power analysis was performed using G*Power 3.1.9.6 for Mac OS X [11, 12].

Randomization and allocation concealment

After written informed consent 70 patients were randomized via envelope method. Allocation concealment was achieved using sealed opaque envelopes. Performance blinding was not possible in this study design. Patients and postoperative outcome assessors (anesthetists, ENT specialist, dentist) were unaware of the randomization results. Statistical analysis was performed blinded to study allocation.

Patients were pre-medicated with 3.75–7.5 mg oral midazolam 45 min before surgery. On arrival in the induction area, all participants were blinded, randomly assigned to either direct laryngoscopy (DL) or videolaryngoscopy using the GlideScope® Titanium device (GVL, GlideScope; Verathon Inc., Bothell, WA) by sealed envelope randomisation. In the OR patients were positioned supine, standard monitoring was applied according to current national guidelines and peripheral intravenous access (IV) established. Patients received pre-oxygenation with 100% oxygen through a mask over 5 min. After pre-oxygenation, anaesthesia was induced with $0.3\,\mu g\,kg^{-1}$ sufentanil and $2\,mg\,kg^{-1}$ propofol intravenously. Thereafter, $0.6\,mg\,kg^{-1}$ rocuronium bromide was applied. The neuromuscular monitoring was performed by a relaxometry Train of Four (TOF). DLT intubation was performed when full relaxation status (TOF 0/4) was reached. Maintenance of general anesthesia was performed as total intravenous anaesthesia (TIVA) according to the local standards using propofol (4–6 $mg\,kg^{-1}\,h^{-1}$) and remifentanil (15–25 $\mu g\,kg^{-1}\,h^{-1}$) adjusted according to the measured anesthetic depth using Bispectral Index monitoring (BIS) at a target zone of 40–60.

The size of the DLT (Rüsch Bronchopart; Teleflex Medical GmbH, Dublin, Ireland, 35–41 FR) used was determined for each patient according to the rule of Slinger et al. [13]. Intubation with a DLT was performed using a conventional MacIntosh blade (size 3 or 4) in the DL group or with the hyperangulated GlideScope®-Titanium Single-Use-blade (size 3 or 4) in the GVL group. The original DLT stylet was used for intubation in both groups. It was shaped according to the respective angulation of the blade used (Fig. 1). All intubations were performed by the same three experienced physicians.

Postoperative assessment

The first endoscopic examination was performed at the end of surgery under general anesthesia and before extubation, while the follow-up endoscopic examination was performed the day after surgery under topical anesthesia. Stored endoscopic video clips were postprocessed for anonymisation and blinding. Thereafter, they were evaluated by three independent investigators (2 anaesthesiologists and 1 ENT specialist, investigator-blinded). The video clips of both examinations (postoperative & first postoperative day) were evaluated independently by blinded investigators. The hypopharynx, the vocal cords and the arytenoid cartilage were evaluated on the basis of various criteria. The different criteria were scored from according to the degree of injury (0 = not assessable, 1 = without pathological findings, 2 = minor injuries, 3 = severe injuries). The results were averaged for further analysis. Second, a physician of oral and maxillofacial surgery (investigator blinded) performed a dental examination after DLT intubation in all study patients, examining the patient for lip and dental trauma. Third, the patients first completed a questionnaire (Validated H&N35 Quality of Life Questionnaire Head and Neck Module and NRS) to express their subjective symptoms (hoarseness, etc.). The H&N Score ranged from 0 to 100. A high score correlated with a high degree of complaints and symptoms [14].

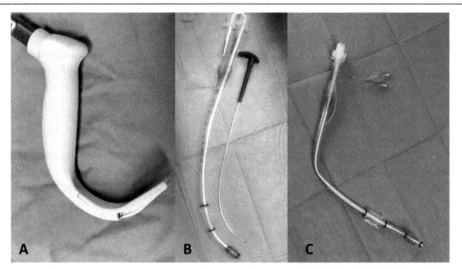

Fig. 1 Comparison DLT used for intubation with GVL or DL. **a** GVL blade used; **b** DLT shaped for GVL; **c**) DLT shaped for DL

Statistical analysis

All values for descriptive statistics and outcome parameters were non normally distributed. All non-normally distributed data were expressed as median and interquartile range (IQR). Dichotomous outcome parameters were expressed as events (percentages). Non-parametric data were analysed using the Mann-Whitney U-test. A $p < 0.05$ was considered being statistically significant. Normally distribution was assessed using Shapiro-Wilk test. Statistical analysis was performed using SPSS (IBM Corp. Released 2016, IBM SPSS Statistics for Windows, Version 24.0, Armonk, NY: IBM Corp.). Data are presented as tables and box-and-whisker diagrams.

Results

Demographics and biometric data

After written informed consent, 70 patients were recruited. Out of 70 patients 65 completed the study and were included in the final intention-to treat analysis (Fig. 2). Four patients in the MacIntosh group (DL) and one patient in the GlideScope® group (GVL) were excluded from the final analysis. In two participants randomised to the DL group, the conventional DLT intubation attempts failed and the experienced examiner changed the method using videolaryngoscopy. Finally intubation with a single endotracheal tube and a bronchial blocker had to be performed in these two cases because of impossible DLT intubation, with both devices. Two

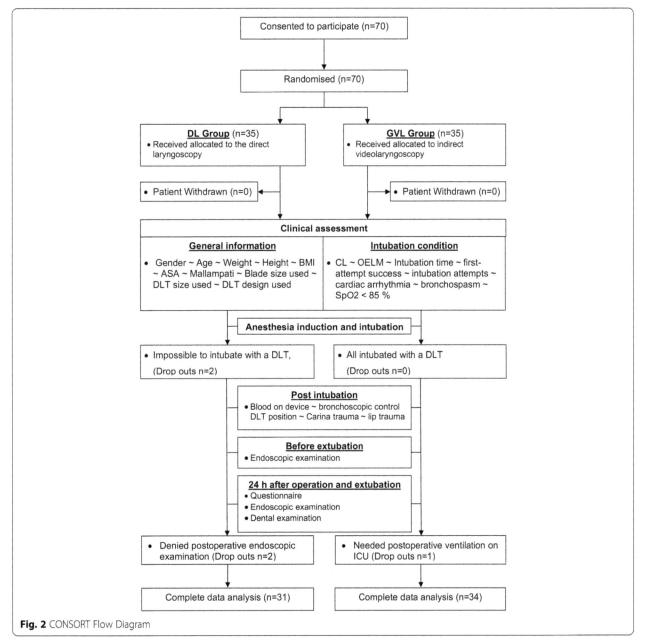

Fig. 2 CONSORT Flow Diagram

participants randomised to DL group refused postoperative nasal endoscopic examination and one participant in GVL group needed long-term postoperative ventilation on the intensive care unit and was lost to follow-up. All five participants were excluded from the final analysis due to relevant study protocol violation as predefined (Fig. 2).

Both groups had no significant differences in biometric data and preoperative airway assessments (Table 1). In almost all cases, a left-sided DLT was used. It was noticeable that all three experienced specialists in thoracic anaesthesia who performed the DLT intubations in the study used smaller blades and tended towards smaller tube sizes in the GVL group. The difference between the two groups was statistically significant [$p < 0.05$] (Table 1).

Primary endpoint

Our primary endpoint duration of the successful completion of DLT intubation was significantly [$p = 0.044$]

longer in the GVL group 93 s (63–160) compared to the DL group 74 (58–94) (see Table 2 and Fig. 3).

Secondary endpoints

Regarding the secondary endpoints our data showed better visualisation of the larynx with GVL. CL grade of 1 was with 97% more frequent in the GVL group. For the CL grade 1–4, a statistically significant difference in our data could be shown between the groups [$p = 0.008$]. In 32% of the patients in GVL group and 45% in the DL group, the OELM manoeuvre was necessary to achieve better conditions for endobronchial intubation [$p > 0.05$] (Table 2).

The first-attempt success did not differ significantly between GVL group (85%) and DL group (90%) [$p > 0.05$]. There was no statistically significant difference between both groups in the frequency of intubation attempts [$p > 0.05$]. None of the participants from DL group included in the analysis required more than three intubation attempts (Table 2).

Table 1 Biometric data and descriptive data of patients enrolled in the study. Data are presented as median (25th–75th percentile) or numbers (percentage), respectively

Parameter	DL (n 31)	GVL (n 34)	Mann Whitney U-test (p-Value)
Gender (male/female)	25/6	25/9	0.50
Age (years)	60 (52–65)	66 (58–75)	0.087
Weight (kg)	83 (75–95)	80 (68–90)	0.207
Height (cm)	178 (172–181)	173 (165–178)	0.038*
Body mass index (kg m^{-2})	25.7 (24.2–30.8)	25.2 (24.1–29.1)	0.604
ASA n (%):			
I	0 (0%)	1 (3%)	0.824
II	10 (32%)	9 (26%)	
III	19 (61%)	24 (71%)	
IV	2 (7%)	0 (0%)	
Mallampati score n (%):			
I	11 (35%)	14 (41%)	0.819
II	16 (52%)	14 (41%)	
> II	4 (13%)	6 (18%)	
Blade size used n (%):			
size 3	1 (3%)	16 (47%)	< 0.001*
size 4	30 (97%)	18 (53%)	
DLT size used n (%):			
35 French	1 (3%)	1 (3%)	0.023*
37 French	6 (19%)	18 (53%)	
39 French	17 (55%)	10 (29%)	
41 French	7 (23%)	5 (15%)	
DLT design used n (%):			
left-sided	31 (100%)	33 (97%)	0.340
right-sided	0 (0%)	1 (3%)	

*Statistically significant

Table 2 DLT intubation data: Assessment of difficulty and complications. Data are presented as median (25th - 75th percentile) or number (percentage)

Parameter	DL (n 31)	GVL (n 34)	Mann Whitney U-test (p-Value)
time to successful intubation (s)	74 (58–94)	93 (63–160)	0.044*
Cormack-Lehane score n (%):			
I°	23 (74%)	33 (97%)	0,008*
II°	7 (23%)	1 (3%)	
III°	1 (3%)	0 (0%)	
IV°	0 (0%)	0 (0%)	
OELM maneuver n (%):			
yes	14 (45%)	11 (32%)	0,293
no	17 (55%)	23 (68%)	
first-attempt success n (%):			
yes	28 (90%)	29 (85%)	0,287
no	3 (10%)	5 (15%)	
DLT intubation attempts n (%):			
1	28 (90%)	29 (85%)	0,497
2	2 (7%)	2 (6%)	
3	1 (3%)	1 (3%)	
> 3	0 (0%)	2 (6%)	
SpO2 < 85% n (%):			
yes	2 (6%)	2 (6%)	0,925
no	29 (94%)	32 (94%)	
Bronchospasm n (%):			
yes	2 (6%)	0 (0%)	0,135
no	29 (94%)	34 (100%)	
Cardiac arrhythmia n (%):			
yes	0 (0%)	0 (0%)	1,000
no	31 (100%)	34 (100%)	
blood on device n (%):			
yes	4 (13%)	3 (9%)	0,599
no	27 (87%)	31 (91%)	
Correct DLT position n (%):			
yes	24 (77%)	18 (53%)	0,041*
no	7 (23%)	16 (47%)	
Carina trauma n (%):			
yes	0 (0%)	1 (3%)	0,340
no	31 (100%)	33 (97%)	
Lip trauma n (%):			
yes	0 (0%)	0 (0%)	1,000
no	31 (100%)	34 (100%)	
Dental trauma n (%):			
yes	0 (0%)	0 (0%)	1,000
no	21 (100%)	26 (100%)	
Enamel fractures n (%):			
yes	0 (0%)	0 (0%)	1,000
no	21 (100%)	26 (100%)	

*Statistically significant

During bronchoscopic control a correct DLT position directly after successful endobronchial intubation was reported in 77% of the CL group and only 53% of the GVL group. The difference observed between the two groups was statistically significant [$p = 0.041$] (Table 2).

There was no other significant difference in terms of direct complications under DLT intubation between the two groups (Table 2). Furthermore, lip and dental trauma, as well as enamel fractures examined by the dental follow-up, were not significantly different in both groups (Table 2).

When analysing the postoperative questionnaires (H&N35 and NRS Score) to record the subjective symptoms after DLT-Intubation, no significant differences were found between both groups [$p > 0.05$] (Tables 3 and 4).

In contrast to the subjective symptoms, endoscopic examinations revealed significant differences in the GVL group compared to the DL group in the objectifiable trauma red-blooded vocal cord [$p = 0.004$], vocal cord haematoma [$p = 0.022$] and vocal cord haemorrhage [$p = 0.002$] (Table 5).

Discussion

We compared the insertion of a double-lumen tube using a conventional MacIntosh laryngoscope with a thin blade videolaryngoscope. Intubation time was significantly prolonged for the videolaryngoscopy group. However, intubation conditions were improved but there were more malpositioned double-lumen tubes in the GVL group.

Despite an objective reduction in 3 of 17 predefined airway trauma parameters evaluated by follow-up endoscopy, patients in both groups showed comparable subjective wellbeing.

Prolonged intubation times for GVL videolaryngoscopy for DLT intubation were shown in previous studies [8, 15, 16]. Prolonged intubation times inevitably have a greater risk of hypoxia and could be harmful to patients with pulmonary comorbidities. In a prior study by Russell et al., anaesthetists found that GVL was more difficult to use than DL blade and DLT intubation took longer. In their study all DLT intubations were performed by less experienced anaesthetists [8], whereas in our study, all DLT intubations were performed by three consultants of anaesthesiology well experienced with DLT intubations in thoracic anaesthesia and GlideScope® videolaryngoscopy.

Contrary, a recent meta-analysis in 2018 by Liu et al., showed no difference in intubation time. The meta-analysis included studies with various videolaryngoscopes like Airtraq, McGrath Series 5, McGrath MAC - not all of these provide hyperacute angled devices [10]. Considering only the four studies using GlideScope® videolaryngoscopy included in the meta-analysis, our results are consistent with three of these four studies [8, 9, 15, 16]. Only Hsu et al. were able to show shorter intubation times with Glidescope videolaryngoscopy for DLT intubation [9]. From a clinical point of view, the intubation time differences between our groups are modest and potentially have no

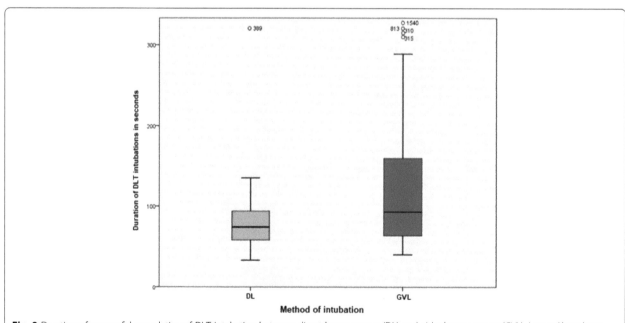

Fig. 3 Duration of successful completion of DLT intubation between direct laryngoscopy (DL) and videolaryngoscopy (GVL). Legend:boxplot x-axis: methods Macintosh-DL (green) and GlideScope-VL (blue), y-axis: Duration of successful DLT intubation in seconds

Table 3 Results of relevant selected parameters from evaluation of the H&N35 Quality of Life Questionnaire Head and Neck Module (H&N Score). Data are presented as median (25th- 75th percentile)

Parameter (H&N Score)	DL (n 31)	GVL (n 34)	Mann Whitney U-test (p-Value)
Sore throat	0 (0–33)	0 (0–0)	0,402
Dysphagia	0 (0–0)	0 (0–33)	0,115
Cough	0 (0–33)	0 (0–33)	0,532
Hoarseness	0 (0–33)	0 (0–33)	0,640
Dry mouth	33 (0–100)	33 (0–67)	0,735
Viscous mucus	0 (0–67)	0 (0–33)	0,628
Paresthesia	0 (0–0)	0 (0–0)	0,340
Language problems	0 (0–0)	0 (0–0)	0,457
Mouth opening problems	0 (0–0)	0 (0–0)	1,000
Toothache	0 (0–0)	0 (0–0)	0,295

impact on morbidity but only demonstrate a more technically challenging situation using GVL instead of DL for DLT insertion.

The first attempt success rate reported here using GVL for DLT intubation was 85%. Our reported failure rate of 15% at the first attempt using GVL is similar to most of the results reported by other groups [8, 17, 18]. We were also unable to show a 100% first pass success rate with GVL, as showed by the group of Hsu et al. [9]. In the study of Hsu et al., all DLT intubations were performed by two experienced anaesthetists, who had both performed over 300 intubations using DLT with GVL. In addition, a external laryngeal manipulation was not required for successful DLT intubations with GVL [9].

The procedural step of advancing the DLT past the vocal cords seems to be the main sticking point for using hyper-angulated videolaryngoscopy [8, 19]. Multiple attempts may prolong the intubation time. Our findings support that DLT tube delivery and advancement into the trachea is the most difficult step in the procedure using videolaryngoscopy with hyper-angulated non-channelled blades for DLT intubations which causes prolonged intubation times for GVL. This assumption is supported by our data. The anaesthetists in our study needed a OELM manoeuvre in 32% of all DLT intubations with GVL and we reported significantly more

malpositions of the DLT (in 47% of cases). Presumably caused by the rotation manoeuvre, which is needed for the advancement into the trachea, there is a higher incidence of main bronchus malposition of the DLT. Caused by the required bending of the DLT-tube for hyper-angulated blades, the tip of the DLT often hits the ventral wall of the trachea when advancing the tube past the vocal cords. Usually, a OELM manoeuvre is first performed to adjust the trachea, positioning it more posterior and more in line. Second, a rotation manoeuvre could be necessary. Such a rotation manoeuvre was described by Bustamante and Hernandez [20, 21]. Rotation manoeuvre more often results in the incorrect position of the DLT. Liu et al. concluded that the use of videolaryngoscopes, especially with a hyper-angulated blade for DLT intubation, complicates the already complicated DLT intubation technique through rotation manoeuvres [10]. Our data support the thesis that these sequential rotation manoeuvres are probably the reason why videolaryngoscopy increases the incidence of mispositioning of DLT. However, further studies are needed in the future to investigate this issue. We could not confirm our hypothesis that a thinner hyper-angulated blade provides better visibility and in consequence more space for a rotation manoeuvre and therefore a lower incidence of sore throat and hoarseness. Hsu et al. were able to show

Table 4 Results of parameters additionally examined with numerical rating scale (NRS). NRS scores 1–3 correspond to mild, scores of 4–6 to moderate and scores ≥7 to severe symptoms. Values are expressed as the number of patients or as the total number in percent

Parameter NRS Score	DL (n 31)	GVL (n 34)	U-test (p-Value)
Sore throat n (mild/ moderate/ severe) (total in %)	7/2/0 (29%)	6/3/1 (29%)	0,430
Dysphagia n (mild/ moderate/ severe) (total in %)	4/3/0 (23%)	6/3/2 (32%)	0,289
Cough n (mild/ moderate/ severe) (total in %)	9/3/1(42%)	10/3/1 (41%)	0,782
Hoarseness n (mild/ moderate/ severe) (total in %)	7/5/0 (39%)	4/6/1 (32%)	0,477

Table 5 Data of the reported intubation related injuries from two transnasal endoscopic examinations; before and 24 h after DLT extubation. All different criteria were scored from 0 to 3. (0 = not assessable, 1 = without pathological findings, 2 = minor injuries, 3 = severe injuries). Values are expressed as median (25th - 75th percentile)

Parameter	DL pre-extubation	GVL pre-extubation	U-Test (*p*-Value)	DL 24 h post-extubation	GVL 24 h post-extubation	U-Test (*p*-Value)
Vocal cord swelling	1,00 (1,00-1,50)	1,00 (1,00-1,50)	0,310	1,33 (1,00-1,67)	1,33 (1,00-1,67)	0,478
Vocal cord redness	1,00 (1,00-1,33)	1,00 (1,00-1,00)	0,402	1,33 (1,00-1,33)	1,00 (1,00-1,00)	0,004*
Vocal cord oedema	1,00 (1,00-1,00)	1,00 (1,00-1,00)	0,309	1,00 (1,00-1,00)	1,00 (1,00-1,00)	0,589
Vocal cord erythema	1,00 (1,00-1,00)	1,00 (1,00-1,00)	1,0	1,00 (1,00-1,00)	1,00 (1,00-1,00)	0,624
Vocal cord hematoma	1,00 (1,00-1,00)	1,00 (1,00-1,00)	0,436	1,33 (1,00-1,67)	1,00 (1,00-1,33)	0,022*
Vocal cord hemorrhage	1,00 (1,00-1,50)	1,00 (1,00-1,00)	0,070	1,33 (1,00-1,33)	1,00 (1,00-1,00)	0,002*
Vocal cord granuloma	1,00 (1,00-1,00)	1,00 (1,00-1,00)	1,0	1,00 (1,00-1,00)	1,00 (1,00-1,00)	0,182
Vocal cord mobility	–	–	–	1,00 (1,00-1,00)	1,00 (1,00-1,00)	0,294
Arytenoid cartilage trauma	1,00 (1,00-1,00)	1,00 (1,00-1,00)	0,517	1,00 (1,00-1,00)	1,00 (1,00-1,00)	0,705
Hypopharynx redness	1,33 (1,00-1,33)	1,00 (1,00-1,42)	0,467	1,33 (1,33-1,67)	1,33 (1,00-1,50)	0,162
Hypopharynx oedema	1,00 (1,00-1,00)	1,00 (1,00-1,33)	0,149	1,00 (1,00-1,33)	1,00 (1,00-1,33)	0,433
Hypopharynx hematoma	1,00 (1,00-1,33)	1,0 (1,00-1,00)	0,323	1,33 (1,00-1,67)	1,00 (1,00-1,33)	0,226
Hypopharynx hemorrhage	1,00 (1,00-1,67)	1,17 (1,00-1,50)	0,895	1,00 (1,00-1,33)	1,00 (1,00-1,33)	0,777
Subglottic redness	–	–	–	1,00 (1,00-1,00)	1,00 (1,00-1,33)	0,072
Subglottic oedema	–	–	–	1,00 (1,00-1,00)	1,00 (1,00-1,00)	0,313
Subglottic hematoma	–	–	–	1,00 (1,00-1,50)	1,00 (1,00-1,67)	0,844
Subglottic hemorrhage	–	–	–	1,00 (1,00-1,00)	1,00 (1,00-1,33)	0,052

*Statistically significant

a lower incidence of sore throat and hoarseness [9]. There are controversial results in the literature. Russell et al. were unable to identify any significant differences in their study [8]. Due to the controversial results in the current literature and our results, the question remains whether the questionnaires used are sensitive enough to record differences in subjective symptoms.

With regard to the incidence of dental trauma, a study by Lee et al. (2011) comparing DL and GVL showed that less force is exerted on the teeth of the upper jaw when using GVL [22, 23]. This is in accordance with the results of the current study situation [8, 16]. Our dental follow up showed no significant differences in DLT intubation-related injuries. However, our study was not powered to detect that the incidence of dental trauma is different.

Limitations

This study was randomised but has some limitations. First, the operators were not blinded to the intubation device used; however, it is difficult to circumvent this problem when evaluating different laryngoscopy devices. Nevertheless, the patient and follow-up endoscopic examinations were anonymised and blinded.

A further limitation of our study is the small number of patients with a supposed difficult airway (Mallampati 3 and 4, 13% in the DL group vs. 17% in the GVL group)

and the low incidence of predicted difficult airways (CL 3 and 4, 3% in the DL group vs. 0% in the GVL group).

In addition, an appropriate rigid stylet for the DLT intubation with the GlideScope, like the GlideRite® Rigid Stylet, which is standardly used for the single lumen tube intubation, was not available at the start of the study [17]. Instead, we used the original rigid GlideRite® stylet for the single-lumen endotracheal tube as a template to shape the inner stylet of the DLT. A technique like the one developed and described by Bussier et al. and Bustamante et al. was not mandatory for our anaesthetists [17, 20].

DLT intubation with the GlideScope®-Titanium might be improved if the users are given some additional training and use the adequate rigid stylet for DLT, which keeps its shape and is better adapted to the hyperangulated blade of the GVL.

There are currently many different videolaryngoscopes with varying designs and quality available on the market. For these reasons, our study results should not be generalised, and further investigation regarding videolaryngoscopy for double lumen tube insertion is needed.

Conclusions

In conclusion, our randomized controlled trial showed faster intubation time using a conventional laryngoscope compared to the GlideScope® Titanium videolaryngoscopy for double-lumen tube insertion. Additionally, malposition of the DLT was more common in the video-laryngoscopy group. Despite some improvements in objectivable airway injuries during the postoperative course, there was no subjective difference for the patient as a relevant patient-centered outcome parameter. Further studies are needed to increase the number of first-pass optimal placement of DLT using videolaryngoscopy.

Abbreviation
BIS: Bispectral Index Monitoring; CL: Cormack and Lehane; DL: Direct Laryngoscopy; DLT: Double Lumen Tube; GVL: GlideScope Videolaryngoscopy; IQR: Interquartile range; NRS: Numeric Rating Scale; OELM: Optimal external laryngeal manipulation; OR: Operating room; SD: Standard deviation; TIVA: Total intravenous anaesthesia; TOF: Train of Four

Authors' contributions
JR, AKS, TW and KM analysed and interpreted the patient data. JR, KM wrote the manuscript. AKS and TW revised the manuscript drafts. AH, MZ and DS helped acquire the data, and revised the manuscript. AK and CF helped revise and edit the manuscript. HW helped design the conceptual design and revised the manuscript. ALL authors read and approved the final manuscript.

Authors' information
Our study adheres to CONSORT guidelines and we included with submission a completed CONSORT checklist and CONSORT Diagram.

Author details
[1]Center of Emergency Medicine, University Hospital Essen, Hufelandstrasse 55, 45122 Essen, Germany. [2]Department of Anesthesiology and Intensive Care Medicine, Philipps-University Marburg, Baldingerstraße, 35033 Marburg, Germany. [3]Visceral, Thoracic and Vascular Surgery Clinic, University Hospital Giessen and Marburg GmbH, Baldingerstraße, 35033 Marburg, Germany.

References
1. Meggiolaro KM, Wulf H, Feldmann C, Wiesmann T, Schubert AK, Risse J. Airway management for lung separation in thoracic surgery : an update. Anaesthesist. 2018;67(8):555–67.
2. Defosse J, Schieren M, Böhmer A, von Dossow V, Loop T, Wappler F, et al. A Germany-wide survey on anaesthesia in thoracic surgery. Anaesthesist. 2016; 65(6):449–57.
3. Zhong T, Wang W, Chen J, Ran L, Story DA. Sore throat or hoarse voice with bronchial blockers or double-lumen tubes for lung isolation: a randomised, prospective trial. Anaesth Intensive Care. 2009;37(3):441–6.
4. Liu H, Jahr JS, Sullivan E, Waters PF. Tracheobronchial rupture after double-lumen endotracheal intubation. J Cardiothorac Vasc Anesth. 2004;18(2):228–33.
5. Chen A, Lai HY, Lin PC, Chen TY, Shyr MH. GlideScope-assisted double-lumen endobronchial tube placement in a patient with an unanticipated difficult airway. J Cardiothorac Vasc Anesth. 2008;22(1):170–2.
6. Purugganan RV, Jackson TA, Heir JS, Wang H, Cata JP. Video laryngoscopy versus direct laryngoscopy for double-lumen endotracheal tube intubation: a retrospective analysis. J Cardiothorac Vasc Anesth. 2012;26(5):845–8.
7. Cohen E. Methods of lung separation. Curr Opin Anaesthesiol. 2002;15(1):69–78. https://doi.org/10.1097/00001503-200202000-00011.
8. Russell T, Slinger P, Roscoe A, McRae K, Van Rensburg A. A randomised controlled trial comparing the GlideScope(®) and the Macintosh laryngoscope for double-lumen endobronchial intubation. Anaesthesia. 2013;68(12):1253–8.
9. Hsu HT, Chou SH, Wu PJ, Tseng KY, Kuo YW, Chou CY, et al. Comparison of the GlideScope® videolaryngoscope and the Macintosh laryngoscope for double-lumen tube intubation. Anaesthesia. 2012; 67(4):411–5.
10. Liu TT, Li L, Wan L, Zhang CH, Yao WL. Videolaryngoscopy vs. Macintosh laryngoscopy for double-lumen tube intubation in thoracic surgery: a systematic review and meta-analysis. Anaesthesia. 2018;73(8):997–1007.
11. Faul F, Erdfelder E, Buchner A, Lang AG. Statistical power analyses using G*power 3.1: tests for correlation and regression analyses. Behav Res Methods. 2009;41(4):1149–60.
12. Faul F, Erdfelder E, Lang AG, Buchner A. G*power 3: a flexible statistical power analysis program for the social, behavioral, and biomedical sciences. Behav Res Methods. 2007;39(2):175–91.
13. Lumb AB, Slinger P. Hypoxic pulmonary vasoconstriction: physiology and anesthetic implications. Anesthesiology. 2015;122(4):932–46.
14. Fayers P, Aaronson N, Bjordal K, Sullivan M. The EORTC QLQ-C30 Scoring Manual. 3rd ed; 2001. p. 1–33.
15. Yi JHY, Luo A. Comparison of GlideScope video-laryngoscope and Macintosh laryngoscope for double-lumen tube intubation. Chinese J Anesthesiol. 2013;33:201–4.
16. Bensghir M, Alaoui H, Azendour H, Drissi M, Elwali A, Meziane M, et al. Faster double-lumen tube intubation with the videolaryngoscope than with a standard laryngoscope. Can J Anaesth. 2010;57(11):980–4.
17. Bussières JS, Martel F, Somma J, Morin S, Gagné N. A customized stylet for GlideScope® insertion of double lumen tubes. Can J Anesth. 2012;59(4):424–5.
18. Lin W, Li H, Liu W, Cao L, Tan H, Zhong Z. A randomised trial comparing the CEL-100 videolaryngoscope (TM) with the Macintosh laryngoscope blade for insertion of double-lumen tubes. Anaesthesia. 2012;67(7):771–6.
19. Yao WL, Zhang CH. Macintosh laryngoscopy for double-lumen tube placement - a reply. Anaesthesia. 2015;70(10):1206–8.
20. Bustamante S, Parra-Sánchez I, Apostolakis J. Sequential rotation to insert a left double-lumen endotracheal tube using the GlideScope. Can J Anaesth. 2010;57(3):282–3.
21. Hernandez AA, Wong DH. Using a Glidescope for intubation with a double lumen endotracheal tube. Can J Anaesth. 2005;52(6):658–9.
22. Verelst PL, van Zundert AA. Use of the EZ-blocker for lung separation. J Clin Anesth. 2013;25(2):161–2.
23. Lee RA, van Zundert AA, Maassen RL, Wieringa PA. Forces applied to the maxillary incisors by video laryngoscopes and the Macintosh laryngoscope. Acta Anaesthesiol Scand. 2012;56(2):224–9.

24

The influence of different patient positions during rapid induction with severe regurgitation on the volume of aspirate and time to intubation: A prospective randomised manikin simulation study

Michael St. Pierre[*] ⓘ, Frederick Krischke, Bjoern Luetcke and Joachim Schmidt

Abstract

Background: Aspiration is a main contributor to morbidity and mortality in anaesthesia. The ideal patient positioning for rapid sequence induction remains controversial. A head-down tilt and full cervical spine extension (Sellick) might prevent aspiration but at the same time compromise airway management. We aimed to determine the influence of three different positions during induction of general anaesthesia on the volume of aspirate and on participants' airway management.

Methods: Eighty-four anaesthetic trainees and consultants participated in a prospective randomised simulation study. Anaesthesia was induced in reverse Trendelenburg position (+ 15°) in a manikin capable of dynamic fluid regurgitation. Participants were randomised to change to Trendelenburg position (− 15°) a) as soon as regurgitation was noticed, b) as soon as 'patient' had been anaesthetised, and c) as soon as 'patient' had been anaesthetised and with full cervical spine extension (Sellick). Primary endpoints were the aspirated volume and the time to intubation. Secondary endpoints were ratings of the laryngoscopic view and the intubation situation (0–100 mm).

Results: Combining head-down tilt with Sellick position significantly reduced aspiration ($p < 0.005$). Median time to intubate was longer in Sellick position (15 s [8–30]) as compared with the head in sniffing position (10 s [8–12.5]; $p < 0.05$). Participants found laryngoscopy more difficult in Sellick position (39.3 ± 27.9 mm) as compared with the sniffing position (23.1 ± 22.1 mm; $p < 0.05$). Both head-down tilt intubation situations were considered equally difficult: 34.8 ± 24.6 mm (Sniffing) vs. 44.2 ± 23.1 mm (Sellick; p = n.s).

Conclusions: In a simulated setting, using a manikin-based simulator capable of fluid regurgitation, a − 15° head-down tilt with Sellick position reduced the amount of aspirated fluid but increased the difficulty in visualising the vocal cords and prolonged the time taken to intubate. Assessing the airway management in the identical position in healthy patients without risk of aspiration might be a promising next step to take.

Keywords: Airway management, Aspiration, Rapid sequence induction, Patient safety, Simulation

* Correspondence: michael.st.pierre@kfa.imed.uni-erlangen.de
Anästhesiologische Klinik, Universitätsklinikum Erlangen, Krankenhaustrasse 12, 91054 Erlangen, Germany

Background

Pulmonary aspiration has been a feared complication of anaesthesia from the very start. Currently, the rapid (sequence) induction and intubation is the technique of choice for securing the airway in patients at risk of aspiration [1–3]. However, despite the technique's widespread use, there is still an ongoing debate concerning the quality of evidence supporting its use [4], as well as the components and execution of the technique [3, 5]. In particular, the ideal positioning of the patient at risk of regurgitation and aspiration at the time of induction remains controversial [3, 6]. Historically, a semi-sitting head-up position with a pillow under the occiput [7], a supine position with a slight head-down tilt [8], as well as the head-down position [9] have been suggested. Despite the controversy surrounding the induction, it is sometimes recommended to tilt the patient head-down as soon as an aspiration event during induction has occurred [6, 10, 11].

A few years ago Takenaka and colleagues used an airway management trainer as a static pulmonary aspiration model to determine the optimal head-down tilt and head–neck positions for preventing aspiration[12]. Their results suggest that only a head-down tilt ($\geq 10°$) combined with a full cervical spine extension (Sellick) was suitable to prevent aspiration within a clinically relevant range. They qualified their statement by pointing out that this position may not be the best for laryngoscopy.

Therefore, we wanted to see how the reported benefits of a head-down tilt combined with a full cervical spine extension might translate into a rapid sequence induction in a dynamic model of a regurgitating patient.

Using the design specifications of the static pulmonary aspiration model [12] as a starting point, we developed a manikin-based simulator capable of dynamic fluid regurgitation. The two primary objectives of this study were to a) determine the influence of three different positions during induction of general anaesthesia on the volume of aspirate in the manikin's trachea and bronchi when severe regurgitation occurred and b) the mean time to intubate in the two final head positionings (Trendelenburg position with sniffing position and Trendelenburg with Sellick extension).

The secondary objectives were participants ratings of the difficulty in visualising the vocal cords and the difficulty of the head-down tilt intubation situation, partly with full cervical spine extension.

1 Methods

Participants

After obtaining approval of the study protocol by the ethics committee of the Friedrich-Alexander University Erlangen-Nuremberg (reference number 002_18 B), we enrolled 84 participants into this prospective, randomised controlled trial (Fig. 1). Participants were part of the annual institutional simulation training programme at the authors' department (February – March 2018). Written informed consent was obtained from all participants prior to the scenario.

Study protocol

We did not perform an a priori sample size calculation, but used a convenience sample, targeting all participating consultants and anaesthetic trainees. Using a web-based tool (https://www.randomizer.org) participants were randomly assigned to one of three groups which were defined by a) the position in which regurgitation occurred and b) the presence or absence of full cervical spine extension (Sellick-position; Fig. 2):

Group 1: Induction of anaesthesia in reverse Trendelenburg position (+ 15°). As soon as regurgitation occurred the mannekin was placed in Trendelenburg position (– 15°) and intubated in Trendelenburg position with the head supported by a pillow ('sniffing position').

Group 2: Induction of anaesthesia in reverse Trendelenburg position (+ 15°). As soon as the 'patient' had been anaesthetised the mannekin was placed in Trendelenburg position (– 15°). Thereupon regurgitation occurred and the simulator was intubated in Trendelenburg position with the head supported by a pillow ('sniffing position').

Group 3: Induction of anaesthesia in reverse Trendelenburg position (+ 15°). As soon as the 'patient' had been anaesthetised the mannekin was placed in Trendelenburg position (– 15°) and full cervical spine extension (Sellick). Thereupon regurgitation occurred and the simulator was intubated in Trendelenburg position without the pillow supporting the head and with full cervical spine extension.

The extent of full cervical spine extension was determined by positioning the manikin's neck over the joint of the headrest and then tilting the headrest until the head started to suspend in mid-air. The two positions for reverse Trendelenburg and Trendelenburg position were defined by the maximum tilt of the mobile OR-table (range: + 15° to – 15°) used at our hospital.

Participants from all three groups were briefed on the scenario with a scripted explanation of the purpose and methodology of the study. The script was supplemented with a final passage in which participants received a detailed description on how to proceed with the allocated induction protocol.

Participants were asked to perform a rapid sequence induction in a patient with a suspected acute mesenteric infarction. Once anaesthesia had been induced, the patient was positioned according to the randomisation protocol. Every participant expected to receive a verbal cue when to start with laryngoscopy and was surprised when the mannekin regurgitated fluid instead.

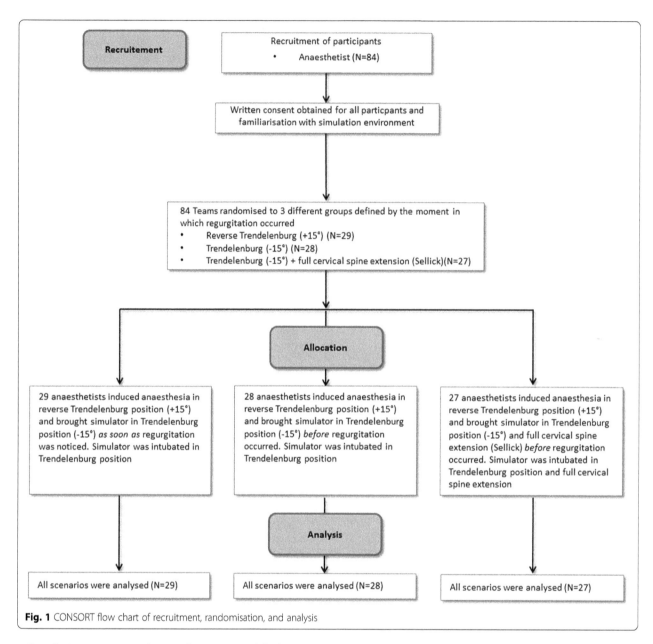

Fig. 1 CONSORT flow chart of recruitment, randomisation, and analysis

Simulations were run by combining a modified resuscitation manikin (HeartSim 4000; Laerdal Norway), capable of regurgitating liquid, with the monitor display of a manikin-based simulator (SimMan; Laerdal Norway).

Haemodynamic and pulmonary variables were programmed as trends into the software of the SimMan. To add time pressure to the induction, the rate of desaturation during apnoea was approximated to a published time course of desaturation in apnoea in obesity [13]. Regurgitation was triggered by the injection of the muscle relaxant with a 20 s delay. Study protocol allowed participants to manage regurgitation at their own discretion (i.e. intubation during regurgitation with simultaneous suctioning or after regurgitation had ceased).

Modification of a resuscitation manikin

The resuscitation manikin was equipped with an airway identical to that used in the static pulmonary aspiration model [12]. The manikin's bronchi were modified with two detachable reservoirs, which collected the regurgitated fluid and allowed quantification of the aspirated volume (Fig. 3). To simulate an elevated intragastric pressure we developed a pneumatic system with a pressure-stable reservoir containing the 'small bowel liquid'. The liquid reservoir was connected to the manikin's esophagus through a large riser 4 cm in diameter. A memory-programmable control controlled two pneumatic 2/3 directional control valves (V1, V2). On activation, both valves allowed pressurised air to flow into the pressure tank, consecutively displacing the fluid towards

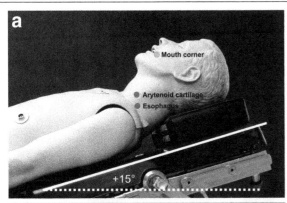
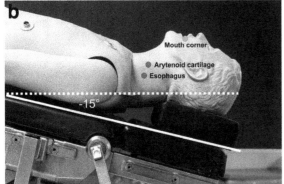
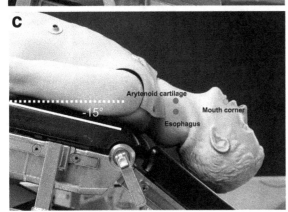

Fig. 2 The three positions of the manikin used: (**a**) Reverse Trendelenburg position (+ 15°) and head supported by a pillow ('sniffing position'); (**b**) Trendelenburg position (− 15°) and 'sniffing position'; (**c**) Trendelenburg position (− 15°) and full cervical spine extension ('Sellick'). Sellick position was determined by tilting the head rest until the head started to suspend in mid-air

the manikin. One second after the liquid had reached the hypopharynx and had created an initial surge, the system turned off V1 and continued to provide a pressure of 25 mbar (18.75 mmHg) via V2, which provided a constant diminished flow of 8 s duration. We chose a pressure of 25 mbar because intra-abdominal measurements have shown that severe abdominal infections can generate pressures up to > 20 mmHg [14]. The dynamics of the regurgitation as well as the amount of regurgitated fluid appeared to be clinically realistic to all four authors. 'Small bowel fluid'

was created by mixing water with soluble coffee powder and vinegar in a predefined ratio. Finally, the dynamics of the regurgitation, as well as the haemodynamic and pulmonary trends, were pretested before study commencement using nonparticipating subjects, and the results served to refine both simulation components.

Data collection

After each scenario the quantity of liquid in the intrapulmonary reservoirs was measured. Multiscreen synchronised video recordings were available for offline evaluation. Time taken to intubate was defined as the interval between the moment the participant started to open the mouth to introduce the laryngoscope and the insertion of the orotracheal tube.

At the end of the simulation session participants were asked to rate the subjective ease in visualising the vocal cords and the difficulty of the head-down tilt intubation situation, partly with full cervical spine extension, on a visual analogue scale (0–100 mm: 0 = not difficult; 100 = worst possible difficulty).

Statistics

Data were analysed with the use of SPSS software version 21.0 (IBM). Homogeneity of variances was assessed with Levene's test. Where variance across groups was equal (e.g. participant characteristics, survey ratings, mean volumes of aspirate) the independent sample t-test and ANOVA were utilised. Where homogeneity of variance was violated (e.g. time to intubation) a non-parametric equivalent of the analysis was conducted (Welch's unequal variance t-test). A Spearman's rank-order correlation was run to determine the relationship between years of clinical experience and the time taken to intubate, the difficulty in visualising the vocal cords, and the difficulty of the intubation situation in all three groups. Visual analogue scale ratings as well as other parametric data are reported as mean ± SD. Non-parametric data are presented as the median and interquartile range [IQR]. All reported p-values are two-sided, and p-values of less than 0.05 were considered statistically significant.

Results

Eighty-four anaesthetic trainees and consultants participated in the study (Fig. 1). There were no group differences in terms of years of clinical experience (Table 1). All participants intubated the manikin after regurgitation had ceased. There was a significant difference in mean volume of aspirate as a function of positioning during induction: 588 ± 157 ml vs. 414 ± 224 ml for group 1 vs. group 2 ($p < 0.005$) and 414 ± 224 ml vs. 43 ± 59 ml for group 2 vs. group 3 ($p < 0.005$) (Fig. 4). In group 3, the bronchial tree and the reservoirs were completely free of aspirated liquid in 48% of cases (13 of 27).

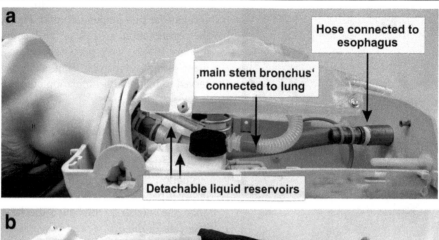
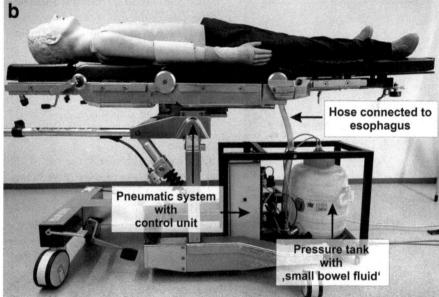

Fig. 3 Setup of the manikin: (**a**) The tracheal tree was modified by inserting two detachable reservoirs that collected the aspirated fluid while leaving ventilation unchanged. The oesophagus was connected to the pneumatically driven liquid reservoir with a flexible hose; (**b**) Operational manikin. During simulations, the pneumatic system and liquid reservoir were hidden from the participants by surgical drapes

Median time to intubate was longer when the head was in full cervical spine extension (group 3) as compared with the head in sniffing position (groups 1 and 2: 15 s [8–30] vs. 10 s [8–12.5]; $p < 0.05$). Intubation times ranged from 7 to 120 s in full cervical spine extension as compared with 5 to 30 s in the sniffing position (Fig. 3).

Participants found it more difficult to visualise the vocal cords during full cervical spine extension (group 3) as compared with the sniffing position (groups 1 + 2: 39.3 ± 27.9 mm vs. 23.1 ± 22.1 mm; $p < 0.05$).

Both head-down tilt intubation situations were considered equally difficult: 34.8 ± 24.6 mm (groups 1 + 2) vs. 44.2 ± 23.1 mm (group 3; p = n.s.).

The years of clinical experience correlated weakly with the time to intubation (groups 1 + 2: $r_s(57) = -0.19$, p = n.s; group 3: $r_s(27) = -0.18$, p = n.s), with participants'

Table 1 Participant characteristics of the randomly assigned groups: sex, age and years of clinical experience

Characteristics	Reverse Trendelenburg (+ 15°) (n = 29)	Trendelenburg (− 15°) (n = 28)	Trendelenburg (− 15°) + Sellick (n = 27)	p
Sex (m:f)	17:12	10:18	16:11	n.s.
Age (yrs)	33.1 (± 6.1)	37.0 (± 7.2)	36.1 (± 8.5)	n.s.
Clinical Experience (yrs)	6.8 (± 5.5)	8.1 (± 6.3)	8.6 (± 7.0)	n.s.

Participants were randomly assigned to one of three groups which were defined by the position in which regurgitation occurred (Reverse Trendelenburg or Trendelenburg) and the presence or absence of full cervical spine extension (Sellick-position) in the Trendelenburg group
Data are mean (±SD)

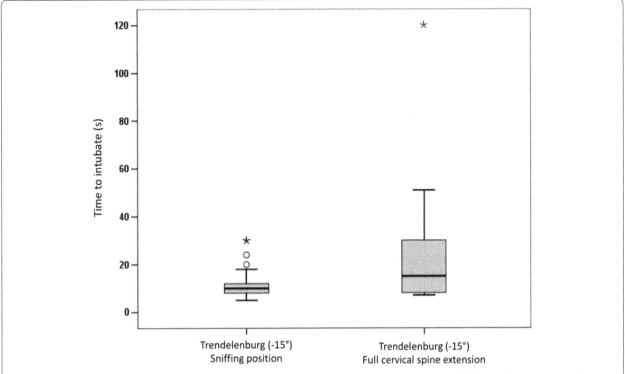

Fig. 4 Intubation position and the resulting time to intubate. Intubation times ranged from 5 to 30 s in the sniffing position as compared to 7 to 120 s in full cervical spine extension

rating of the difficulty in visualising the vocal cords (groups 1 + 2: $r_s(57) = -0.24$, p = n.s; group 3: $r_s(27) = -0.22$, p = n.s), and with their appraisal of the head-down tilt intubation situation (groups 1 + 2: $r_s(57) = -0.32$, p = n.s; group 3: $r_s(27) = -0.37$, p = n.s).

Discussion

Patient positioning during induction and intubation in patients with risk of aspiration has been reviewed in several recent publications [15–18]. Although the head-down (Trendelenburg) position has been advocated together with the supine position and the semi-sitting position as one of three preventive methods against aspiration during rapid induction and intubation for more than 50 years [9] there is little data on the feasibility of such a technique. In a recent German survey reporting on patient positioning in the clinical setting, the majority of respondents preferred a semi-sitting (84%) or a supine (13%) positioning, while the induction in Trendelenburg position was chosen by 3% of anaesthetists [19]. Another German study addressing rapid sequence induction in the prehospital setting found a comparable frequency distribution: the preferred positioning was a semi-sitting (61,8%), followed by a supine (33%), and a moderate Trendelenburg-position (3,5%) [16].

The debate about the ideal position centres around five clinical aspects: the likelihood of passive regurgitation, the

inevitability of aspiration, the quality of preoxygenation, the difficulty in securing the airway, and haemodynamic sequelae.

Proponents of the *head-up position* argue that preoxygenation is improved in both obese and non-obese patients [1, 17, 20]. Furthermore, the likelihood of regurgitation is reduced because the gravitational effect of the head-up position may exceed the intragastric pressure [2, 3]. However, if regurgitation does occur, gastric content may readily enter the trachea and bronchi before the anaesthetist becomes aware of the condition [8].

Supporters of the *supine position* contend that the anaesthetist's familiarity with this position will accelerate endotracheal intubation and that research has provided convincing evidence that regurgitation in the supine position can be prevented as long as cricoid pressure is applied properly [21].

The main advantage of a *head-down position* is that the carina is higher than the larynx and that regurgitated matter does not find its way into the tracheobronchial tree [12]. The main concern with the Trendelenburg position has always been that it may actually predispose to regurgitation by increasing gastric pressure [2, 3]. However, regurgitation may not be a concern in patients without gastrointestinal pathology. In awake, non-fasting volunteers, a change in body position (20° head-up, supine, 20° head-down) had no influence on the frequency of gastroesophageal reflux or on the intragastric-oesophageal barrier pressure [22]. In a similar vein, a 15° head-down tilt caused no change in intragastric and barrier pressure in patients undergoing gynaecologic surgery [23]. In obese patients, too, the intragastric-oesophageal barrier pressure remained positive in the Trendelenburg position (– 20°) [24]. Yet, these results may not apply to patients suffering from acute abdomen conditions with an elevated intra-abdominal pressure. For this reason, we chose acute mesenteric infarction as the clinical scenario for our study. Finally, the Trendelenburg position has been associated with an increased risk of hypoxia, as airway management may be more difficult and may take longer [2, 3]. Furthermore, reduced lung compliance may impair effective mask ventilation should this become necessary [2, 3].

In the attempt to prevent aspiration completely, Takenaka [12] suggested modifying the Trendelenburg position by combining the head-down tilt with the Sellick position [8]. In this position, the height of the corner of the mouth will be lower than the arytenoid cartilage and tracheal bifurcation, allowing liquid to flow freely away from the larynx. However, without the head supported by a pillow the resulting anatomical position has the potential to make tracheal intubation more difficult.

In our study, the mean volume of aspirate was the highest in the group where the manikin was placed head down only after regurgitation had started. These findings corroborate the concern that during passive regurgitation gastric content will enter the trachea and bronchi before the anaesthetist becomes aware of the condition.

The mean volume of aspirate was less in the Trendelenburg position and even less when combined with the Sellick position. In contrast with Takenaka's study, in which a 10° head-down tilt with Sellick position completely prevented aspiration [12], the identical position prevented aspiration in only about half of our cases. We explain this discrepancy by the slightly differing head-down tilt angles in both studies. Whereas Takenaka achieved maximum neck extension by taping the manikin's head to the table, our study protocol required that neck extension stopped as soon as the head started to suspend in mid-air. As a result, the mouth corner might not always have levelled with the arytenoid cartilages.

Placing the simulator in the Trendelenburg position with an elevated head did not delay intubation as compared with the conventional supine position. Our measured intubation times (ranging from 5 to 30 s) are consistent with reported intubation times of 9–30 s when a Macintosh laryngoscope was used in an airway management trainer [25–28].

However, placing the head in full cervical spine extension significantly prolonged mean intubation times from 10 s to 15 s. It is arguable whether this difference of 5 s, despite statistical significance, has any clinical relevance. Clinically relevant, however, is the fact that 5 out of 27 participants (18.5%) needed between 40 and 120 s until the airway was secured (Fig. 3). In a clinical setting with a small bowel ileus, this delay would most certainly put the patient at risk of hypoxia. As presumed, participants found it more difficult to visualise the vocal cords in Sellick position than in the familiar sniffing position. Because no participant had ever intubated a manikin or a patient in Sellick position prior to the study we cannot exclude the possibility that unfamiliarity with the approach rather than genuine anatomical problems account for the difference. Given the learning curve for intubation [29] it is conceivable that repeated intubations in head-down tilt with Sellick position would shorten intubation times and possibly eliminate statistical outliers. If that were the case, the Trendelenburg position with full cervical spine extension would indeed offer protection from aspiration without putting the patient at an unjustifiable risk of hypoxia. In any case, in order to become solid clinical skills, both head-down intubating positions would have to be trained on a regular basis in healthy patients with a normal airway.

Our finding that a head-down tilt (– 15°) with full cervical spine extension can prevent pulmonary aspiration raises the clinical question whether intubation should be delayed until the end of regurgitation with the patient placed in Trendelenburg position or whether the upper airway should be protected as quickly as possible with the aid of a large bore suction. Our preliminary findings in a simulated setting offer the clinician another strategy to consider in case of regurgitation but do not warrant any final conclusion. Rather, this decision will continue to depend upon the anaesthetist's situational assessment of the volume of regurgitating fluid, the dynamic of the regurgitation (continuous oesophageal rise or one short surge) and the effectiveness of the suctioning efforts.

In the setting of aspiration, regurgitation occurs more commonly than active vomiting [30]. General anaesthetic techniques attenuate the protective upper airway reflexes and physiological mechanisms that prevent regurgitation and aspiration. Excessively light depths of anaesthesia in combination with insufficient neuromuscular blockade may evoke gastrointestinal motor responses during laryngoscopy and intubation such as gagging or retching that may increase gastric pressure over and above lower oesophageal sphincter pressure facilitating regurgitation [31]. Allthough study protocol left the choice of drugs at the discretion of the anaesthetist, all participants followed local clinical guidelines for rapid sequence induction which included fentanyl, an induction agent (e.g. etomidate, propofol, or thiopental), and rocuronium as non-depolarizing neuromuscular blocking agent which would have provided an adquate depth of anaesthesia and complete neuromuscular blockade in a real patient.

Limitations of the study

The results of this simulation study indicate that the rapid induction and intubation in Trendelenburg position with full cervical spine extension might be a feasible option to prevent aspiration and to secure the airway in a justifiable time. However, the findings cannot simply be transferred to the clinical context for several reasons.

First, a modified manikin was used as a model for pulmonary aspiration. Although relevant anatomical landmarks in airway trainers (e.g. arytenoid cartilage, oesophagus, mouth corner) may correlate with landmarks in adult human volunteers [12], extrapolating results from the evaluation in manikins to humans is nevertheless problematic. A comparison of computed tomography scans of patients and airway trainers revealed that the pharyngeal airspace of airway trainers is generally wider than a patient's pharyngeal airspace [32]. As a result, the wide pharyngeal airspace could lead to an inappropriately easy airway. This structural feature of airway trainers might explain the fact that we were unable to observe a correlation between years of clinical experience and time to intubate: the airway made intubation easy for both, novices and experts. Furthermore, a single airway trainer does not reflect the multitude of different airways found in real patients. Hence, the time to intubate an airway trainer can be significantly different from the time taken to insert an airway device in humans [33].

Second, the synthetic laryngeal structure of the airway trainer with the vocal chords fixated in abducted position created an unobstructed inflow tract for the regurgitating fluid. Assuming that a volume of 0.8–1 ml/kg (or > 50 ml in a 70 kg adult) with a pH < 3,5 is the critical value for the development of an aspiration pneumonitis [34], this value would have been exceeded in 75% (63/84) of measurements. However, we do not want to draw any clinical conclusions, but rather wish to interpret the trend towards lower mean volumes in the head-down positions as an indication that patients at risk of aspiration may benefit from a Trendelenburg position in combination with a Sellick position. After all, 48% of manikins in group 3 did not experience aspiration and when they did, the mean aspirated volume amounted to 1/15th and 1/10th of groups 1 and 2, respectively.

Third, our model can only simulate the clinical condition of passive aspiration following gravity. However, the clinical consequences of regurgitation may be more severe in a spontaneously breathing patient where respiration efforts may actively suction regurgitated fluid into the airways, hereby increasing the volume of aspirate.

Fourth, the Trendelenburg position may not be an option in obese patients in which an additional head-down position will further reduce functional residual capacity, thereby increasing the risk of hypoxia. Finally, a full cervical spine extension will not be feasible in patients with reduced cervical spine mobility or suspected cervical spine injury.

A major limitation of our study is the fact that it was not conducted as a separate clinical study but instead part of our annual institutional simulation training programme. Time and ressources available only permitted one rapid sequence induction per participant which possibly introduced a bias in each group about experience and technical skills. A cross-over study with the repetition of the three situations for every participant with a randomized order in the groups might have avoided this possibility and would have increased the power of our study.

Normally, manikin studies conclude their discussions by pointing to the fact that further clinical studies are needed to evaluate the results in patients. In an editorial on the uncontrolled proliferation of manikin studies in evaluating new airway equipment, the authors demanded that researchers should follow up their published manikin-based study with a patient-based study, to confirm the initial results [33]. This claim, however, leaves us at an impasse. A follow-up study in patients at risk of aspiration is out of question for ethical reasons. As a result, we do not know how the observed benefits of the two Trendelenburg positions in general, and the Trendelenburg position with full cervical spine extension in particular, could possibly translate into clinical practice, especially as airway management should be informed by the respective national airway management guidelines. Unfortunately, until now few national societies have issued recommendations on rapid-sequence inductions. If they have, they did not usually address the issue of patient positioning [5, 35].

However, assuming that a head-down tilt (– 15°) with full cervical spine extension can prevent pulmonary aspiration, a question worth pursuing might be how the simulated laryngoscopic view and intubation situation correlate with an identical airway management in healthy patients who have no risk of aspiration and who can be effortlessly mask-ventilated.

Conclusions

In a simulated setting, using a manikin-based simulator capable of dynamic fluid regurgitation, the rapid sequence induction in a – 15° head-down tilt with full cervical spine extension reduced the amount of liquid aspirated but increased the difficulty in visualising the vocal cords and prolonged the time taken to intubate. As we cannot confirm the initial results with a patient-based study for ethical reasons, assessing the airway management in Trendelenburg position with full cervical spine extension in healthy patients without risk of aspiration might be a promising next step to take.

Abbreviations
IQR: Interquartile range; RSI: Rapid sequence induction

Acknowledgements
The manuscript was professionally proofread.

Authors' contributions
MS: Study conception, acquisition of data, analysis of video data, drafting of manuscript; FK: Study conception, design and construction of modified resuscitation mannequin; BL: Study conception, acquisition of data, analysis of video data, drafting of manuscript; JS: Study conception, drafting of manuscript; All authors read and approved the final manuscript.

References
1. Wallace C, McGuire B. Rapid sequence induction: its place in modern anaesthesia. Continuing Education in Anaesthesia Critical Care & Pain. 2014;14(3):130–5.
2. Benington S, Severn A. Preventing aspiration and regurgitation. Anaesthesia & Intensive Care Medicine. 2007;8(9):368–72.
3. El-Orbany M, Connolly LA. Rapid sequence induction and intubation: current controversy. Anesth Analg. 2010;110(5):1318–25.
4. Neilipovitz DT, Crosby ET. No evidence for decreased incidence of aspiration after rapid sequence induction. Can J Anaesth. 2007;54(9):748–64.
5. Wetsch WA, Hinkelbein J. Current national recommendations on rapid sequence induction in Europe. How standardised is the 'standard of care'? Eur J Anaesthesiol. 2014;31(8):443–4.
6. Nason KS. Acute intraoperative pulmonary aspiration. Thorac Surg Clin. 2015;25(3):301–7.
7. Stept WJ, Safar P. Rapid induction-intubation for prevention of gastric-content aspiration. Anesth Analg. 1970;49(4):633–6.
8. Sellick BA. Cricoid pressure to control regurgitation of stomach contents during induction of anaesthesia. Lancet. 1961;2(278):404–6.
9. Morton HJV, Wylie WD. Anaesthetic deaths due to regurgitation or vomiting. Anaesthesia. 1951;6(4):190–201.
10. Kluger MT, Visvanathan T, Myburgh JA, Westhorpe RN. Crisis management during anaesthesia: regurgitation, vomiting, and aspiration. Qual Saf Health Care. 2005;14(3):e4.
11. Engelhardt T, Webster NR. Pulmonary aspiration of gastric contents in anaesthesia. Br J Anaesth. 1999;83(3):453–60.
12. Takenaka I, Aoyama K, Iwagaki T. Combining head-neck position and head-down tilt to prevent pulmonary aspiration of gastric contents during induction of anaesthesia: a volunteer and manikin study. Eur J Anaesthesiol. 2012;29(8):380–5.
13. Farmery A, Roe P. A model to describe the rate of oxyhaemoglobin desaturation during apnoea. Br J Anaesth. 1996;76:284–91.
14. Malbrain M, Chiumello D, Cesana B, Blaser A, Starkopf J, Sugrue M, Pelosi P, Severgnini P, Hernandez G. A systematic review and individual patient data meta-analysis on intra-abdominal hypertension in critically ill patients: the wake-up project. World initiative on Abdominal Hypertension Epidemiology, a Unifying Project (WAKE-Up!). Minerva Anestesiol. 2014;80(3):293–306.
15. Eichelsbacher C, Ilper H, Noppens R, Hinkelbein J, Loop T. Rapid sequence induction and intubation in patients with risk of aspiration: recommendations for action for practical management of anesthesia. Anaesthesist. 2018;67(8):568–83.
16. Warnecke T, Dobbermann M, Becker T, Bernhard M, Hinkelbein J. Performance of prehospital emergency anesthesia and airway management : an online survey. Anaesthesist. 2018;67(9):654–63.
17. Sajayan A, Wicker J, Ungureanu N, Mendonca C, Kimani PK. Current practice of rapid sequence induction of anaesthesia in the UK - a national survey. Br J Anaesth. 2016;117(Suppl 1):i69–74.
18. Ehrenfeld JM, Cassedy EA, Forbes VE, Mercaldo ND, Sandberg WS. Modified rapid sequence induction and intubation: a survey of United States current practice. Anesth Analg. 2012;115(1):95–101.
19. Rohsbach CB, Wirth SO, Lenz K, Priebe HJ. Survey on the current management of rapid sequence induction in Germany. Minerva Anestesiol. 2013;79:716–26.
20. Lane S, Saunders D, Schofield A, Padmanabhan R, Hildreth A, Laws D. A prospective, randomised controlled trial comparing the efficacy of pre-oxygenation in the 20 degrees head-up vs supine position. Anaesthesia. 2005;60(11):1064–7.
21. Salem MR, Khorasani A, Zeidan A, Crystal GJ. Cricoid pressure controversies: narrative review. Anesthesiology. 2017;126(4):738–52.
22. Jeske HC, Borovicka J, von Goedecke A, Meyenberger C, Heidegger T, Benzer A. The influence of postural changes on gastroesophageal reflux and barrier pressure in nonfasting individuals. Anesth Analg. 2005;101(2):597–600.
23. Heijke SAM, Smith G, Key A. The effect of the Trendelenburg position on lower oesophageal sphincter tone. Anaesthesia. 1991;46:185–7.
24. de Leon A, Thorn SE, Ottosson J, Wattwil M. Body positions and esophageal sphincter pressures in obese patients during anesthesia. Acta Anaesthesiol Scand. 2010;54(4):458–63.
25. Kim HJ, Chung SP, Park IC, Cho J, Lee HS, Park YS. Comparison of the GlideScope video laryngoscope and Macintosh laryngoscope in simulated tracheal intubation scenarios. Emerg Med J. 2008;25(5):279–82.
26. Maharaj CH, Higgins BD, Harte BH, Laffey JG. Evaluation of intubation using the Airtraq or Macintosh laryngoscope by anaesthetists in easy and simulated difficult laryngoscopy - a manikin study. Anaesthesia. 2006;61(5):469–77.
27. Lim TJ, Lim Y, Liu EHC. Evaluation of ease of intubation with the GlideScope or Macintosh laryngoscope by anaesthesist in simulated easy and difficult laryngoscopy. Anaesthesia. 2005;60:180–3.
28. Hesselfeldt R, Kristensen MS, Rasmussen LS. Evaluation of the airway of the SimMan full-scale patient simulator. Acta Anaesthesiol Scand. 2005;49(9):1339–45.
29. Konrad C, Schüpfer G, Wietlisbach M, Gerber H. Learning manual skills in anesthesiology: is there a recommended number of cases for anesthetic procedures? Anesth Analg. 1998;86:635–9.
30. Cook TM, Woodall N, Frerk C: Major complications of airway management in the United Kingdom. Report and findings. The Royal College of Anaesthetists and the difficult airway Society 2011. https://www.rcoa.ac.uk/nap4 (accessed December 25th 2018).
31. Robinson M, Davidson A. Aspiration under anaesthesia: risk assessment and decision-making. Continuing Education in Anaesthesia Critical Care & Pain. 2014;14(4):171–5.
32. Schebesta K, Hüpfl M, Rössler B, Ringl H, Müller MP, Kimberger O. Airway anatomy of high-fidelity human patient simulators and airway trainers. Anesthesiology. 2012;116(6):1204–9.
33. Rai MR, Popat MT. Evaluation of airway equipment: man or manikin? Anaesthesia. 2011;66:1–3.
34. Rocke DA, Brock-Utne JG, Rout CC. At risk for aspiration: new critical values of volume and pH? Anesth Analg. 1993;76:666.
35. Jensen AG, Callesen T, Hagemo JS, Hreinsson K, Lund V, Nordmark J. Scandinavian clinical practice guidelines on general anaesthesia for emergency situations. Acta Anaesthesiol Scand. 2010;54(8):922–50.

Supraglottic jet oxygenation and ventilation for obese patients under intravenous anesthesia during hysteroscopy

Hansheng Liang[1], Yuantao Hou[1], Liang Sun[1], Qingyue Li[1], Huafeng Wei[2] and Yi Feng[1]* ⓘ

Abstract

Background: Supraglottic jet oxygenation and ventilation (SJOV) can effectively maintain adequate oxygenation in patients with respiratory depression, even in apnea patients. However, there have been no randomized controlled clinical trials of SJOV in obese patients. This study investigated the efficacy and safety of SJOV using WEI Nasal Jet tube (WNJ) for obese patients who underwent hysteroscopy under intravenous anesthesia without endotracheal intubation.

Methods: A single-center, prospective, randomized controlled study was conducted. The obese patients receiving hysteroscopy under intravenous anesthesia were randomly divided into three groups: Control group maintaining oxygen supply via face masks (100% oxygen, flow at 6 L/min), the WNJ Oxygen Group with WNJ (100% oxygen, flow: 6 L/min) and the WNJ SJOV Group with SJOV via WNJ [Jet ventilator working parameters:100% oxygen supply, driving pressure (DP) 0.1 MPa, respiratory rate; (RR): 15 bpm, I/E; ratio 1:1.5]. SpO_2, $P_{ET}CO_2$, BP, HR, ECG and BIS were continuously monitored during anesthesia. Two-Diameter Method was deployed to measure cross sectional area of the gastric antrum (CSA-GA) by ultrasound before and after SJOV in the WNJ SJOV Group. Episodes of SpO_2 less than 95%, $P_{ET}CO_2$ less than 10 mmHg, depth of WNJ placement and measured CSA-GA before and after jet ventilation in the WNJ SJOV Group during the operation were recorded. The other adverse events were collected as well.

Results: A total of 102 patients were enrolled, with two patients excluded. Demographic characteristics were similar among the three groups. Compared with the Control Group, the incidence of $P_{ET}CO_2 < 10$ mmHg, $SpO_2 < 95\%$ in the WNJ SJOV group dropped from 36 to 9% ($P = 0.009$),from 33 to 6% ($P = 0.006$) respectively,and the application rate of jaw-lift decreased from 33 to 3% ($P = 0.001$), and the total percentage of adverse events decreased from 36 to 12% ($P = 0.004$). Compared with the WNJ Oxygen Group, the use of SJOV via WNJ significantly decreased episodes of $SpO_2 < 95\%$ from 27 to 6% ($P = 0.023$), $P_{ET}CO_2 < 10$ mmHg from 33 to 9% ($P = 0.017$), respectively. Depth of WNJ placement was about 12.34 cm in WNJ SJOV Group. There was no significantly difference of CSA-GA before and after SJOV in the WNJ SJOV Group ($P = 0.234$). There were no obvious cases of nasal bleeding in all the three groups.

(Continued on next page)

* Correspondence: fengyimzk@163.com
[1]Department of Anesthesiology, Peking University People's Hospital, Beijing100044, Beijing, China

(Continued from previous page)
Conclusions: SJOV can effectively and safely maintain adequate oxygenation in obese patients under intravenous anesthesia without intubation during hysteroscopy. This efficient oxygenation may be mainly attributed to supplies of high concentration oxygenation to the supraglottic area, and the high pressure jet pulse providing effective ventilation. Although the nasal airway tube supporting collapsed airway by WNJ also plays a role. SJOV doesn't seem to increase gastric distension and the risk of aspiration. SJOV can improve the safety of surgery by reducing the incidence of the intraoperative involuntary limbs swing, hip twist and cough.

Keywords: Jet ventilation, Supraglottic, Obesity, Anesthesia, Gastric antrum, Ultrasound, Hysteroscopy

Background

It is estimated that more than 100,000 patients receive hysteroscopy each year in China. Usually, hysteroscopy is accomplished under intravenous (IV) anesthesia or sedation without endotracheal intubation, primarily with IV propofol and remifentanil [1]. Endoscopic sedation and analgesia by propofol/remifentanil have been significantly increased during the past 10 years [2]. Remedial oxygenation by the jaw lift or pressurized mask ventilation is usually performed to manage anesthesia/sedation mediated respiratory depression, especially in obese patients. Supraglottic jet oxygenation and ventilation (SJOV) is aimed at oxygenation and ventilation in patient with depressed respiration or apnea, and have been demonstrated effective in difficult airway management without significant complications [3]. However, it is unclear whether SJOV can be used effectively and safely to maintain adequate oxygenation/ventilation in obese patients during hysteroscopy under intravenous sedation. The efficacy and safety of SJOV via nasopharyngeal approach in the obese patients needs further elucidated, although recent case reports [4, 5] and several clinical trials [6–8] delineated effectiveness of SJOV maintaining oxygenation in the non-obese patients. The Wei Nasal Jet Tube (WNJ, Well Lead Medical Co. Ltd., Guangzhou, China. number: 20170501) with an inner diameter of 5.0 mm, outer diameter of 7.5 mm, and a length of 18 cm is a newly invented nasal tube [9]. Here, we conducted a single-blind, prospective, randomized controlled study, and hypothesized SJOV using WNJ can reduce adverse events of hypoxia and hypoventilation in obese patients under IV anesthesia with propofol and remifentanil during hysteroscopy, without tracheal intubation.

Methods

Ethics, consent and permissions

This study was approved by the local Ethics Committee of Peking University People's Hospital (No. 2018PHB036–01). Informed written consent was obtained from the obese patients who underwent hysteroscopy between July and September 2018. This study adhered to the Consolidated Standards of Reporting Trials (CONSORT) guidelines.

Study design

Patients were randomized to the mask oxygen group (Control Group) maintaining oxygen absorption via face mask (100% oxygen, flow at 6 L/min), the WNJ oxygen group with WNJ (100% oxygen, flow at 6 L/min) and the WNJ SJOV group with SJOV via WNJ [Jet ventilator working parameters:100% oxygen supply, driving pressure (DP) 0.1 MPa, respiratory rate (RR): 15 bpm, I/E ratio 1:1.5]. The Sample Size was calculated by SAS, considering at least a 90 and 60% reduction in patients with SpO$_2$ reduction in WNJ SJOV group and WNJ oxygen group compared to that in control group by the preliminary test. With a standard deviation of 0.8, and bilaterally equal to 0.05, or even 0.2 (power = 0.8), estimated value of each group should be 34 cases ($n = 2(\mu_\alpha + \mu_\beta)^2\sigma^2/\delta^2$ with 20% shedding rate). The randomization was performed by random number table from the SPSS23.0, and the blinding was completed by one medical student and two anesthesiologists. Patients were labeled with WNJ SJOV, WNJ or Control by One anesthesiologist, and the other anesthesiologist administered the intravenous anesthesia and maintained oxygenation. The flow diagram of this study was shown in Fig. 1.

Patients

In-patients receiving routine hysteroscopy under IV anesthesia with propofol and remifentanil were recruited. Inclusion criteria were as follows: (1) 18 yrs. < age < 65 yrs.; (2) BMI > 30 kg/m^2; (3) Fasting for 8 h and no water for 4 h before surgery; (1) ASA class: I-II classes. Exclusion criteria were as follows: (1) Epistaxis; (2) Nasal stenosis; (3) Long-term use of anticoagulants; (4) Rhinitis episodes; (5) Severe reflux disease; (6) History of severe respiratory, cardiovascular and cerebrovascular diseases.

Anesthesia

Induction of anesthesia was conducted by IV injection of propofol (1.5–2 mg/kg) and remifentanil (0.5 μg/kg). Anesthesia was maintained by continuous IV infusion of propofol (3-5 mg/kg/h) and remifentanil (0.05–0.08μg/kg/ min). After anesthesia induction, the face

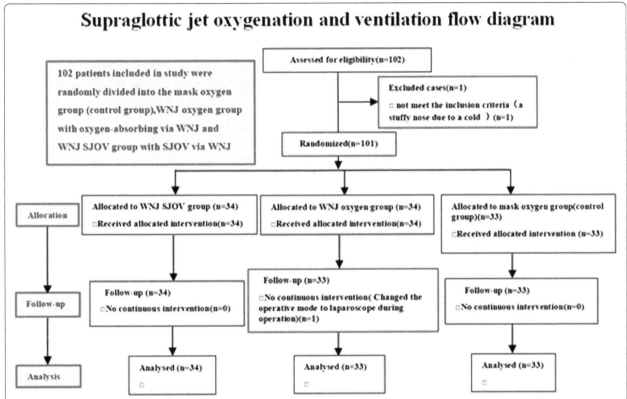

Fig. 1 Supraglottic jet oxygenation and ventilation flow diagram. A total of 102 patients with BMI > 30 receiving hysteroscopy were randomly divided into three groups: the mask oxygen group (control group) maintaining oxygen absorption via face mask (N = 33), the WNJ oxygen group maintaining oxygen absorption via WNJ(N = 33) and the WNJ SJOV group maintaining SJOV via WNJ(N = 34). One patient in the control group was excluded because of stuffy nose due to a cold(N = 1). The other patient in WNJ oxygen group was abandoned intervention due to change of the operative mode during operation(N = 1)

mask in control group, the WNJ in WNJ oxygen group and WNJ SJOV group were placed appropriately straightway. Before putting WNJ into the unobstructed nostril of patients, a paraffin oil cotton swab was used to clear the nasal cavity and about 1 ml lidocaine ointment was smeared on the tip of WNJ (the depth was equivalent to the distance from the alar to the ipsilateral earlobe [3]. The jet catheter of the WNJ was connected to an automated jet ventilator-TKR-400 (Well Lead Medical Equipment Ltd. Guangzhou, China.) (Fig. 2). Bispectral index (BIS) was maintained at 45–60 [additional propofol (0.3–0.5 mg/kg) was given with one bolus infusion if needed] and SpO_2 was maintained above 95%. A dose of ephedrine (3–6 mg) was administered as needed in order to maintain the mean arterial pressure above 55 mmHg. Remedial measures were executed immediately in the setting of oxygen saturation (SpO_2) < 95%, including adjusting the WNJ position (1 cm deep or shallow) in the WNJ SJOV group and the WNJ oxygen group, and taking jaw-lift maneuver in the three groups. Mask pressurized ventilation was used to provide oxygen only when SpO_2 < 90% happened in all the three groups.

Intraoperative monitoring

We continuously monitored following parameters during the anesthesia: pulse SpO_2, End-tidal carbon dioxide partial pressure $(P_{ET}CO_2)$, mean blood pressure (MBP), heart rate (HR), electrocardiogram (ECG) and BIS. SpO_2 < 95% and $P_{ET}CO_2$ < 10 mmHg were considered hypoxic adverse event and hyperventilation, respectively [10]. Two-Diameter Method was used to measure antral cross-sectional area of gastric antrum (CSA-GA) by ultrasound [Vivid, GE MEDICAL SYSTEMS CO.,LTD, China] with patients in the supine position before and after SJOV in the WNJ SJOV group, using the sagittal plane measurement at the xiphoid process level, with the help of the anatomical markers (the superior mesenteric artery,the left liver lobe and abdominal aorta) (Fig. 3). The diameter of antero-posterior and cranio-caudal antral was expressed as AP and CC, respectively, with a π of 3.1416 during $CSA = (AP \times CC \times \pi)/4$. Stomach volume was estimated and calculated by estimated stomach volume (ESV) = 27.0 + 14.6 × CSA-1.28 × age (yrs) [11, 12].

Episodes of SpO_2 less than 95% and $P_{ET}CO_2$ less than 10 mmHg during the operation were recorded. The other adverse events such as hip twist, cough, nasal bleeding

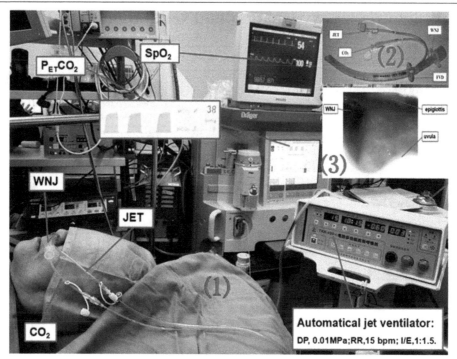

Fig. 2 (1) The scene of supraglottic jet oxygenation and ventilation (SJOV) via WNJ with or without spontaneous breathing. SJOV could maintain oxygen saturation and carbon dioxide exhalation. $P_{ET}CO_2$ = End-tidal carbon dioxide partial pressure; SpO_2 = pulse oxygen saturation;DP = driving pressure;RR = respiratory rate; I/E ratio = inhalation/exhalation ratio. (2) Wei Nasal Jet tube (WNJ), which has two channels built inside the tube wall for jet ventilation and the end-tidal pressure of CO_2 monitoring, respectively. FVD = fixed valve of depth. (3) The position of the WNJ into the laryngopharynx observed by nasal fiberoptic scope. The depth of placement of the WNJ was about equivalent to the distance from the alar to the ipsilateral earlobe. The best site for WNJ insertion under fiber bronchoscope was between the epiglottis and uvula

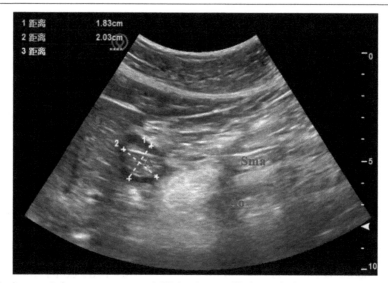

Fig. 3 Two-Diameter Method was carried out to measure antral CSA by ultrasound before and after SJOV in the WNJ SJOV group. GA = Gastric antrum, Ao = aorta, Sma = superior mesenteric artery, L = liver. The antero-posterior (AP) antral diameter was expressed as dotted line 1,The cranio-caudal (CC) antral diameter was represented by dotted line 2,and π was 3.1416 during CSA = $(AP \times CC \times \pi)/4$

and remedial interventions such as jaw-lift, pressure mask, depth of WNJ placement were also noted. Types and time of surgery, recovery time of anesthesia, dose of anesthetics, measured CSA-GA before and after jet ventilation in the WNJ SJOV group were also recorded.

Statistical analysis

The measurement data was expressed as mean ± SD and the count data was presented as the number and percentage. Kruskal-wallis single factor ANOVA test was used to compare the difference of time of surgery, recovery time of anesthesia, dosage of anesthetics between different groups. The data about depth of WNJ placement between the WNJ SJOV and the WNJ oxygen groups was analyzed by Wilcoxon rank sum test. Independent sample t-test was used for comparing the CSA-GA and ESV before and after jet ventilation in the WNJ SJOV group. Categorical variables as the cases of SpO_2 less than 95%, $P_{ET}CO_2$ less than 10 mmHg, hip twist, nasal bleeding, and patients requiring jaw-lift, pressured mask ventilation, as well as other perioperative adverse reactions were all analyzed withchi-square test and Fisher's exact test. All data was analyzed with SPSS23.0 statistical software (SPSS Inc., Chicago, IL, USA). A value of $p < 0.05$ was considered the difference was statistically significant.

Results

A total of 102 patients were enrolled. One patient in the control group was excluded because of stuffy nose due to catching a cold, and another patient in WNJ oxygen group was removed because of change of the operative mode during operation. All the patients tolerated the hysteroscopy well. There were no serious adverse events (i.e. aspiration, laryngospasm, nasal bleeding post operation, barotrauma and death).

Clinical characteristics of study population

The clinical characteristics of patients was represented in Table 1. Age, height, weight, BMI, ASA classification, airway-related parameters, (including mouth opening degree, thyromental distance, neck circumference, Mallampati class), snore history, and obstructive sleep apnea hypoventilation syndrome (OSAHS) were compared. Data of the surgical and anesthesia procedure, adverse events and remedial interventions were analyzed in Table 2.

Primary outcome
Adverse events of hypoxia and hypoventilation

The majority of patients had shown good wave form and good values of $P_{ET}CO_2$ during SJOV. Compared with the Control Group, the incidence of $P_{ET}CO_2 < 10$ mmHg, $SpO_2 < 95\%$ in the WNJ SJOVgroup dropped from 36 to 9% ($P = 0.009$), from 33 to 6% ($P = 0.006$) respectively, and the application rate of jaw-lift decreased from 33 to 3%

Table 1 General information of patients in the three groups and the surgical types. The differences among the three groups and between each two groups were not statistically significant($p > 0.05$)

Characteristic (mean ± SD)	mask oxygen(I) (N = 33)	WNJ oxygen (II) (N = 33)	WNJ SJOV (III) (N = 34)
Age (yr.)	44.7 ± 11.65	44.1 ± 12.86	43.8 ± 15.22
Height (cm)	155.6 ± 5.56	154.4 ± 7.23	156.3 ± 8.23
Weight (kg)	80.3 ± 6.05	79.2 ± 10.34	80.5 ± 5.17
BMI (kg.m^{-2})	33.18 ± 2.87	33.23 ± 3.22	32.97 ± 2.36
mouth opening(I)(II)(III)(IV)	(32)(1)(0)(0)	(33)(0)(0)(0)	(33)(1)(0)(0)
thyromental Distance(I)(II)(III)	(27)(5)(1)	(28)(5)(0)	(30)(4)(0)
neck circumference(I)(II)(III)	(11)(19)(3)	(13)(18)(2)	(10)(20)(4)
mallampati class (I)(II)(III)(IV)	(8)(23)(2)(0)	(7)(22)(4)(0)	(8)(22)(4)(0)
Snore history [n (%)]	11 (33%)	13 (39%)	13 (38%)
OSAHS [n (%)]	0 (0%)	0 (0%)	1 (3%)
ASA(I)(II)	(28)(5)	(30)(3)	(30)(4)
surgical types of hysteroscopy			
TCRP [n(%)]	4 (12)	5 (15)	6 (18)
TCRM [n(%)]	6 (18)	5 (15)	6 (18)
TCRS [n(%)]	11 (33)	12 (36)	11 (32)
TCRA [n(%)]	12 (36)	11 (33)	11 (32)

BMI body mass index; Mouth opening(I/II/III/IV):I > 4.0 cm, II 2.5–3.0 cm, III 1.2–2.0 cm, and IV < 1.0 cm; Thyromental distance (I/II/III): I > 6.5 cm, II 6–6.5 cm, and III < 6 cm; Neck circumference(I/II/III): I < 35 cm, II 35–41 cm, and III > 41 cm; *OSAHS* obstructive sleep apnea hypoventilation syndrome, *SJOV* supraglottic jet oxygenation and ventilation, *WNJ* Wei nasal jet tube, *TCRP* transcervical polyp resection, *TCRM* transcervical hysteroscopy fibroid resection, *TCRS* transcervical resection of septa, *TCRA* transcervical resection of adhesions

Table 2 Data about the procedure, drugs dosage, adverse events and remedial interventions. Compared with the mask oxygen or WNJ oxygen groups, the use of SJOV via WNJ during the surgery significantly decreased the total percentage of adverse events and surgical time, cases of SpO$_2$ < 95% and P$_{ET}$CO$_2$ < 10 mmHg, and the application rate of jaw-lift

Monitored variables [n (%)]	mask oxygen(I) (N = 33)	WNJ oxygen (II) (N = 33)	WNJ SJOV (III) (N = 34)	P-Value (I VS II)	P-Value (I VS III)	P-Value (II VS III)	P
Surgical time (min)	24.28 ± 10.18	23.19 ± 9.72	22.56 ± 5.91	0.053	0.013	0.053	0.027 (Kruskal-wallis)
Anesthesia recovery (min)	14.73 ± 5.59	13.22 ± 3.73	13.97 ± 4.12	0.068	0.217	0.866	0.061 (Kruskal-wallis)
WNJ placement depth (cm)	–	12.22 ± 0.54	12.34 ± 0.47	–	–	0.087[a]	–
Propofol dose (mg)	207.01 ± 62.85	212.57 ± 51.44	225.01 ± 48.63	1.000	0.002	< 0.001	< 0.001 (Kruskal-wallis)
Remifentanil dose (μg)	32.28 ± 6.18	33.02 ± 8.27	33.21 ± 4.97	0.059	0.244	0.196	0.079 (Kruskal-wallis)
Ephedrine dose (mg)	5.14 ± 1.03	5.23 ± 1.16	5.25 ± 1.10	0.516	0.417	0.975	0.022 (Kruskal-wallis)
Total adverse events	12 (36)	13 (39)	4 (12)	1.000	0.004	0.002	0.013
Intra-operation							
SpO$_2$ < 95%	11 (33)	9 (27)	2 (6)	0.789	0.006	0.023	0.017
P$_{ET}$CO$_2$ < 10 mmHg	12 (36)	11 (33)	3 (9)	1.000	0.009	0.017	0.019
Jaw-lift	11 (33)	10 (30)	1 (3)	1.000	0.001	0.003	0.004
Mask pressurized ventilation	5 (15)	3 (9)	0 (0)	0.708	0.025	0.114	0.071
Oropharyngeal tube	2 (6)	0 (0)	0 (0)	0.492	0.239	–	0.126
Nasal bleeding	0 (0)	1 (3)	2 (6)	1.000	0.493	1.000	0.369
Cough	3 (9)	1 (3)	1 (3)	0.613	0.356	1.000	0.420
Laryngospasm	0 (0)	0 (0)	0 (0)	–	–	–	–
Aspiration	0 (0)	0 (0)	0 (0)	–	–	–	–
Hip twist	2 (6)	1 (3)	0 (0)	1.000	0.239	0.493	0.348
Bradycardia	9 (27)	8 (24)	4 (12)	1.000	0.132	0.217	0.254
Tachycardia	2 (6)	1 (3)	0 (0)	1.000	0.239	0.493	0.348
Hypertension	5 (15)	4 (12)	1 (3)	1.000	0.105	0.197	0.221
Hypotension	1 (3)	1 (3)	3 (9)	1.000	0.614	0.614	0.453
Post-operation							
Nausea or Vomiting	1 (3)	2 (6)	1 (3)	1.000	1.000	0.614	0.761
Pharyngalgia	2 (6)	3 (9)	3 (9)	1.000	1.000	1.000	0.881
Xerostomia	2 (6)	3 (9)	4 (12)	1.000	0.427	0.709	0.488
Nasal bleeding	0 (0)	0 (0)	0 (0)	–	–	–	–
Barotrauma	0 (0)	0 (0)	0 (0)	–	–	–	–

SpO$_2$: pulse oxygen saturation; P$_{ET}$CO$_2$: End-tidal carbon dioxide partial pressure; SJOV:supraglottic jet oxygenation and ventilation; WNJ: Wei nasal jet tube

($P = 0.001$), and the total percentage of adverse events decreased from 36 to 12% ($P = 0.004$). Compared with the WNJ Oxygen Group, the use of SJOV via WNJ significantly decreased episodes of SpO$_2$ < 95% from 27 to 6% ($P = 0.023$), P$_{ET}$CO$_2$ < 10 mmHg from 33 to 9% ($P = 0.017$), respectively. There were no significant differences in episodes of SpO$_2$ < 95% and P$_{ET}$CO$_2$ < 10 mmHg between the WNJ Oxygen Group and the Control Group ($P = 0.789$ and $P = 1.000$). (Table 2).

Secondary outcome
Incidence of the nasal bleeding, cough and hip twist
There were three cases of nasal bleeding (a small amount of blood attached WNJ) during operation in this study.

One occurred in WNJ oxygen group, the other two cases happened in WNJ SJOV group. On the second day after surgery, these three patients had no other symptoms except feeling slight dry and itching in the throat.

There were no significant differences in the cough and hip twist among three groups ($P = 0.420$ and $P = 0.348$). However, compared with the Control Group, SJOV could slightly decrease the incidence of cough from 9 to 3% ($P = 0.356$) and hip twist from 6 to 0% ($P = 0.239$) (Table 2).

Incidence of the nausea or vomiting, pharyngalgia, and xerostomia after surgery, changes of CSA-GA and ESV
There were no significant differences in the nausea or vomiting, pharyngalgia and xerostomia among three groups

after surgery ($P = 0.761$, $P = 0.488$ and $P = 0.881$).(Table 2). The changes of the CSA-GA and ESV were not significant before and after supraglottic jet ventilation in the WNJ SJOV Group ($P = 0.234$ and $P = 0.777$). (Table 3).

Propofol dosage

Compared with the Control Group and the WNJ Oxygen Group, respectively, the dosage of propofol in the WNJ SJOV Group increased significantly ($P = 0.002$, $P < 0.001$).

Discussion

Hysteroscopy is one of the most common procedures in gynecology [1]. Involuntary limbs swing and hip twist should be avoided during hysteroscopy surgery [13], considering that it not only increases potential risk of uterine perforation but adding extra burden to operation. Therefore, sufficient depth of anesthesia and analgesic intensity is required. Admittedly, intraspinal anesthesia can provide adequate analgesia and satisfactory patient cooperation, but it is not conducive to rapid postoperative recovery of patients [14]. With the application of propofol and remifentanil in clinical practice, short IV anesthesia is possible and can be easily accepted by surgeons and patients. At present, IV anesthesia becomes a trend in hysteroscopy [1]. Majholm, an obstetrician and gynecologist in Denmark, believed that although the time of hysteroscopy surgery under non-intubation IV anesthesia was similar to that under intraspinal anesthesia or intubation general anesthesia, the length of hospital stay reduced and patients' satisfactions were improved [15]. However, while providing satisfactory anesthesia and rapid patients' recovery, anesthesiologists must guarantee a difficult task, that is adequate oxygenation and ventilation of patients. Therefore, the key to anesthesia management in hysteroscopy surgery is how to balance the short time, analgesic intensity and anesthesia depth with airway safety of patients. Shallow anesthesia is unable to meet surgery needs, however, deep anesthesia may lead to significant airway collapse. When the depth of anesthesia is sufficient for the operation, supplemental oxygen was proved to be an effective intervention measure to improve oxygenation and ventilation. These common measures include nasal catheter, mask, jaw-lift, or pressurized mask ventilation, which require the patient to maintain an autonomous breathing. Usually, pressurized mask ventilation is used as the last attempt in the settings of non-artificial airway assisted-

ventilation [2]. However, this ventilation mode is easy to make stomach flatulence, and increase the risk of gastric reflux and aspiration [16]. Obesity is a multisystem, chronic, proinflammatory disorder, and specific care is needed for airway management [17]. Leakage is likely to occur when airway pressure is more than $20cmH_2O$ for the patients with obesity under intravenous general anesthesia using laryngeal mask, and ventilation and oxygenation are affected. When the airway pressure exceeds $25cmH_2O$, it is easy to increase gastric distension and the risk of aspiration [18].

Transnasal humidified rapid insufflation ventilatory exchange (THRIVE) is a new approach to enhance oxygenation [19]. THRIVE has the advantage of increasing oxygen concentration, removing carbon dioxide from the ineffective chamber, and maintaining positive airway pressure, thus improving lung compliance and reducing upper airway obstruction [20]. However, in terms of upper airway obstruction, jet ventilation, which was developed in 1967, has the same enhanced oxygenation advantage as THRIVE, although they work in different ways [21, 22].

Jostrand from Sweden first introduced the technology of using 60 to 100 breaths per minute, which was called high frequency positive pressure ventilation (HFPPV) [23]. Klein studied the HFPPV and renamed the system as high frequency jet ventilation (HFJV) [24]. Since then, HFJV has become a technique to maintain ventilation. The application of this technique enables rapid pulsation gas to enter the respiratory tract through a narrow jet tube under low pressure [25, 26]. HFJV has three characteristics [27–29], open system, high-frequency (> 60 bpm) and low tidal volume. Transtracheal jet ventilation (TTJV) is one of the popular methods of emergency airway management in the ASA guide, but barotrauma is a severe complication that damper the excitement to use it [30–32]. The characteristics of supraglottic jet ventilation (SJV) are that can be used as the ventilation of emergency airway, and auxiliary oxygenation of difficult airway, with more open ventilating system, less complications, and low requirement for spontaneous breathing [33]. Advantages of WNJ are jetting ventilation via side hole, releasing gas from the main hole and surrounding upper airway space, and reduction of barotrauma.

In addition to observing chest fluctuation, $P_{ET}CO_2$ can also be monitored [34] [Fig. 2(2)]. In this study, we successfully applied SJOV via WNJ to decrease the episodes

Table 3 Two-Diameter Method was used to measure CSA-GA by ultrasound. Stomach volume was estimated and calculated by $ESV = 27.0 + 14.6 \times CSA-1.28 \times age$ (years). Compared with before jet ventilation, CSA-GA and ESV after jet ventilation had not been increased in the WNJ SJOV group ($p > 0.05$)

Monitored variables	Before WNJ SJOV ($N = 34$)	After WNJ SJOV ($N = 34$)	P-Value (before VS after)
CSA-GA (cm^2)	3.32 ± 0.59	3.34 ± 0.56	0.234
ESV (ml)	18.78 ± 6.68	18.89 ± 6.59	0.777

CSA-GA cross sectional area of the gastric antrum, *ESV* Estimated stomach volume, *SJOV* supraglottic jet oxygenation and ventilation, *WNJ* Wei nasal jet tube

of hypoxia and hypoventilation for the patients receiving hysteroscopy surgery under IV anesthesia by propofol and remifentanil. This efficient oxygenation may be accomplished primarily by jet ventilation, though nasal airway tube supporting collapsed airway also plays a role. Additionally, SJOV was seemed to improve the safety of surgery by reducing the incidence of the intraoperative involuntary limbs swing and hip twist, cough, and stomach flatulence.

The scene of SJOV via WNJ was shown in Fig. 2(1). With or without spontaneous breathing, both oxygenation and carbon dioxide exhalation were well maintained. The depth of placing the WNJ was equivalent to the distance from the alar to the ipsilateral earlobe. Meanwhile, we located the front-end of WNJ by fibro bronchoscope and found that the best site for WNJ oxygenation was between epiglottis and uvula in the WNJ SJOV Group. The distance was about 12.34 cm [Fig. 2(3)]. Oxygenation effect can be maintained better in the WNJ SJOV Group than that in the WNJ Oxygen Group, although the same WNJs were used for the patients in both groups. Accordingly, we believe the role of maintaining oxygenation was mainly jet ventilation rather than propping up the collapsed airway with or without spontaneous respiration. For obese patients, it was usually difficult to perform hysteroscopy surgery under general IV anesthesia without intubation and maintain proper intensity of spontaneous breathing without respiratory depression under the guarantee of surgical safety. Therefore, WNJ SJOV had more advantages in enhancing oxygenation than WNJ alone.

Theoretically, SJV can make the WNJ front end swing, which may cause damage to the throat soft tissue. However, we did not find such kind of swing under the fiberoptic bronchoscopy. The possible reasons were that the curved part of the nasal cavity of WNJ weakened the airflow impact, and the jet ventilation through the WEJ side hole reduced the airflow and the airflow pressure. SJV via WNJ (WNJ SJV) could provide adequate ventilation, although it is less effective than transtracheal jet ventilation (TTJV). However, WNJ SJV could significantly reduce the complications of TTJV, such as barotrauma. WNJ SJV within 25 min did not increase incidence of postoperative laryngopharyngeal pain, cough and ability of discharge of sputum, suggesting that this technique may not produce inflammatory reaction caused by damage of airway mucosa and throat soft tissue.

Although the mechanisms about the respiratory depressant effect of propofol have not been fully explained, it is clear that propofol causes the respiratory depressant effect in a dose-dependent manner [35]. When mask/nasopharyngeal tube oxygen is used to maintain oxygenation under propofol sedation, propofol dosage is often reduced involuntary due to respiratory depressant, which

will increase the incidence of the intraoperative involuntary limbs swing, hip twist and cough. The respiratory depressant effect may be not worried with/without spontaneous respiration during SJOV via WNJ to maintain oxygenation under propofol sedation. The short duration of hysteroscopy and the small total dosage of propofol which did not lead to the difference in anesthesia recovery, although there were differences in the dosage of propofol among the three groups.

Although it had been reported that SJV can maintain 1 h oxygenation, but it was not suitable for longer time application [8]. Appropriate use time and whether it will cause airway mucosal inflammation remains to be observed in large-sample multi-center randomized controlled trials in the future. Previous anesthesiologists criticize that this methods may not be sensitive enough to monitor gastric volume and extension by ultrasound. The CSA-GA in the evaluation of gastric flatulence may seemed to have poor quantitative accuracy, but it could provide some qualitative reference value in clinical application, so making efforts to explore this field was required in the future work.

The shortcomings of this trial are reflected in the small sample size, which cannot fully reflect the real situation of adverse reactions. The position of the patient during ultrasound examination is not the optimal position.

Conclusions

SJOV can effectively and safely maintain adequate oxygenation in obese patients under intravenous anesthesia without intubation during hysteroscopy. This efficient oxygenation may be mainly attributed to supplies of high concentration oxygen to the supraglottic area, and the high pressure jet pulse providing effective ventilation. Although the nasal airway tube supporting collapsed airway by WNJ also plays a role. SJOV doesn't seem to increase gastric distension and the risk of aspiration. SJOV can improve the safety of surgery by reducing the incidence of the intraoperative involuntary limbs swing, hip twist and cough.

Abbreviations

Ao: aorta; AP: Antero-posterior; ASA: American Society of Anesthesiologists; BIS: Bispectral index; BMI: body mass index; CC: cranio-caudal; CONSORT: Consolidated standards of reporting trials; CSA-GA: Cross sectional area of the gastric antrum; DP: Driving pressure; ECG: Electrocardiogram; ESV: Estimated stomach volume; FVD: Fixed valve of depth; GA: Gastric antrum; HFJV: High frequency jet ventilation; HR: Heart rate; I/E ratio: Inhalation/exhalation ratio; IV: Intravenous; L: Liver; MBP: Mean blood pressure; OSAHS: Obstructive sleep apnea hypoventilation syndrome; $P_{ET}CO_2$: End-tidal carbon dioxide partial pressure; RR: Respiratory rate; SJOV: Supraglottic jet oxygenation and ventilation; SJV: Supraglottic jet ventilation; Sma: Superior mesenteric artery; SpO₂: Pulse oxygen saturation; TCRA: Transcervical resection of adhesions; TCRM: Transcervical hysteroscopy fibroid resection; TCRP: Transcervical polyp resection; TCRS: Transcervical resection of septa; THRIVE: Transnasal humidified rapid insufflation ventilatory exchange; TTJV: Transtracheal jet ventilation; WNJ: Wei Nasal Jet tube

Acknowledgements
We thank Dr. Xin Yang, Dr. Xudong Liang and Dr. Yi Li from department of gynaecology, Peking University people's hospital for their understanding, support and cooperation in this clinical trial, and for making some pertinent suggestions.

Authors' contributions
Study conception: YF, HL, HW. Study design: YF, HL. Study conduct: YF, HL, QL. Data analysis: HL,YH, LS. Data interpretation: HW, YH, LS, QL. Drafting of the manuscript: YF, HL. All authors approved the final version of the manuscript.

Author details
[1]Department of Anesthesiology, Peking University People's Hospital, Beijing100044, Beijing, China. [2]Department of Anesthesiology and Critical Care, Hospital of the University of Pennsylvania, Philadelphia, PA 19104, USA.

References
1. Sloth SB, Schroll JB, Settnes A, et al. Systematic review of the limited evidence for different surgical techniques at benign hysterectomy: a clinical guideline initiated by the Danish health authority. Eur J Obstet Gynecol Reprod Biol. 2017;216(2):169–77.
2. Mazanikov M, Udd M, Kylänpää L, et al. Patient-controlled sedation with propofol and remifentanil for ERCP: a randomized, controlled study. Gastrointest Endosc. 2011;73(2):260–6.
3. Wei HF. A new tracheal tube and methods to facilitate ventilation and placement in emergency airway management. Resuscitation. 2006;70:438–44.
4. Xie P, Li Q, Wei H, et al. Supraglottic jet oxygenation and ventilation saved a patient with 'cannot intubate and cannot ventilate' emergency difficult airway. J Anesth. 2017;31(1):144–7.
5. Dziewit JA, Wei H. Supraglottic jet ventilation assists intubation in a Marfan's syndrome patient with a difficult airway. J Clin Anesth. 2011;23:407–9.
6. Qin Y, Li LZ, Su DS, et al. Supraglottic jet oxygenation and ventilation enhances oxygenation during upper gastrointestinal endoscopy in patients sedated with propofol: a randomized multicentre clinical trial. Br J Anaesth. 2017;119(1):158–66.
7. PENG J, YE J, ZHAO Y, et al. Supraglottic jet ventilation in difficult airway management. J Emerg Med. 2012;43:382–90.
8. Wu CN, Ma WH, Wei JQ, et al. Laryngoscope and a new tracheal tube assist lightwand intubation in difficult airways due to unstable cervical spine. PLoS One. 2015;10(3):e0120231.
9. LEVITT C, WEI H. Supraglotic pulsatile jet oxygen ventilation during deep propofol sedation for upper gastrointestinal endoscopy in a morbidly obese patient. J Clin Anesth. 2014;26:157–9.
10. Athayde RAB, Oliveira Filho JRB, Lorenzi Filho G, et al. Obesity hypoventilation syndrome: a current review. J Bras Pneumol. 2018;44(6):510–8.
11. Van de Putte P, Vernieuwe L. When fasted is not empty: a retrospective cohort study of gastric content in fasted surgical patients. Br J Anaesth. 2017;118(3):363–71.
12. Van de Putte P, Vernieuwe L, Perlas A. Term pregnant patients have similar gastric volume to non-pregnant females: a single-centre cohort study. Br J Anaesth. 2019;122(1):79–85.
13. Cai HL, Pan LY, Wang SF, et al. Discussion on operative skills in the embolization of hydrosalpinx by hysteroscopic placement of a microcoil. Medicine. 2019;98(11):e14721.
14. Munmany M, Gracia M, Nonell R, et al. The use of inhaled sevoflurane during operative hysteroscopy is associated with increased glycine absorption compared to intravenous propofol for maintenance of anesthesia. J Clin Anesth. 2016;31:202–7.
15. Majholm B, Bartholdy J, Clausen HV, et al. Comparison between local anaesthesia with remifentanil and total intravenous anaesthesia for operative hysteroscopic procedures in day surgery. Br J Anaesth. 2012;108(2):245–53.
16. An X, Ye H, Chen J, Lu B. Effect of positive end-expiratory pressure on overlap between internal jugular vein and carotid artery in mechanically ventilated patients with laryngeal mask airway (LMA) insertion - a prospective randomized trial. Med Sci Monit. 2019;25:2305–10.
17. Petrini F, Di Giacinto I, Cataldo R, et al. Perioperative and periprocedural airway management and respiratory safety for the obese patient: 2016 SIAARTI consensus. Minerva Anestesiol. 2016;82(12):1314–35.
18. Wang H, Gao X, Wei W, et al. The optimum sevoflurane concentration for supraglottic airway device blockbuster™ insertion with spontaneous breathing in obese patients: a prospective observational study. BMC Anesthesiol. 2017;17(1):156.
19. George S, Humphreys S, Williams T, et al. Transnasal Humidified Rapid Insufflation Ventilatory Exchange in children requiring emergent intubation (Kids THRIVE): a protocol for a randomised controlled trial. BMJ Open. 2019;9(2):e025997.
20. Hermez LA, Spence CJ, Payton MJ, et al. A physiological study to determine the mechanism of carbon dioxide clearance during apnoea when using transnasal humidified rapid insufflation ventilatory exchange (THRIVE). Anaesthesia. 2019;74(4):441–9.
21. Toussaint M, Gonçalves M, Chatwin M. Effects of mechanical insufflation-exsufflation on the breathing pattern in stable subjects with duchenne muscular dystrophy: a step in a wrong direction. Respir Care. 2019;64(2):235–6.
22. Philips R, deSilva B, Matrka L.Jet ventilation in obese patients undergoing airway surgery for subglottic and tracheal stenosis. Laryngoscope. 2018;128(8):1887–92.
23. Altun D, Çamcı E, Orhan-Sungur M, et al. High frequency jet ventilation during endolaryngeal surgery: Risk factors for complications. Auris Nasus Larynx. 2018;45(5):1047–52.
24. Buchan T, Walkden M, Jenkins K, et al. High-frequency jet ventilation during cryoablation of small renal tumours. Cardiovasc Intervent Radiol. 2018;41(7):1067–73.
25. Bialka S, Copik M, Rybczyk K, et al. Assessment of changes of regional ventilation distribution in the lung tissue depending on the driving pressure applied during high frequency jet ventilation. BMC Anesthesiol. 2018;18(1):101.
26. Abedini A, Kiani A, Taghavi K, et al. High-frequency jet ventilation in nonintubated patients. Turk Thorac J. 2018;19(3):127–31.
27. Engstrand J, Toporek G, Harbut P, et al. Stereotactic CT-guided percutaneous microwave ablation of liver tumors with the use of high-frequency jet ventilation: An accuracy and procedural safety study. AJR Am J Roentgenol. 2017;208(1):193–200.
28. Mowes A, de Jongh BE, Cox T, et al. A translational cellular model to study the impact of high- frequency oscillatory ventilation on human epithelial cell function. J Appl Physiol (1985). 2017;122(1):198–205.
29. Barry RA, Fink DS, Pourciau DC, et al. Effect of increased body mass index on complication rates during laryngotracheal surgery utilizing jet ventilation. Otolaryngol Head Neck Surg. 2017;157(3):473–7.
30. Mokra D, Kosutova P, Balentova S, et al. Effects of budesonide on the lung functions, inflammation and apoptosis in a saline-lavage model of acute lung injury. J Physiol Pharmacol. 2016;67(6):919–32.
31. Wheeler CR, Smallwood CD, O'Donnell I, et al. Assessing initial response to high-frequency jet ventilation in premature infants with hypercapnic respiratory failure. Respir Care. 2017;62(7):867–72.
32. Carpi MF. High-frequency jet ventilation in preterm infants: Is there still room for it? Respir Care. 2017;62(7):997–8.
33. Yang ZY, Meng Q, Wei HF, et al. Supraglottic jet oxygenation and ventilation during colonoscopy under monitored anesthesia care: a controlled randomized clinical trial. Eur Rev Med Pharmacol Sci. 2016;20:1168–73.
34. Liang H, Hou Y, Wei H, Feng Y. Supraglottic jet oxygenation and ventilation assisted fiberoptic intubation in a paralyzed patient with morbid obesity and obstructive sleep apnea: a case report. BMC Anesthesiol. 2019;19(1):40.
35. Doğanay F, Ak R, Alışkan H, et al. The effects of intravenous lipid emulsion therapy in the prevention of depressive effects of propofol on cardiovascular and respiratory systems: An experimental animal study. Medicina (Kaunas). 2018;55(1):1–10.

26

Case report of neonate Pierre Robin sequence with severe upper airway obstruction who was rescued by finger guide intubation

Li Zhang, Jian Fei*⬦, Jian Jia, Xiaohua Shi, Meimin Qu and Hui Wang

Abstract

Background: Pierre Robin Sequence (PRS) patients are known for their triad of micrognathia, glossoptosis, and airway obstruction. Their airway can be a challenge even for the most experienced pediatric anesthesiologist.

Case presentation: We report the case of a 9 day old 3.5 kg boy diagnosed with PRS, cleft palate, and a vallecular cyst with severe upper airway obstruction. The combination of PRS, cleft palate and the presence of vallecular cyst made this a cascade reaction of difficult airway. Due to his unique anatomy, we didn't appreciate how difficult his airway was until multiple attempts with high-tech equipment failed. Ultimately it was the finger guide intubation, this old technique without any equipment, that rescued this patient from lose of airway.

Conclusions: The boy was successfully rescued by finger guided intubation. Finger guide intubation should be added to the anesthesiologist's newborn rescue intubation training.

Keywords: Pierre Robin sequence, Upper airway obstruction, Finger guide intubation

Background

Pierre Robin Sequence(PRS)patients are known for their triad of micrognathia, glossoptosis, and airway obstruction [1]. In addition to positioning and nasal pharyngeal airway (NPA), newborns with PRS may require surgical treatments including tongue lip adhesion (TLA), mandibular distraction osteogenesis (MDO), subperiosteal release of the floor of the mouth (SPRFM), tracheostomy if their airway obstruction deteriorates or they failure to thrive [2]. To have those procedures done, their airway need to be secured first. Their airway can be a challenge even for the most experienced pediatric anesthesiologist. We describe the case of an anatomical abnormality associated with PRS which complicated attempts at airway management, and the ultimate technique that enabled placement of an endotracheal tube.

* Correspondence: 18951769690@189.cn
Department of Anesthesiology, Children's Hospital of Nanjing Medical University, Nanjing 210008, Jiangsu Province, China

Case presentation

A 9 day old 3.5 kg boy was referred to our tertiary care hospital with diagnosed of PRS. Other than atrial septal defect (ASD), aspiration pneumonia and unilateral complete cleft palate with a maximum width of about 0.8 cm. There are no cleft lip or alveolar cleft or any other comorbidity. Upon admission, he presented with cyanosis with venous carbon dioxide pressure (PvCO$_2$) 87.8 mmHg, multiple bedside direct laryngoscopy and GlideScope (UE Medical, China) attempts were made however none were successful. His saturation was improved to 95% by facial mask. The next morning he had thin sliced Computed Tomography (CT, Philips) with craniofacial as well as airway reconstruction (Fig. 1a, b).

The same night he deteriorated again. We attempted intubation with GlideScope which revealed grade 4 view. Next we tried a blind intubation with endotracheal tube loaded with stylet, however, this failed as well. Then we tried size 1 laryngeal mask airway (LMA, Well Lead Medical, China), however, we felt the LMA was blocked by an occupying lesion at the left side of tongue's base

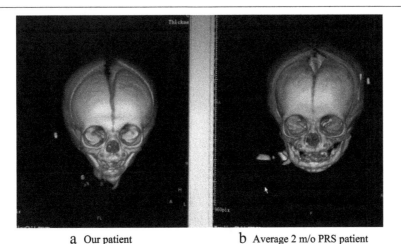

a Our patient   b Average 2 m/o PRS patient

Fig. 1 a shows the Craniofacial CT reconstruction of our patient. **b** shows the Craniofacial CT reconstruction of a normal 2-months-old PRS patient

so we decided not to force it through for fear it might further aggravate his airway. His respiratory distress was improved after we placed a NPA and saturation returned to 100%.

The third morning he was brought to operating room for MDO placement. After giving Penehyclidine to dry his secretion, we slowed dialed Sevoflurane to 6% then back to 3% to maintain his spontaneous breathing. Placement of a glidescope revealed no identifiable glottic structures. Fiberoptic scope (Olympus, Japan) revealed the epiglottis lying on the posterior pharynx, which could not be maneuvered beneath. Size 1 LMA and lighted wand (CLARUS Medical, MN) cannot be placed in the right place, multiple attempts with high-tech equipment failed to establish his airway. Since NPA could maintain his saturation, we decided to abort the procedure. Upon arrival in surgery intensive care unit (SICU), his $PvCO_2$ was 119.4 mmHg. A TLA procedure was performed with sedation. The fourth night his $PvCO_2$ was elevated to 183.8 mmHg. We reviewed his airway CT again with a different radiologist. We found he had large lesion with size of 21.1 mm X 11.7 mm occupying his base of tongue extending from left all the way to middle. Most likely it was thyroglossal cyst per the second radiologist. (Fig. 2a, b).

Knowing his hypercarbia could get even worse, on day 5 we brought him back to the operating room. After inducing patient with ketamine and sevoflurane, operator

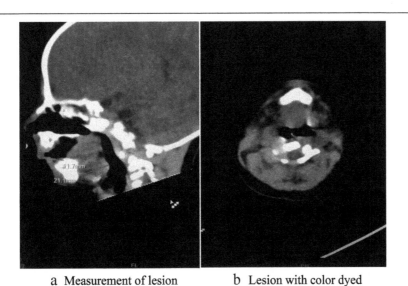

a Measurement of lesion   b Lesion with color dyed

Fig. 2 a shows the airway CT of our patient. we found he had large lesion with size of 21.1 mm X 11.7 mm occupying his base of tongue extending from left all the way to middle. **b** shows the same lesion with color dyed

gloved then advanced nondominant middle finger along the tongue, once patient's epiglottis was touched, middle finger was bent slightly to lift epiglottis, dominant hand then passed the lubricated and bent endotracheal tube based on 3D reconstruction right next to the middle finger into his trachea. Tube position was confirmed with capnography with endotidal CO_2 of 120 mmHg. Once airway secured, patient had MDO procedure without any problem. He was sent back to SICU and successfully extubated there on postoperative day 5.

Discussion

The concept of finger guide intubation was first described in 1543 when Vesalius mentioned how to place a tube into the trachea for control of ventilation. In 1941 Ross and Strong reported using this concept for neonatal resuscitation. Sensing it was not gaining traction among clinicians, in 1968 Woody and Woody advocating this technique again arguing in experienced hands it only took 3–5 s [3]. In 1992 Hancock reported their experiences with finger intubation in newborns and stated it was their preferred method of intubation among physician or nurse once learned [4]. In 2011 Xue pointed out that finger guided intubation in newborns and infants with difficult airways is a possible ignored technique [5].

Nanjing Children's hospital is one of the largest PRS treatment centers in China. In 2017 alone, we treated 225 patients with PRS including 8 neonates, 24 infants aged 1~3 months, 54 infants aged 3~6 months, as well as 98 infants aged 6~12 months. We are well versed in direct laryngoscopy as well as all advanced airway equipment such as GlideScope, fiberoptic scope, lighted wand, LMA or combination of those instruments. This patient was born by G4P3 mother with 2 normal siblings. We didn't anticipate too much of difficulty when it was time to secure his airway thinking he was just another patient with PRS. The combination of PRS, cleft palate and the presence of vallecular cyst made this into a cascade reaction of difficult airway. The cyst pushed patient's epiglottis downward which almost completely obscured the view of patient's vocal cord. Direct laryngoscopy, glidescope, size 1 LMA, fiberoptic scope as well as lighted wand all failed to establish his airway. Ultimately it was the finger guide intubation, this old technique without any equipment, that eventually rescued this patient from lose of airway. Tracheostomy would have been plan B had digital intubation failed, however, tracheostomy has its own complication such as sudden airway obstruction from accidental decannulation, or mucous plugging; airway infections, tracheal obstruction and inhibition of proper speech and swallowing development.

After this, we made a point to teach this technique to our trainees and junior attending physicians. The contents of the course include guided learning in neonates with normal anatomy/abnormal anatomy and guided learning using manikin models. Familiarity with the technique makes it possible to quickly confirm intubation where unexpected anatomic abnormalities emerges with no immediate availability of hightech airway equipment. Sometimes neonates born with meconium aspiration are hard to be intubated due to poor visualization because of meconium soiling of larynx. Likewise, in ruptured airway vascular abnormality, digital intubation might be the only means to secure patient's airway when blood gushing out of patient's mouth. For newborns, the fingers are more flexible than the laryngoscope therefore easier to touch the position of the epiglottis. Plus, there is no need to stoop or bend to adjust eye level, no need for equipment not even lighting source. Having said that, an obvious limitation factor for newborns is the size (airway versus clinician's finger), it might be very difficult to do digital intubation by a beefy hand trying to negotiate inside a neonate's very small upper airway.

At a tertiary Children's Hospital specialized in treating pediatric Pierre Robin Sequence, we had to resort to old fashioned digital intubation to finally secure the airway of this PRS neonate due to unique anatomy. Therefore, perhaps there should be a role of this technique so future anesthesia providers will have one more weapon in their armamentarium of airway management. The anesthesiologist's newborn rescue intubation training should include the finger guide intubation.

Abbreviations

ASD: Atrial septal defect; CT: Computed tomography; LMA: Laryngeal mask airway; MDO: Mandibular distraction osteogenesis; NPA: Nasal pharyngeal airway; PRS: Pierre robin sequence; PvCO2: Venous carbon dioxide pressure; SICU: Surgery intensive care unit; SPRFM: Subperiosteal release of the floor of the mouth; TLA: Tongue lip adhesion

Acknowledgements

We want to thank Dr. John Wei Zhong from Children's Medical Center Dallas, for his helps not only on proof reading our manuscript with standard English language, but also on giving essential comments to improve our work.

Authors' contributions

LZ performed the data analyses and wrote the manuscript. JF conceived of the study. XS helped perform the analysis with constructive discussions. JJ and MQ helped the data collection. HW participated in the work's design and coordination. All authors read and approved the final manuscript.

References

1. Bookman LB, Melton KR, Pan BS, et al. Neonates with tongue-based airway obstruction: a systematic review. Otolaryngol Head Neck Surg. 2012;146:8–18.
2. Cladis FP, Kumar AR, Grunwaldt LJ, et al. Pierre Robin sequence: a perioperative review. Anesth Analg. 2014;119:400–12.
3. Woody NC, Woody HB. Direct digital intratracheal intubation for neonatal resuscitation. J Pediatr. 1968;73:903–5.
4. Hancock PJ, Peterson G. Finger intubation of the trachea in newborns. Pediatrics. 1992;89:325–6.
5. Shan XF, Ping LH, Liao X, et al. Finger guided intubation in newborns and infants with difficult airways: a possible ignored technique. Paediatr Anaesth. 2011;21:701–2.

27

Ultrasound-guided versus Shikani optical stylet-aided tracheal intubation

Yuanyuan Ma[1], Yan Wang[1,2*], Ping Shi[1], Xue Cao[1] and Shengjin Ge[1*] ⓘ

Abstract

Background: To compare ultrasound-guided tracheal intubation (UGTI) versus Shikani optical stylet (SOS)-aided tracheal intubation in patients with anticipated normal airway.

Methods: Sixty patients aged 18–65 years old who presented for elective surgery under general anesthesia were recruited in this prospective randomized study. They were assigned into two equal groups, either an ultrasound-guided group (Group UG, $n = 30$) or an SOS-aided group (Group SOS, $n = 30$). After the induction of anesthesia, the tracheal intubation was performed by a specified skilled anesthesiologist. The number of tracheal intubation attempt and the duration of successful intubation on the first attempt were recorded. Complications relative to tracheal intubation including desaturation, hoarseness and sore throat were also recorded.

Results: The first-attempt success rate is 93.3% (28/30) in Group UG and 90% (27/30) in Group SOS ($P = 0.640$). The second-attempt was all successful for the 2 and 3 patients left in the two groups, and the overall success rate of both groups was 100%. The duration of successful intubation on the first attempt of Group UG was not significantly different from that of Group SOS (34.0 ± 20.8 s vs 35.5 ± 23.2 s, $P = 0.784$). One patient in Group SOS had desaturation ($P = 0.313$), and there was none hoarseness in the two groups. Sore throat was detected in both group (4 in Group UG, 5 in Group SOS, $P = 0.718$).

Conclusion: Ultrasound-guided tracheal intubation was as effective as Shikani optical stylet-aided tracheal intubation in adult patients with anticipated normal airway.

Keywords: Ultrasound, Shikani optical Stylet, Tracheal intubation, Anesthesia

Background

Nowadays, ultrasound is used to manage the airway in anesthesia and intensive care as a non-invasive tool. Real-time surface ultrasound-guided tracheal intubation (UGTI) was firstly reported by Fiadjoe et al. [1] on a 14-month-old child. They provided a new perspective of endotracheal intubation: from the outside rather than

the inside. Optical stylet is also a nonconventional intubation tool, which integrates flexible fiberoptic imaging features in a rigid intubating stylet. The Shikani optical stylet (SOS) (Clarus Medical, Minneapolis, MN) is one of the most commonly used fiberoptic stylets for intubation. It not only has the characteristics of a fiberoptic bronchoscope but also very light and convenient [2, 3]. UGTI and SOS-aided tracheal intubation have some similar manipulations in the intubation: opening the mouth with hands, placing the styletted tube, and inserting the tube with the guidance of ultrasound or light

* Correspondence: 53987816@qq.com; ge.shengjin@fudan.edu.cn
[1]Department of Anesthesia, Zhongshan Hospital, Fudan University, No. 180 Fenglin Road, Shanghai 200032, China

spot and optical stylet. And they are particularly effective for some special patients, who has limitation of mouth opening or difficult visualization of the airway obscured by secretions or blood.

The purpose of this study was to compare UGTI with SOS-aided tracheal intubation in patients with anticipated normal airway undergoing elective surgery under general anesthesia.

Methods

Ethics approval and registration

This prospective randomized study was approved by the Ethical Committee of Zhongshan Hospital, Fudan University (Approval No: B2016-099R). The study was registered at chictr.org.cn (ChiCTR-IIC-17010875). Written informed consent was obtained from all participants.

Patient population

This study adhered to CONSORT guidelines for randomized trials. Sixty patients aged 18–65 years old who presented for elective surgery under general anesthesia were recruited at Zhongshan Hospital, Fudan University. Inclusion criteria included a body mass index (BMI) of 18.5–25 $kg \cdot m^{-2}$, American Society of Anesthesiologists (ASA) physical status I-II, and Mallampati Grade I-II. Exclusion criteria included any sign of difficult airway such as mouth and neck mass or infection, allergy to the study drugs, drug or alcohol abuse, and pregnancy.

Anesthetic technique

Using a computer-generated table and a sealed envelope with sequence of numbers, patients were randomly divided into two equal groups: an ultrasound-guided group (Group UG, $n = 30$) and an SOS group (Group SOS, $n = 30$).

A specified attending anesthesiologist conducted the pre-anesthetic interview to the patients. All participants were fasting according to the rules of Zhongshan Hospital without preoperative medications. After patients arrived at the operating room, an 18G peripheral venous catheter was established, and oxygen ($8 L \cdot min^{-1}$) was supplemented via face mask. Intraoperative monitoring included pulse oxygen saturation (SpO_2), electrocardiogram (lead II and V_5), heart rate, noninvasive blood pressure, and capnography.

After pure oxygen with a flow rate of $8 L \cdot min^{-1}$ was inhaled for 3 min via a sealed mask, plasma target-controlled infusion of propofol 4 $\mu g \cdot ml^{-1}$, intravenous fentanyl 2 $\mu g \cdot kg^{-1}$, remifentanil 0.2 $\mu g \cdot kg^{-1} \cdot min^{-1}$ and dexamethasone 5 mg were given. After loss of consciousness, rocuronium 0.6 $mg \cdot kg^{-1}$ and lidocaine 1.5 $mg \cdot kg^{-1}$ were administered. Ninety seconds later, the tracheal intubation was carried out according to the randomly

allocation by a specified anesthesiologist who had performed UGTI or SOS-aided tracheal intubation for more than 50 times, respectively.

Before the manipulation of tracheal intubation in the two groups, the ready-to-use stylet was lubricated and bent to imitate the shape and structure of the airway from the central incisors to the cricoid cartilage, then an endotracheal tube (7.0 mm ID for female, 7.5 mm ID for male) was mounted on it.

Group UG

A 6–13 MHz linear ultrasound probe (Sonosite EDGE ultrasound) was put transversely on the patient's neck at the level of the cricothyroid membrane to guide intubation. The probe cloud been moved cephalad to obtain a clear image of the vocal cords that were shown as an isosceles triangle with a central tracheal shadow. The specified anesthesiologist opened patient's mouth and maintained manual inline stabilization and jaw thrust while inserting the pre-shaped styletted tracheal tube. The tube should be kept in the midline of the mouth during the operation. Hypoechoic shadowing and widening of the vocal cords were the certification of successful placement of the tube into the trachea. When the tube was to be stuck in the midline using the ultrasound, then it was withdrawn outside from the mouth and reshaped by bending its tip downwards. Once the tracheal tube passed posterolateral of the airway to the esophagus which was a hyperechoic structure with posterior shadowing in the image of ultrasound, it should be withdrawn. Then, the tip of tube required to be bent upwards and then reinserted [1, 4].

Group SOS

The specified anesthesiologist held and elevated the mandible using the left hand; the stylet was introduced from the right side of the mouth. Thereafter, a significant light spot was seen through the front of neck, the tip was inserted into the glottis under direct vision, the "tube stop" was released. The tube was uninstalled into the trachea, then the stylet was removed.

After the correct position of the tube was confirmed by the end-tidal of carbon dioxide ($ETCO_2$) monitoring and stethoscope, the anesthesia machine was connected and parameters were set to maintain the partial pressure of $ETCO_2$ at 30–40 mmHg. The failure of intubation attempt defined as the time > 180 s or desaturation ($SpO_2 < 93\%$). To ensure patient safety, the intubation attempt must be stopped and ventilated with pure oxygen for 3 min to perform another attempt. Failure of intubation was considered as 2 failed attempts of insertion, then intubation was executed with a ready video laryngoscope.

The time of the intubation was from passage of the mounted tracheal tube between the teeth until the tracheal tube was confirmed in place by the capnography, and the number of tracheal intubation attempt were recorded. Complications relative to tracheal intubation including desaturation, hoarseness and sore throat were also recorded.

Data collection

Our null hypothesis was: the success rate of UGTI at the first attempt is equal to that of SOS-aided tracheal intubation in patients with anticipated normal airway undergoing elective surgery under general anesthesia. Then, the primary outcome was to compare the success rate of intubation of the two groups on the first attempt. The secondary outcomes were to detect the overall success rate, the time of the intubation with a first-attempt success, and complications related to each method, such as desaturation and trauma.

The sample size was calculated using the PASS software version 11: Two-Sample T-Test Power Analysis. It was estimated that a sample size of 34 patients ($n_1 = n_2 = 17$) would achieve a power of 80% ($\beta = 0.2$) to detect a clinical significant difference of 5% with standard deviations of 5% between the two groups as regards the success rates at the first attempt using a T-Test with significance level at 0.05 ($\alpha = 0.05$).

Statistical analysis

Data were analyzed by using IBM SPSS version 24 software. Qualitative data were described using number and were compared using the Chi-square test and the Fisher exact test, whereas normally distributed quantitative data were expressed as mean ± SD and were compared using T-Test for two independent groups, non-normally distributed quantitative data were expressed as median (Inter-Quartile Range) and were compared using Mann-Whitney U test. $P < 0.05$ was considered statistically significant.

Results

Demographic data in both groups are presented in Table 1. There was no statistically significant difference between the two groups about demographics including sex, age, height, weigh (P = 0.301, 0.273, 0.835, and 0.726, respectively).

The first-attempt success rate is 28/30 in Group UG and is 27/30 in Group SOS ($P = 0.640$). The reason of the failure at the first-attempt in both 2 patients in the two groups was taking time > 180 s, and in another 1 patient in Group SOS was $SpO_2 < 93\%$. The second-attempts were all successful for the 2 and 3 patients left in the two groups ($P = 0.640$), then the overall success rate of both groups was 100%. Comparing the time of the intubation with a first-attempt success between the two groups, there was no significant difference (34.0 ± 20.8 s in Group UG and 35.5 ± 23.2 s in Group SOS, respectively) with a P value of 0.784.

All patients successfully underwent the intraoperative period and were extubated uneventfully at the end of the operations. One patient in Group SOS had desaturation ($P = 0.313$), none hoarseness happened, and sore throat was observed in 4 patients (13.3%) in Group UG and 5 (16.7%) in Group SOS ($P = 0.718$).

Discussion

At present, there are many kinds of endotracheal intubation assistant tools, the most used are video laryngoscope (bladed laryngoscope) and ordinary direct laryngoscope. In the treatment of difficult airway, the flexible fiberoptic bronchoscope is the classical and universally accepted choice. Optical stylets integrate flexible fiberoptic imaging features in a rigid intubating stylet. Not only can it be applied to normal airway intubation, but also shows the prospect of assisting difficult intubations. The SOS, one of the most used intubating fiberoptic stylets, has the unique advantages and characteristics. Firstly, it has a portable and reusable scope with a shapeable stainless-steel stylet and adjustable tube stop. Secondly, a special port allowed to delivery oxygen to the patient. Furthermore, the high-resolution eyepiece with light source can be used independently, or connected with a camera or a monitor. It has been widely used in clinic because of its fast, effective and little effect on hemodynamics [2, 3].

Ultrasound technology is more and more used in clinical anesthesia due to its safe, reliable, repeatable and easy to realize characteristics. In the case of endotracheal intubation, using ultrasound image, we can determine the endotracheal tube size [5–7], observe the position of cricothyroid membrane and glottis [1, 4, 5, 8], guide tracheal intubation [1, 4, 5], judge whether the tracheal tube enters the trachea [1, 4, 5, 9], and judge whether

Table 1 Demographic data in the two groups

Group	n	M/F	Age (years old)	Height (cm)	Weight (kg)	Mallampati Grade (I / II)
UG	30	16/14	49.3 ± 11.3	164.7 ± 8.6	63.6 ± 10.8	15/15
SOS	30	12/18	45.8 ± 13.1	164.3 ± 7.5	62.6 ± 11.2	15/15

the position of tracheal tube is correct [5, 10–12]. At present, portable ultrasound is the standard equipment in many hospitals, which is easy to get, and is very suitable for promotion and application in basic hospitals.

UGTI is still a relatively new method in China and aboard. As mentioned above, real-time surface UGTI and SOS-aided tracheal intubation are similar in their operational procedures and applicable patients. To our knowledge, there is no study comparing these two methods. The purpose of this study is to compare UGTI with SOS-aided tracheal intubation, to explore the feasibility and practicability of UGTI, and to provide reference for clinical airway management. As the results showed, both ultrasound and SOS were successfully applied to endotracheal intubation with comparable first-attempt success rate and time for tracheal intubation.

In this study, we selected the anesthetized adult patients with normal airways to perform UGTI. We found that the tracheal tube and stylet were not hyperechoic, but their characteristic hypoechoic shadow in the pharynx could be immediately identified and then guided into the trachea with ultrasonography. The characteristic of UGTI is to be guided by the external view of the airway rather than the internal visualization of the airway. What's more, the operator could evaluate the relationship between the tracheal tube tube with the glottic structures in the whole process of intubation. The visual information of ultrasound could assist to identify the location of the resistance either on the arytenoid cartilages or the vocal cords during advancing the styletted tube. Then, the operator could make some adjustments to bypass the resistance [1, 4, 5].

There are some limitations of UGTI. Firstly, two anesthesiologists are required to complete UGTI, one of them to obtain ultrasound visualization and the other to intubate. Secondly, the poor ultrasound images might affect its application. Thirdly, it is necessary for the operator to have the basic knowledge of ultrasound machine in order to perform the typical controls and adjustments. Notably, it is essential to conduct clinical training in visualization of the airway structures and sonographic features of successful tracheal intubation using ultrasound before attempting UGTI [4]. Fourthly, further evaluation is required to determine the optimal stylet structure, although the stylet has been bent to simulate the shape of airway from the central incisors to the cricoid cartilage. Fifthly, this technique has the potential for airway injury, although accurate the ultrasound image was necessary for correct intubation. Regardless of the intubation method, the anesthesiologist should stop inserting the tracheal tube once resistance appeared. Inappropriate strength might increase the risk of airway injury during the procedure of intubation. Sixthly, it is worth mentioning that experience and

capability are critical to the successful of any techniques in clinical application. In terms of the possible bias in a randomized controlled trial, the operators must be able to be proficient in the techniques studied [13], even all of the tracheal intubation in this study were performed by a specified anesthesiologist who were skilled in using the ultrasound and SOS in tracheal intubation. Finally, this study was performed in a single center on a relatively small number of patients and the results need to be confirmed by multicenter studies.

Conclusions
This study validated that ultrasound-guided tracheal intubation was as effective as Shikani optical stylet-aided tracheal intubation in patients with anticipated normal airway.

Acknowledgements
The authors acknowledge the staff of anesthesia nurses at the department of Anesthesia, ZhongShan Hospital, Fudan University.

Authors' contributions
All authors have read and approved the final manuscript. YYM, YW and SJG conceived and designed the study. YW performed the statistical analyses. YYM wrote the first draft of the manuscript, which was revised by SJG. YYM, YW, PS, XC, SJG participated in data collection.

Author details
[1]Department of Anesthesia, Zhongshan Hospital, Fudan University, No. 180 Fenglin Road, Shanghai 200032, China. [2]Kashgar Regional Second People's Hospital, Kashi City, Xinjiang Uygur Autonomous Region, China.

References
1. Fiadjoe JE, Stricker P, Gurnaney H, Nishisaki A, Rabinowitz A, Gurwitz A, McCloskey JJ, Ganesh A. Ultrasound-guided tracheal intubation: a novel intubation technique. Anesthesiology. 2012;117(6):1389–91.
2. Mahrous RSS, Ahmed AMM. The Shikani optical stylet as an alternative to awake fiberoptic intubation in patients at risk of secondary cervical spine injury: a randomized controlled trial. J Neurosurg Anesthesiol. 2018;30(4): 354–8.
3. Phua DS, Mah CL, Wang CF. The Shikani optical stylet as an alternative to the GlideScope(R) videolaryngoscope in simulated difficult intubations--a randomised controlled trial. Anaesthesia. 2012;67(4):402–6.
4. Moustafa MA, Arida EA, Zanaty OM, El-Tamboly SF. Endotracheal intubation: ultrasound-guided versus fiberscope in patients with cervical spine immobilization. J Anesth. 2017;31(6):846–51.
5. Osman A, Sum KM. Role of upper airway ultrasound in airway management. J Intensive Care. 2016;4:52.
6. Gupta K, Gupta PK, Rastogi B, Krishan A, Jain M, Garg G. Assessment of the subglottic region by ultrasonography for estimation of appropriate size endotracheal tube: a clinical prospective study. Anesth Essays Res. 2012;6(2): 157–60.
7. Pillai R, Kumaran S, Jeyaseelan L, George SP, Sahajanandan R. Usefulness of ultrasound-guided measurement of minimal transverse diameter of subglottic airway in determining the endotracheal tube size in children with congenital heart disease: a prospective observational study. Ann Card Anaesth. 2018;21(4):382–7.
8. You-Ten KE, Wong DT, Ye XY, Arzola C, Zand A, Siddiqui N. Practice of ultrasound-guided palpation of neck landmarks improves accuracy of external palpation of the cricothyroid membrane. Anesth Analg. 2018;127(6): 1377–82.
9. Muslu B, Sert H, Kaya A, et al. Use of sonography for rapid identification of esophageal and tracheal intubations in adult patients. J Ultrasound Med. 2011;30(5):671–6.

10. Chun R, Kirkpatrick AW, Sirois M, et al. Where's the tube? Evaluation of hand-held ultrasound in confirming endotracheal tube placement. Prehosp Disaster Med. 2004;19(4):366–9.

11. Blaivas M, Tsung JW. Point-of-care sonographic detection of left endobronchial main stem intubation and obstruction versus endotracheal intubation. J Ultrasound Med. 2008;27(5):785–9.

12. Hosseini JS, Talebian MT, Ghafari MH, et al. Secondary confirmation of endotracheal tube position by diaphragm motion in right subcostal ultrasound view. Int J Crit Illn Inj Sci. 2013;3(2):113–7.

13. Wang SY, Xue FS, Liu YY. Comparing ultrasound-guided and fiberscope-guided intubation. J Anesth. 2018;32(1):147.

28

Emergent airway management outside of the operating room: A retrospective review of patient characteristics, complications and ICU stay

Uzung Yoon[1]*[iD], Jeffrey Mojica[1], Matthew Wiltshire[1], Kara Segna[2], Michael Block[1], Anthony Pantoja[1], Marc Torjman[1] and Elizabeth Wolo[1]

Abstract

Background: Emergent airway management outside of the operating room is a high-risk procedure. Limited data exists about the indication and physiologic state of the patient at the time of intubation, the location in which it occurs, or patient outcomes afterward.

Methods: We retrospectively collected data on all emergent airway management interventions performed outside of the operating room over a 6-month period. Documentation included intubation performance, and intubation related complications and mortality. Additional information including demographics, ASA-classification, comorbidities, hospital-stay, ICU-stay, and 30-day in-hospital mortality was obtained.

Results: 336 intubations were performed in 275 patients during the six-month period. The majority of intubations ($n = 196$, 58%) occurred in an ICU setting, and the rest 140 (42%) occurred on a normal floor or in a remote location. The mean admission ASA status was 3.6 ± 0.5, age 60 ± 16 years, and BMI 30 ± 9 kg/m^2. Chest X-rays performed immediately after intubation showed main stem intubation in 3.3% ($n = 9$). Two immediate (within 20 min after intubation) intubation related cardiac arrest/mortality events were identified. The 30-day in-hospital mortality was 31.6% ($n = 87$), the overall in-hospital mortality was 37.1% ($n = 102$), the mean hospital stay was 22 ± 20 days, and the mean ICU-stay was 14 days (13.9 ± 0.9, CI 12.1–15.8) with a 7.3% ICU-readmission rate.

Conclusion: Patients requiring emergent airway management are a high-risk patient population with multiple comorbidities and high ASA scores on admission. Only a small number of intubation-related complications were reported but ICU length of stay was high.

Keywords: Emergent airway, Outside the operating room, Intubation, Mortality, Cardiac arrest

Background

Emergent airway management is required outside of the operating room (OR) in every hospital setting. It is an inherently higher risk procedure when compared to controlled OR settings [1]. In the OR, most intubations are done under an elective, controlled environment and under supervision of attending anaesthesiologists. Intubations outside of the OR are performed under less ideal conditions which can lack appropriate personnel, equipment and monitoring devices. Outside OR intubations are performed in the ICU, general floor, emergency room or remote locations. Very little is known about the number of intubations performed and subsequent outcome of those patients.

Patients requiring emergent intubation are frequently hemodynamically unstable, hypoxic, and rarely NPO. History, physical exam, and information handoff by the primary care team is often incomplete or limited in an emergent airway setting. There is also limited time to perform an adequate airway exam.

* Correspondence: uzyoon@gmail.com
[1]Department of Anesthesiology, Thomas Jefferson University Hospital, Suite 8290 Gibbon, 111 South 11th Street, Philadelphia PA 19107, USA

Emergent intubation complications often result from compromised patient's physiologic status, limited reserve, limited airway evaluation, difficult airway management, and inability to pre-oxygenate the patient. A 3% mortality rate within 30 min of intubation has been reported in the intensive care unit (ICU) setting [2]. Several studies have documented an 8–12% incidence of difficult intubation in the emergent setting [3–5] compared to an incidence of 5.8% during elective intubation in the OR [6].

Limited data exist about outside OR intubations including patient comorbidity on admission and physiologic state at the time of intubation and shortly thereafter. Also little is known about the length of ICU-stay and in-hospital mortality of those patient population.

The objective of this study was to evaluate the patient characteristics, intubation performance and outcome after emergent airway management occurring outside of the OR.

Methods

Following institutional review board approval and waived consent, data for all airway intubations were collected retrospectively over a 6-month period. At our institution, the anaesthesiology department is responsible for all airway management outside of the OR except in the emergency department. This includes the acute care floors (587 beds), medical-ICU (23 beds), surgical-ICU (17 beds), cardiac-ICU (17 beds), neurosurgery-ICU (14 beds), and remote locations (CT, MRI, cardiac-catheterization-laboratory, interventional-radiology, endoscopy).

The airway response resident responded to the emergent airway when there is a page received to an emergency pager. This included code blue, rapid response (RRT), Anaesthesia STAT, level 1 trauma, or elective intubation request which were defined as:

Code blue was announced for cardiopulmonary arrest or other life-threatening events.

RRT was announced for non-life threatening but significant change in physiologic status and/or vital signs that requires urgent intervention by the RRT team. Anesthesia STAT was announced for urgent intubation in a hemodynamically stabile patient. (e.g. self extubation, GI bleeding). Elective intubation was announced in patients with stable vital signs requiring non-urgent intubation (e.g. elective procedure outside of the OR, anticipation of potential respiratory failure, airway protection).

Level 1 trauma was announced for injury with signs of shock or respiratory distress, penetrating injury to head, neck, torso, fascial or neck injury with actual or potential airway compromise or traumatic cardiac arrest.

For intubation an anaesthesia attending and/or any training level resident was available for assistance in airway management. The induction medication kit was centralized by pharmacy and brought by the nursing staff to the bedside. Induction kit medications contained etomidate, rocuronium, succinylcholine, phenylephrine, and ephedrine. Sugammadex was not available at this time as part of the standard induction medication kit.

Intubation was confirmed by 6 breath trial capnometer color change and bilateral breath sounds. After intubation, documentation was completed by the anaesthesia resident performing or supervising the intubation. Defined data points were time of intubation, location, indication for intubation, number of attempts, laryngoscopic view, $ETCO_2$ detection, medication use, vital signs, and complications. Additionally, we retrospectively performed a complete search of the electronic health and imaging records for every intubated patient.

Immediate intubation-related mortality was defined as the event that occurred during or within 30 min of intubation without clear indication of other causes. Extubation was defined as either endotracheal extubation or tracheostomy placement. The primary outcome measure of the study was immediate intubation related complication and mortality (< 30 min). Secondary outcome measures were ICU stay, ICU readmission rate, hospital stay, 30-day in-hospital mortality. Additionally, demographics including age, sex, BMI, ASA status and comorbidity were collected on initial admission. No recalculation was performed for patients who had reintubation events. Cerebral performance category was upon cischarge was calculated to measure the extent and severity of neurological impairment and disability (1. Full recovery, 2. Moderate cerebral disability but independent in activities of daily living 3. Severe cerebral disability, dependent in activities of daily living, 4. Persistent vegetative state, 5. Brain dead).

Arithmetic mean, standard deviations, and 95% confidence intervals was used to report the patient's demographics. Data were also reported as medians with interquartile range (IQR) when indicated. Statistical analyses were performed using Chi-Square, Fisher, and independent 2 tailed t-tests. Systat (Systat Software Inc., San Jose, CA) version 13 software was used.

Results
Demographics and clinical details
Data for 352 emergent intubations were collected and reviewed. Due to lack of documentation, 16 patients were excluded. The final analysis included 336 intubations in 275 patients during the 6-month period. Reintubation occurred in 51 patients (18.5%). Overall 58% of the patients were male aged 59 ± 15 years with a mean admission ASA status of 3.6 ± 0.5 and BMI if $30 \pm 9 \text{ kg/m}^2$ (Table 1). The most common comorbidity was hypertension, followed by sepsis, hyperlipidaemia, and malignancy (Fig. 1). Airway management was requested for the

Table 1 Characteristics of patients requiring emergent intubation outside the OR. (*n* = 275)

Demographics	
Age (years)	59.4 ± 15.4
Male	159 (57.8%)
Female	116 (42.2%)
Ethnicity	
White	179 (65.1%)
Black	65 (4.4%)
Hispanic	12 (1.5%)
Unknown	11 (23.6%)
Asian	4 (4%)
Height	169.7 ± 12.3 cm
Weight	86 ± 28.1 kg
BMI (overall)	30 ± 8.8 (kg/m^2)
< 18.5 (underweight)	12 (4.4%)
18.5–24.9 (normal)	73 (26.5%)
25–29.9 (overweight)	85 (30.9%)
30–34.9 (moderate obese)	50 (18.2%)
35–39.9 (severely obese)	23 (8.4%)
≥ 40 (very severely obese)	32 (11.6%)
ASA classification on admission	3.6 ± 0.5
ASA 1	1 (0.3%)
ASA 2	4 (1.5%)
ASA 3	94 (34%)
ASA 4	176 (64%)
ASA 5	0 (0%)
Comorbidity on admission	
Hypertension	163 (48.5%)
Sepsis	99 (29.5%)
Hyperlipidemia	87 (25.9%)
Malignancy	87 (25.9%)
Diabetes	78 (23.2%)
Chronic kidney disease	74 (22%)
Coronary artery disease	62 (18.5%)
Atrial fibrillation	50 (14.9%)
Congestive heart failure	47 (14%)
Cerebrovascular accident	47 (14%)
Acute hepatic failure	42 (12.5%)
Hemodialysis	38 (11.3%)
Myocardial infarction	36 (10.7%)
Seizure	34 (10.1%)
Hepatic encephalophaty	34 (10.1%)
Anticoagulation (active)	33 (9.8%)
Chronic obstructive lung disease	32 (9.5%)
Pulmonary embolism (history)	31 (9.2%)

Table 1 Characteristics of patients requiring emergent intubation outside the OR. (*n* = 275) *(Continued)*

Demographics	
Age (years)	59.4 ± 15.4
Pulmonary hypertension	31 (9.2%)
Gastroesophageal reflux disease	30 (8.9%)
Obstructive sleep apnea	17 (5.1%)
Pulmonary embolism (actively)	16 (4.8%)
Asthma	11 (3.3%)

following reasons: code blue (*n* = 28; 8.3%), rapid response team (*n* = 66; 19%), anaesthesia STAT (*n* = 106; 31.5%), and urgent intubation (*n* = 137; 40.8%). More than half of the intubations occurred in an ICU setting (*n* = 196; 58%), and the rest (*n* = 140; 42%) occurred on a normal floor or in a remote location.

Indication for intubation

The most common indication for intubation was acute respiratory failure in 254 (75.6%) patients, followed by the need for intubation to perform an urgent or elective procedure outside of the OR in 36 (10.7%), airway protection in 24 (7.1%), self extubation in 19 (5.7%), and endotracheal tube exchange in 3 (0.9%). Intubation performance included location, time of event, oxygenation upon arrival, induction, medication used, ventilation, intubation device, grade, attempt, difficulty, and placed ETT size (Table 2).

Post induction hemodynamics and intubation related complications

After induction, there was an average decrease of 2 mmHg (2.3 ± 1.6, CI – 5.3-0.8) in systolic blood pressure and an average increase in heart rate of 5 bpm (4.9 ± 1, CI 2.9–6.9) (Table 3). Chest X-rays performed immediately after intubation showed main stem intubations in 3.6% (*n* = 10). No dental injuries or unrecognized oesophageal intubations were identified. One new onset of a small apical pneumothorax was reported in one patient, with spontaneous resolution within 24 h. Intubation was atraumatic for most patients (*n* = 325; 96.7%). Intubation-related complications were reported in 5 (1.5%) of the intubated patients, and these complications consisted of: lip laceration (*n* = 2; 0.6%), tongue injury (*n* = 1; 0.3%), vomiting during induction (n = 1; 0.3%), and other (n = 1; 0.3%).

Immediate complication and mortality after intubation

Two immediate complications events occurred wihtin 30 min of intubation. The first patient experienced ventricular fibrillation arrest 4 min after intubation with a CPR time of 45 min until expiration. The patient had a history of cardiomyopathy, EF 45%, severe pulmonary

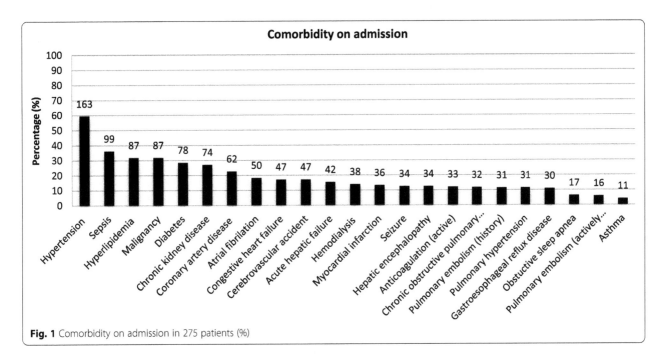

Fig. 1 Comorbidity on admission in 275 patients (%)

hypertension, COPD, coronary artery disease and was admitted for CHF exacerbation.

The second patient had pulseless electrical activity 17 min after intubation with a CPR time of 25 min until expiration. The patient had a history of non-ischemic cardiomyopathy status post multiple cardioversion, cryoablation and ICD placement, atrial fibrillation, aortic value replacement (for bicuspid aortic valve and aortic insufficiency), transient ischemic attack, and pericarditis. This patient was admitted with worsening heart failure, EF 15% complicated by stroke and ventricular tachycardia during their hospital stay.

Intubation related morbidity and in-hospital mortality

33 (12%) patients had newly diagnosed pneumonia after intubation, and 64 patients (23.3%) required a tracheostomy placement after an average of 9.2 ± 7.4 days of intubation. The 30-day in-hospital mortality was 31.6% (n = 87), the overall in-hospital mortality was 37.1% (n = 102), the mean hospital stay was 22 ± 20 days, and the mean ICU-stay was 14 days (13.9 ± 0.9, CI 12.1–15.8) with a 7.3% ICU-readmission rate (Table 4). The most common reason for death was multi-organ dysfunction followed by cardiac and respiratory reasons (Fig. 2).

Discussion

Intubation performance and difficult intubation

In this study, we found 88.1% of the intubations were accomplished on the first attempt. Stauffer et al. reported difficult airway management in 30% of intubations and Willich et al. in 20% [7, 8]. Martin et al. reported difficult airway management in 10% in of patients managed

outside of the OR [9]. Most likely the lower incidence in this study is explained by the extensive airway training and simulation program we perform to prepare physcians for emergent airway managements outside the OR. The importance of airway education for airway management outside th eopreating room has been described by Rochlen et al. [10] In general, repeated attempts at tracheal intubation should be avoided because they increase the incidence of airway obstruction, leading to serious airway complications [11, 12].

Intubation related complications

The immediate intubation-related outcome was low. Traumatic intubation was reported in only less than 1%. Our study showed bronchial intubation rate of 3.6%. The literature reports an ETT misplacement rate ranging from 4 to 28% [13–15]. Several studies have suggested inaccuracy of auscultation of bilateral breath sounds in determining proper ETT position. Anatomical variations such as large breasts, obesity, or barrel chests may make the assessment of auscultation and chest expansion more difficult. Additionally, with partial blockage of the mainstem bronchus breath sounds may be normal. To minimize the risk of bronchial intubation the top of the cuff should be seen to have just passed through the cords, the length of the tube noted at the lips and then secured. Cuff palpation at the sternal notch has been shown to effectively confirm ETT location [16]. Chest x-ray should be performed immediately after intubation to confirm the correct placement of the ETT.

Twelve percent of patients had newly diagnosed pneumonia after intubation. This could be due to the underlying

Table 2 Intubation performance (n = 336)

	Number of patients (N = 336)	Percentage (%)
Indication for Intubation		
Acute respiratory failure	254	(75.6%)
Need for intubation to perform an urgent or elective procedure outside of the OR	36	(10.7%)
Airway protection	24	(7.1%)
Self extubation	19	(5.7%)
Endotracheal tube exchange	3	(0.9%)
Location		
ICU	196	(58%)
Non ICU (ward, remote location, trauma room)	140	(42%)
Timing of events		
6:00 AM - 6:00 PM	193	(57.4%)
6:00 PM - 6:00 AM	139	(41.4%)
Attending Present	13	(3.9%)
Oxygenation (upon arrival to scene)		
Non rebreather face mask	118	(35.1%)
Nasal cannula	87	(25.9%)
Bag mask ventilation	50	(14.9%)
BIPAP (Bilevel Positive Airway Pressure)	42	(12.5%)
Room air	14	(4.2%)
CPAP (Continuous Positive Airway Pressure)	3	(0.9%)
Face tent	1	(0.3%)
Patient was already Intubated	1	(0.3%)
Not documented	20	(6%)
Induction		
Standard intravenous induction	131	(39.0%)
RSI (rapid sequence induction)	176	(52.4%)
Ventilation (after induction)		
Easy ventilation	162	(48.2%)
Easy with airway adjunct	55	(16.4%)
Moderate difficult with airway adjunct	10	(3.0%)
Difficult	4	(1.2%)
Two person ventilation	24	(7.1%)
Unable to ventilate	2	(0.6%)
Not indicated	91	(27.1%)
Cricoid Pressure applied	170	(50.6%)
Cricoid Pressure not applied	159	(47.3%)
Medication		
Etomidate	281	(83.6%)
Propofol	24	(7.1%)
Ketamine	1	(0.3%)
No sedation medication for induction	31	(9.2%)
Rocuronium	277	(82.4%)
Succinylcholine	28	(8.3%)
No muscle relaxant for induction	28	(8.3%)

Table 2 Intubation performance (n = 336) *(Continued)*

	Number of patients (N = 336)	Percentage (%)
Phenylephrine	40	(11.9%)
Ephedrine	4	(1.2%)
Other	5	(1.5%)
Intubation device		
Mac blade	236	(70.2%)
MAC 3	86	(36.4%)
MAC 4	144	(61.0%)
Not reported	6	(2.5%)
Miller	0	(0%)
Video laryngoscope	92	(27.4%)
Glidescope® blade 3	63	(68.5%)
Glidescope® blade 4	25	(27.2%)
Not reported	4	(4.3%)
Laryngeal Mask Airway (LMA)	1	(0.3%)
Awake fiberoptic	5	(1.5%)
Surgical Airway	2	(0.6%)
Bougie	2	(0.6%)
Intubation Grade (Cormack-Lehane Grading)		
Grade 1. Full view of glottis	252	(75.0%)
Grade 2. Partial view of glottis	56	(16.7%)
Grade 3. Only epiglottis seen, none of glottis seen	20	(6.0%)
Grade 4. Neither glottis nor epiglottis seen	5	(1.5%)
Intubation attempt		
Attempts 1	296	(88.1%)
Attempts 2	31	(9.2%)
Attempts 3	7	(2.1%)
Attempts > 3	0	(0%)
Difficulty (Intubation Difficulty Scale)		
Easy	290	(86.3%)
Mod difficult	35	(10.4%)
Difficult	6	(1.8%)
Impossible	1	(0.3%)
Attempt aborted	0	(0%)
Intubation achieved	333	(99.1%)
ETT size (mm)		
5	1	(0.3%)
5.5	0	(0%)
6	1	(0.3%)
6.5	4	(1.2%)
7	48	(14.3%)
7.5	184	(54.8)
8	88	(26.2)
8.5	1	(0.3%)
Unknown	9	(2.7%)

Table 3 Hemodynamic changes pre- and post-induction/ intubation

	(n = 336)			
	Pre intubation	Post intubation		
Systolic blood pressure (SBP)	130 ± 1.8	128 ± 1.8	Decreased 2.3 ± 1.6 mmHg, (CI −5.3-0.8)	$P = 0.079$
Diastolic blood pressure (DBP)	74 ± 0.9	74 ± 1	Decreased 0.4 ± 1.1 mmHg, (CI −2.5-1.7)	$P = 0.411$
Heart rate (HR)	105 ± 1	110 ± 1	Increased 4.9 ± 1 BPM, (CI 2.9–6.9)	$P < 0.001$

respiratory failure or micro-aspiration after intubation. Visible aspiration was not reported on initial intubation in all patients.

Immediate complication and mortality after intubation

Cardiac arrest was reported within 30 min of intubation in 2 patients. Both patients had an extensive cardiac and non-cardiac medical history. Additionally, both patients had exacerbation of their underlying disease requiring intubation. Patients were both induced with etomidate and rocuronium, were easily ventilated, and had an atraumatic intubation on first attempt without significant hypoxia that might have caused cardiac arrest. Most likely, the underlying disease was causing hemodynamic collapse and death.

Cardiac arrest during induction is reported to occur 0.7–11% of patients [5]. It is possible that cardiac arrest is a result of difficult intubation, leading to multiple attempts, resulting in hypoxia-driven bradycardia and possibly cardiac arrest. Additionally, Schwartz et al.

Table 4 Long-term outcome of patients after outside OR airway management

Complications and outcome	(n = 275)
Pneumonia	33 (12%)
Average intubation days	7.1 ± 8.8
Tracheostomy	64 (23.3%)
Average time until tracheostomy	9.2 ± 7.4
Hospital stay	22.3 ± 19.6 days
ICU stay	13.7 ± 15.3 days
ICU readmission rate	7.3%
Reintubations	112 out of 336 intubations (33.3%)
Reintubated patients	51 out of 275 patients (18.5%)
Mortality	
Overall mortality	102 (37.1%)
30-day in hospital mortality	87 (31.6%)
Cerebral performance category upon discharge	3.1 ± 1.6

Cerebral performance category:
1.Full recovery
2.Moderate cerebral disability but independent in activities of daily living
3.Severe cerebral disability, dependent in activities of daily living
4.Persistent vegetative state
5.Brain dead

reported a 3% mortality within 30 min of intubation [15] not necessarily related to the intubation itself. Most of the time the progression of underling disease was the major factor in mortality.

In-hospital mortality and comorbidity on admission

The 30-day in-hospital mortality was 31.6% and the overall in-hospital mortality rate was 37.1% in our study population. The mortality rate reflects the overall very sick patient population and is most likely not associated with our intubation. There is no data in the literature about 30-day mortality or hospital stay of this specific patient population and we believe that this new data is important for hospital management and quality improvement.

In general, according to multicentre studies, the ICU mortality ranges from 8 to 17% [17–19]. Additionally, patients who are admitted to ICUs and survive hospitalization have a 1.3-times higher (14.1% vs. 10.9%) mortality rate in the six months after discharge. ICU survivors receiving mechanical ventilation had substantially increased 3-year mortality (57.6%) compared to non-ventilated patients (32.8%). Similarly, for those receiving mechanical ventilation, the risk was concentrated in the first 6 months after hospital discharge (6-month mortality, 30.1%). Additionally, patients who received mechanical ventilation during their hospitalization were more likely to have greater comorbidities compared with those who did not receive mechanical ventilation [20]. We believe that the mortality seen in our study is higher than the ICU mortality because the patients who required emergent intubation were overall more decompensated and had multiple comorbidities on admission. Further analysis comparing the comorbidity of the general admitted population to the comorbidity of the in-hospital intubated population might be helpful to identify the severity of disease and enable comparison with other data.

Hospital and ICU stays

In our study, the mean hospital stay was 22 ± 20 days, and the mean ICU-stay was 14 days (13.9 ± 0.9, CI 12.1–15.8) with a 7.3% ICU-readmission rate which is significantly higher than the average ICU-stay reported in other studies. By comparison, Rosenberg et al. reported a mean ICU-stay of 4.6 days and hospital stay of 11.8 days [21]. Finkielman reported the median ICU-stay of

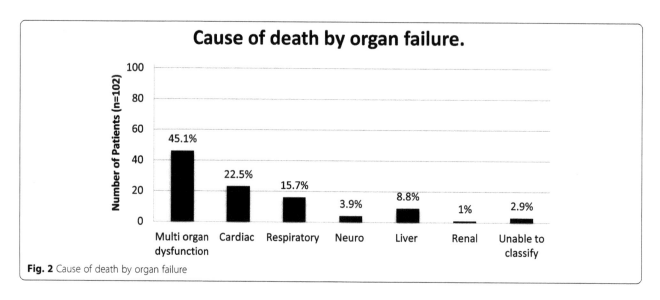

Fig. 2 Cause of death by organ failure

6.5 days [18] and Knaus et al. 3.3 to 7.3 days in a multi-centre analysis including 42 ICUs [22]. Our study finding indicates that patients requiring emergent intubation have significantly longer ICU and hospital stays compared to the general ICU population. The aggregation of several diseases, complications, and operations could have accounted for the prolonged ICU-stay, in addition to prolonged mechanical ventilation. Factors that have been reported to influence ICU-stay include specific medical conditions, like sepsis or acute respiratory distress syndrome, the hospital discharge policy, and ICU staffing. ICU accounts for approximately 7% of total U.S. hospital beds and 20 to 30% of the hospital costs. Although differences in the intensity of treatment may lead to discrepancies, ICU-stay may be used as a surrogate measure of cost [23]. Identifying risk factors to decrease ICU-stay might help saving cost in the future.

Airway management devices and technique

A supraglottic airway device was used in only 1 patient as a bridge to intubation. Supraglottic airway devices have been shown to be effective for airway rescues in emergent airway management. Sorbello M et al. reviewed different types supraglottic airway device use in different situations [24]. A bougie was used in 2 patients. Driver et el. described the use of bougie compared with an endotracheal tube and stylet resulted in significantly higher first-attempt intubation success among patients undergoing emergency endotracheal intubation [25]. The use of video-laryngoscopes for emergent airway management is associated with a lower number of intubation attempts and with a lower frequency of esophageal intubation [26] and thus, may reasonably be regarded as the first choice in emergent airway management. Like other airway management techniques, the use of rapid sequence intubation or cricoid pressure requires preparatory instruction and periodic training. The current

literature is controversial and ss per Salem et al. investigations are warranted to determine the characteristics of the CP technique that maximize its effectiveness while avoiding the risk of airway-related complications in the various patient populations [27]. Ultimately the anesthesiologist needs to judge which device is most suitable by identifying the cause of difficult intubation in each patient. Additionally, anesthesiologist should use the airway technique that they are most experienced with and that is best for the individual situation. As with any intubation, practice and routine use will improve performance.

Airway education

Airway education plays a crucial role preparing for emergent intubations in the hospital setting. Crisis management training, communication, leadership, team coordination, and shared understanding of roles has been shown to improve the success of airway management in emergency settings. We believe that the low complication rate of immediate airway-related complications, such as esophageal intubation, aspiration, and dental trauma, is most likely due to the extensive airway education and training at our institution. Early exposure to real situations combined with simulation and discussion sessions to review every possible scenario in non-operating room emergent airway management will train first responders to use appropriate clinical judgement. Additionally, upon response to an emergent airway management advanced planning, proper positioning, patient preparation, coupled with a strategy for both the intubation procedure and its rescue, are essential to minimize the complication rate.

Beyond that, the nontechnical aspect is important as well. The Difficult Airway Society (DAS) 2015 guidelines clearly introduce the concept of 'stop-and-think' magic words in their algorithm [28]. This concept is to be perceived as a handbrake encouraging us to slow down to automatic (intuitive) thinking in favor of the rational one, aimed at avoiding cognitive biases and to ignite the thinking out-of-the-box process [24].

Limitations

It is difficult to generalize these findings since the approach to the airway management outside the OR is highly dependent on the hospital or institutional settings. Depending on institution, it could be an attending anaesthesiologist, a resident or a CRNA responding to an airway.

Although abundant information was collected on these patients, the retrospective nature of the analysis reveals some interesting relationships however causality of independent variables and risk factors cannot be inferred. The mortality analysis in this study was purely descriptive without analysis of causality or association to intubation we performed. Additionally, mortality is a poor measurement for causality because of the complexity of diseases in addition to many unidentifiable confounders.

Data collection from the intubation notes was a limiting factor. Only information that was pre-created as a check-off box was collected and analysed. There is a risk of underreporting of complications: the quality of the laryngoscopic view obtained, and the actual number of laryngoscopic attempts performed. Additionally, demographics like BMI, ASA status, comorbidity was recorded only on initial admission. There is potential that those demographics might have changed over the hospital course. Whether the demographic change is associated with worsening outcome should be evaluated in future studies.

Conclusion

Emergent airway management outside of the OR is performed in a high-risk patient population with multiple comorbidities with high ASA scores on admission. Only a small number of intubation-related complications were reported. Most of the complications were related to the deconditioning of the patient's physiologic state rather than the intubation procedure itself. Overall, with adequate training and education in the fundamentals of airway management, emergent airway management can be performed safely outside of the OR. Further studies are needed to identify individual predictors of reintubation rate, adverse outcome, and mortality for quality improvement.

Abbreviations

ASA: American Society of Anesthesiologist; BMI: Body Mass Index; CRNA: Certified Registered Nurse Anesthetist; EF: Ejection Fraction; ETT: Endotracheal Tube; ICD: Implantable Cardioverter Defibrillator; ICU: Intensive Care Unit; NPO: Nil Per Os; OR: Operating Room

Authors' contributions

UY designed the study, collected data, interpretation of results and wrote the manuscript. JM collected data and wrote the manuscript. MW collected data and wrote the manuscript. KS collected data and wrote the manuscript. MB collected data and wrote the manuscript. AP collected data and wrote the manuscript. MT statistical analysis and review of the manuscript. EW Principal investigator and review of the manuscript. All authors read and approved the final manuscript.

Author details

[1]Department of Anesthesiology, Thomas Jefferson University Hospital, Suite 8290 Gibbon, 111 South 11th Street, Philadelphia PA 19107, USA. [2]Department of Anesthesiology, Johns Hopkins University Hospital, Baltimore, MD, USA.

References

1. Asai T. Airway management inside and outside operating rooms-circumstances are quite different. Br J Anaesth. 2018 Feb;120:207–9.
2. Divatia JV, Khan PU, Myatra SN. Tracheal intubation in the ICU: life saving or life threatening? Indian J Anaesth. 2011;55:470–5.
3. Benedetto WJ, Hess DR, Gettings E, et al. Urgent tracheal intubation in general hospital units: an observational study. J Clin Anesth. 2007;19:20–4.
4. Jaber S, Amraoui J, Lefrant JY, et al. Clinical practice and risk factors for immediate complications of endotracheal intubation in the intensive care unit: a prospective, multiple-center study. Crit Care Med. 2006;34:2355–61.
5. Mort TC. Emergency tracheal intubation: complications associated with repeated laryngoscopic attempts. Anesth Analg. 2004;99:607–13.
6. Shiga T, Wajima Z, Inoue T, Sakamoto A. Predicting difficult intubation in apparently normal patients: a meta-analysis of bedside screening test performance. Anesthesiology. 2005;103:429–37.
7. Stauffer JL, Olson DE, Petty TL. Complications and consequences of endotracheal intubation and tracheostomy. Am J Med. 1981;70:65–76.
8. Zwillich CW, Pierson DJ, Creagh CE, Sutton FD, Schatz E, Petty TL. Complications of assisted ventilation. Am J Med. 1974;57:161–9.
9. Martin LD, Mhyre JM, Shanks AM, Tremper KK, Kheterpal S. 3,423 emergency tracheal intubations at a university hospital: airway outcomes and complications. Anesthesiology. 2011;114:42–8.
10. Rochlen LR, Housey M, Gannon I, Mitchell S, Rooney DM, Tait AR, Engoren M. Assessing anesthesiology residents' out-of-the-operating-room (OOOR) emergent airway management. BMC Anesthesiol. 2017 Jul 15;17:96.
11. Cook TM, Woodall N, Frerk C. Fourth National Audit Project: major complications of airway management in the UK: results of the fourth National Audit Project of the Royal College of Anaesthetists and the difficult airway society. Part 1: Anaesthesia. Br J Anaesth. 2011;106:617–31.
12. Tachibana N, Niiyama Y, Yamakage M. Incidence of cannot intubate-cannot ventilate (CICV): results of a 3-year retrospective multicenter clinical study in a network of university hospitals. J Anesth. 2015;29:326–30.
13. McCoy EP, Russell WJ, Webb RK. Accidental bronchial intubation. An analysis of AIMS incident reports from 1988 to 1994 inclusive. Anaesthesia. 1997;52: 24–31.
14. Dronen S, Chadwick O, Nowak R. Endotracheal tip position in the arrested patient. Ann Emerg Med. 1982;11:116–7.
15. Schwartz DE, Matthay MA, Cohen NH. Death and other complications of emergency airway management in critically ill adults. A prospective investigation of 297 tracheal intubations. Anesthesiology. 1995;82:367–76.
16. Pollard RJ, Lobato EB. Endotracheal tube location verified reliably by cuff palpation. Anesth Analg. 1995;81:135–8.
17. Zimmerman JE, Kramer AA, Knaus WA. Changes in hospital mortality for United States intensive care unit admissions from 1988 to 2012. Crit Care. 2013;27:17.
18. Finkielman JD. Morales IJ. Peters SG et al Mortality rate and length of stay of patients admitted to the intensive care unit in July Crit Care Med. 2004;32: 1161–5.
19. Kuijsten HA, Brinkman S, Meynaar IA, et al. Hospital mortality is associated with ICU admission time. Intensive Care Med. 2010;36:1765–71.
20. Wunsch H, Guerra C, Barnato AE, Angus DC, Li G, Linde-Zwirble WT. Three-year outcomes for Medicare beneficiaries who survive intensive care. JAMA. 2010;303:849–56.

21. Rosenberg AL, Zimmerman JE, Alzola C, Draper EA, Kmaus WA. Intensive care unit length of stay: recent changes and future challenges. Crit Care Med. 2000;28:3465–73.
22. Knaus WA, Wagner DP, Zimmerman JE, Draper EA. Variations in mortality and length of stay in intensive care units. Ann Intern Med. 1993;15(118): 753–61.
23. Rapoport J, Teres D, Zhao Y, Lemeshow S. Length of stay data as a guide to hospital economic performance for ICU patients. Med Care. 2003;41:386–97.
24. Sorbello M, Petrini F. Supraglottic airway devices: the search for the best insertion technique or the time to change our point of view? Turk J Anaesthesiol Reanim. 2017;45:76–82.
25. Driver BE, Prekker ME, Klein LR, et al. Effect of use of a Bougie vs endotracheal tube and Stylet on first-attempt intubation success among patients with difficult airways undergoing emergency intubation: a randomized clinical trial. JAMA. 2018 Jun 5;319:2179–89.
26. Rombey T, Schieren M, Pieper D. Video versus direct laryngoscopy for inpatient emergency intubation in adults. A Systematic Review and Meta-Analysis of Randomized Controlled Trials Dtsch Arztebl Int. 2018;115:437–44.
27. Salem MR, Khorasani A, Zeidan A, Crystal GJ. Cricoid pressure controversies: narrative review. Anesthesiology. 2017;126:738–52.
28. Sorbello M, Afshari A, De Hert S. Device or target? A paradigm shift in airway management with implications for guidelines, clinical practice and teaching. Eur J Anaesthesiol. 2018;35:811–4.

29

Clinical performance of the LMA Protector™ airway in moderately obese patients

Ina Ismiarti Shariffuddin[1], Sook Hui Chaw[1]*(iD), Ling Wei Ng[1], Ching Hooi Lim[1], Mohd Fitry Zainal Abidin[1], Wan A. Wan Zakaria[1] and Wendy H. Teoh[2]

Abstract

Background: The 4th National Audit Project of The Royal College of Anaesthetists and The Difficult Airway Society (NAP4) reported a higher incidence of supraglottic airway device (SAD) related pulmonary aspiration in obese patients especially with the first-generation SADs. The latest single-use SAD, the Protector™ provides a functional separation of the respiratory and digestive tracts and its laryngeal cuff with two ports allowing additional suction in tandem with the insertion of a gastric tube. The laryngeal cuff of LMA Protector™ allows a large catchment reservoir in the event of gastric content aspiration.

Methods: We evaluated the performance characteristics of the LMA Protector™ in 30 unparalysed, moderately obese patients. First attempt insertion rate, time for insertion, oropharyngeal leak pressure (OLP), and incidence of complications were recorded.

Results: We found high first and second attempt insertion rates of 28(93%) and 1(33%) respectively, with one failed attempt where no capnography trace could be detected, presumably from a downfolded device tip. The LMA Protector™ was inserted rapidly in 21.0(4.0) seconds and demonstrated high OLP of 31.8(5.4) cmH2O. Fibreoptic assessment showed a clear view of vocal cords in 93%. The incidence of blood staining on removal of device was 48%, postoperative sore throat 27%, dysphagia 10% and dysphonia 20% (all self-limiting, resolving a few hours postoperatively).

Conclusions: We conclude that the LMA Protector™ was associated with easy, expedient first attempt insertion success, demonstrating high oropharyngeal pressures and good anatomical position in the moderately obese population, with relatively low postoperative airway morbidity.

Keywords: Supraglottic airway devices, Moderately obese, Oropharyngeal leak pressures, Airway management

* Correspondence: sh_chaw@yahoo.com
[1]Department of Anesthesiology, Faculty of Medicine, University of Malaya, 50603 Kuala Lumpur, Malaysia

Background

Obesity is a known risk factor associated with many complications in anaesthesia, including difficult airway. The Fourth National Audit Project of the Royal College of Anaesthetist and Difficult Airway Society (NAP4) has reported a higher incidence of supraglottic airway device (SAD) associated pulmonary aspiration in obese patients, especially with the first-generation SAD [1].

The LMA Protector™ is the latest single-use second-generation SAD made from medical-grade silicone. It has a preformed-fixed curved structure for easy insertion. It provides access and functional separation of the respiratory and digestive tracts. The respiratory channel can be used as a direct intubation conduit. Uniquely, the LMA Protector contains two drain channels, which emerge as separate ports proximally. A suction tube may be attached to the male drainage port around the laryngeal region or a well-lubricated gastric tube may be passed through the female drainage port to the stomach. The high leakage pressures, the optimal fit of the airway device, and dual gastric ports offer better protection from aspiration [2]. Besides, these features support high ventilation pressures and this would be ideal for obese patients.

Currently, there are limited reports on the outcome of the LMA Protector in airway management and its use in the obese patients. Hence, we conducted this study to evaluate the performance of the LMA Protector in obese (BMI 30–35) patients who required general anaesthesia for surgical procedures.

Methods

Approval from the University of Malaya Medical Centre's Institutional Review Board (201755–5215) and the Australian New Zealand Clinical Trials Registry (ACTR N12617001152314) were obtained before the conduct of the study.

We recruited moderately obese ($30 \, \text{kg/m}^2 \leq \text{BMI} \leq 35 \, \text{kg/m}^2$) patients who were scheduled for elective open surgical procedures under general anaesthesia amenable to supraglottic airway device insertion. Exlusion criteria were patients with American Society of Anaesthesiologists (ASA) physical status IV, those at high risk of aspiration (symptomatic gastroesophageal reflux and hiatus hernia), recent upper respiratory tract infection, previous head and neck surgery or radiotherapy and small mouth opening.

The patients were not premedicated preoperatively. They were positioned supine on the operating table, with the head resting on a head ring. Standard monitoring were applied before induction of anaesthesia. The insertion of LMA Protector was done based on manufacturer's recommendation. The LMA Protector cuff was completely deflated and a water-based lubricant was applied to the posterior part of cuff and airway tube. Only the LMA protector size 3 or 4 was selected for use in our patients, size 3 for woman and size 4 for man.

After pre-oxygenation, anaesthesia was induced with fentanyl 1.5–2 mcg/kg, propofol 2–3 mg/kg, and anaesthesia were maintained with sevoflurane (end tidal concentration of 2 to 3%) in 100% oxygen until minimum alveolar concentration (MAC) of 1.2 and patient's jaw was considered relaxed at the discretion of the investigators, before insertion of the LMA. Under direct vision, the tip of the device was pressed flat against the hard palate and the LMA Protector was inserted until resistance was felt. The cuff was then inflated with air until the marker of the pilot balloon was within the green zone (indicative of 40-60 cm H_2O, with an upper limit of clear zone where the pressure does not exceed 70cmH_2O). The amount of air inflated was recorded, and the intra-cuff pressure was confirmed with a handheld aneroid manometer (Portex® Pressure Gauge; Smiths Medical Intl Ltd., Kent, UK) to achieve an intra-cuff pressure of 40- 60cmH_2O.

The time of insertion was measured from when the tip of the LMA entered the patient's mouth to the time of appearance of first square end tidal carbon dioxide ($ETCO^2$), denoting successful establishment of effective ventilation. Otherwise, the device was removed for another insertion attempt. Each attempt was defined as reinsertion of the airway device into the mouth. A maximum of three insertion attempts were allowed. "Insertion failure" occurred when the investigators failed 3 attempts of insertion or if the entire process of insertion exceeded 120 s. In case of insertion failure, the attending anaesthesiologists would decide the subsequent airway management.

Once the airway device was in place, the SAD was fixed by taping over the patient's cheek. A gel plug was placed in the male gastric drain outlet whilst closing the female port of the gastric drain and the suprasternal notch test was done to confirm placement (gently tapping the suprasternal notch causes the gel to pulsate, confirming the tip location behind the cricoid cartilage). Then, a pre-lubricated 14 French gauge gastric tube was inserted through the female port gastric drain, and graded 1 to 3 (1-easy, 2-difficult, 3-impossible). Confirmation of correct placement of the gastric tube was done by auscultating the epigastrium as air was injected, and by aspiration of gastric contents. We decompressed the stomach and the amount of gastric fluid aspirated was documented, and the fasting duration recorded.

The anatomical airway position of the LMA Protector was then assessed by fibreoptic bronchoscopy (3.7 mm bronchoscope, Karl Storz™, Tuttlingen, Germany) via the airway channel and scored as follows: grade 4, only vocal cords seen; grade 3, vocal cords and posterior epiglottis seen; grade 2, vocal cords and anterior epiglottis seen; and grade 1, vocal cords not seen [3].

Oropharyngeal leak pressure (OLP) was measured after closing the adjustable pressure-limiting (APL) valve with a fresh gas flow of 3 L min^{-1}, noting the airway pressure at equilibrium or when there was an audible air leak from the throat. The epigastrium was also auscultated when measuring the OLP to detect any air entrainment in the stomach. The blood pressure and heart rate were also recorded every minute for the first 5 minutes from beginning of insertion of the LMA Protector™. Airway manoeuvres to facilitate the insertion of the LMA were also documented.

Anaesthesia was maintained with an oxygen and air mixture in sevoflurane to achieve MAC of 1.0–1.2. Patients were placed in supine or lithotomy position based on the types of procedures. All intraoperative complications, such as desaturation to less than 95%, regurgitation or aspiration, bronchospasm, dental, lip or tongue injury, were recorded. At the end of surgery, the airway device was removed upon the adequate spontaneous breathing and eye opening of the patient. The airway device was inspected for the presence of blood. Forty-five minutes later, an independent observer assessed the patients for post-operative sore throat, dysphonia, and dysphagia.

All SAD insertions were performed by anaesthesiologists with more than 10-years' experience in supraglottic airway management and had performed at least ten LMA Protector™ insertion before the study commencement (IIS, CSH and MFZA) [4]. Data collection was done by another independent investigator.

Statistical analysis

Our primary measure was "first attempt success rate". Sample size was based on assumption that 95% of the subjects in the population have first attempt success rate insertion of LMA Protector. Hence, the study would require a sample size of 19 with 10% margin of error relative to the expected proportion and 95% confidence [5]. Therefore, we recruited 30 patients to account for dropouts and protocol breaches. The data that was collected was analysed using SPSS 24 (SPSS Inc., Chicago, IL, USA). Mean and standard deviation was used to describe normally distributed continuous variables; median and interquartile ranges (IQR) were used for non-normally distributed continuous variables. Categorical variables were expressed as number and percentage.

Results

Thirty patients were recruited from August 2017 to August 2018. The performance of LMA protector was evaluated. The patients' baseline demographics, airway anthropometric features, and duration of surgery is depicted in Table 1.

Insertion of the LMA Protector™ was successful in 28 patients (93%) at first attempt and one patient (3%) at second attempt. However, there was an insertion failure in one patient, despite application of rescue manoeuvres. This patient was subsequently managed with another SGA for ventilation. We excluded this patient from the analysis. (Fig. 1).

Table 1 Baseline demographic and airway anthropometric features

Parameters (n = 30)	Results
Age, years	43.3 (16.7)
Body Mass Index, kg/m2	31.7 (1.4)
Gender	
Male	10 [33.3%]
Female	20 [66.7%]
ASA status	
1	15 [50%]
2	15 [50%]
Types of surgery (Open surgeries)	
General surgery	10 [33.3%]
Orthopaedic surgery	9 [30.0%]
Gynaecology	6 [20.0%]
Urology	5 [16.7%]
Mallampati	
1	12 [40.0%]
2	14 [46.7%]
3	4 [13.3%]
4	0 [0%]
Thyromental distance	
> 60 mm	29 [96.7%]
< 60 mm	1 [3.3%]
Interincisor distance	
> 40 mm	30 [100%]
< 40 mm	0 [0%]
Neck flexion	
Full	29 [96.7%]
< 50% limited	0 [0%]
> 50% limited	1 [3.3%]
Neck extension	
Full	29 [96.7%]
< 50% limited	0 [0%]
> 50% limited	1 [3.3%]
Duration of surgery, minutes	71.8 (39.8)

Data expressed as mean (standard deviation) or number [percentage]
ASA American Society of Anesthesiologists

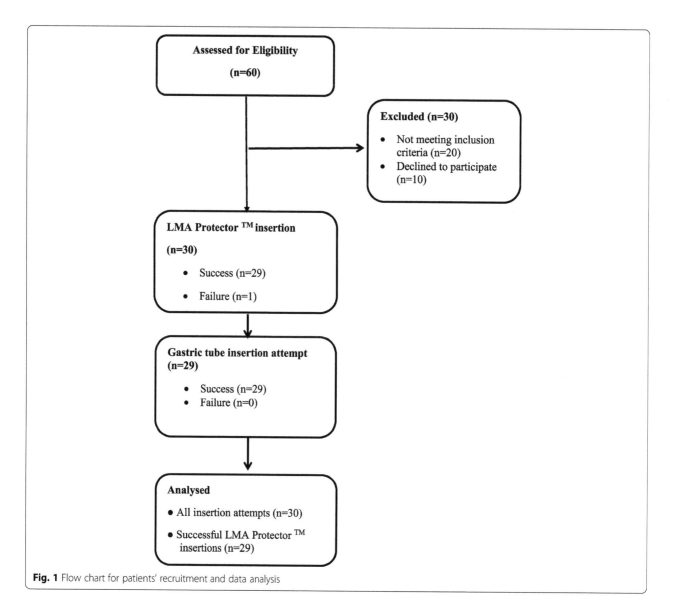

Fig. 1 Flow chart for patients' recruitment and data analysis

The mean time taken for insertion was 21.0 (4.0) seconds. For all the successful LMA insertions, the ease of LMA Protector™ insertion was graded as easy in 26 patients and fair in 3 patients.

The LMA protector™ was found to provide a good seal with mean OLP of 31.8 (5.4) mmHg. Insertion of a gastric tube was easy in 23 patients (79%), while 6 (21%) patients had a difficult gastric tube insertion. On examination of fibreoptic view, 27 patients had a clear view of their vocal cords (93%), 1 had view of arytenoids only, and 1 had view of epiglottis only (Table 2).

There were no airway complications related to SAD insertion during maintenance of anaesthesia. (Table 3) Mucosal injury as evidenced by blood stains on the LMA Protector™ was documented in 48% of patients. Delayed complications were post-operative sore throat (28%), post-operative dysphagia (21%), and post-

operative dysphonia (10%). The degree of post-operative sore throat, dysphagia and dysphonia were described to be mild in nature and lasted for less than 24 h. Most patients did not have any increase in heart rate and mean arterial pressure of more than 20% when compared to baseline, except in 2 patients (7%) (Table 4). There was no incidence of desaturation in all patients.

Discussion

In our study, we found a high first attempt success rate (93%) of LMA Protector™ insertion in thirty moderately obese patients which was comparable to previous studies using LMA Protector™ in non-obese patients [6, 7]. Use of second-generation SADs with a gastric channel and design that allow fibreoptic guided tracheal intubation is crucial in obese patients as it provides efficient airway protection from gastric aspiration, as well as a conduit

Table 2 Parameters for the clinical performance of LMA Protector™

Parameters (n = 30)	Results
Size of LMA protector	
Size 3	10 [63.3%]
Size 4	11 [36.7%]
Number of attempts	
1	28 [93.4%]
2	1 [3.3%]
Failed	1 [3.3%]
Ease of insertion	
Easy	26 [86.7%]
Fair	3 [10.0%]
Difficult	0
Very Difficult	0
Impossible	1 [3.3%]
Time to successful insertion, seconds	21.0 (3.9)
Oropharyngeal leak pressure, OLP, cmH20	31.8 (5.4)
Cuff volume, mls	14.6 (5.6)
Ease of gastric tube insertion	
Easy	23 [79.3%]
Difficult	6 [20.7%]
Impossible	0
Volume of gsastric fluid aspirated, ml	6.9 (13.1)
Duration of fasting, hours	11.7(2.6)
Fibreoptic view	
Only vocal cords seen	27 [93.1%]
Vocal cords and posterior epiglottis	1 [3.4%]
Vocal cords and anterior epiglottis	1 [3.4%]
Vocal cord not seen	0

Data expressed as mean (standard deviation) or number [percentage]

Table 3 Complications related to LMA Protector insertions

Complications	Percentage
Immediate	
Desaturation	0
Bronchospasm	0
Gross regurgitation/aspiration	0
Intraoperative gastric distension	0
Dental injury	0
Lip or tongue injury	0
Mucosal injury/blood on LMA	14 [48.4%]
Delayed	
Post operative sore throat	8 [27.6%]
Post operative dysphonia	3 [10.3%]
Post operative dysphagia	6 [20.7%]

Data expressed as mean (standard deviation) or number [percentage]

Table 4 Patients' haemodynamic response to LMA Protector™ airway insertion

Parameters (n = 30)	Results
Heart Rate	
Increase of 0–10%	18 [62.1%]
Increase of 10–20%	9 [31.0%]
Increase of > 20%	2 [6.9%]
Mean arterial pressure	
Increase of 0–10%	23 [79.3%]
Increase of 10–20%	2 [6.9%]
Increase of > 20%	2 [6.9%]

Data expressed as mean (standard deviation) or number [percentage]

for intubation in case of an unexpected difficult airway [8, 9].

The average BMI in our study was 32. All female patients received the size 3 LMA Protector, and males the size 4. Their ideal mean (SD) body weights of males 66.9 (4.4) kg and females 46.5 (7.3) kg suggested a nice fit according to manufacturer recommendations that we followed e.g., size 3 for less than 50 kg and size 4 for patients weighing in between 50 to 70 kg ^{2}. Previous studies using Proseal LMA™ that had utilised the size 4 for females and size 5 for males, found that despite yielding higher oropharyngeal leak pressures, the larger mask tended to rise up within the mouth more often, predisposing these patients to increased risk of sore throat and lingual nerve damage [10].

The insertion of the LMA Protector™ was graded easy/ fair for 97% of our patients. The LMA Protector™ was inserted expediently in a mean time of 21.0 (4.0) seconds which is comparable to studies using LMA Supreme™ and Ambu® AuraGain™ [11]. The comparable device insertion times shows that there is no increased difficulty in insertion in obese patients compared to non-obese patients despite its bulkier profile with the 2 gastric ports. This is reassuring, as the LMA Protector™ is a new airway device and investigators had only 10 insertions before commencing the study; it is possible that increased usage and experience with the LMA Protector™ could further improve the success rate and insertion timings [4, 6, 12].

We had one failed insertion where despite an easy insertion, we could not obtain a capnograph tracing after 3 attempts. For the first and second insertion attempt, the investigator (CSH) had used the index finger to guide insertion of the LMA Protector™ which was totally deflated and generously lubricated according to manufacturer's recommendations. The entry of the device was smooth but there was absence of end tidal carbon dioxide trace and chest rise upon commencing ventilation. Prior to the third insertion attempt, the patient's head and neck was repositioned, laryngospasm was ruled out, and adequate depth of anaesthesia was confirmed, but again failed to yield an end tidal carbon dioxide trace. Insertion failure was declared, and the airway was successfully rescued with an Ambu® AuraGain™. Being made from medical grade silicone that renders the LMA Protector™ softer and more pliable in nature compared to the polyvinyl chloride (PVC) tip of the Ambu AuraGain, we postulated that the tip of the LMA Protector™ had folded over in the posterior pharynx during insertion. In hindsight, a diagonal shift of the mask during insertion may have been helpful to avoid this downfolding [2].

We found a high OLP of 31.8 (5.4) cmH_2O in this study, which is higher than that reported in non-obese patients. Moser et al. reported an OLP of 28.3 (7.0) cmH_2O while Sng et al. reported an OLP of 25.5 cmH_2O (IQR 23.0 to 29.0 cmH_2O) [6, 7]. This high OLP is similar to the OLP of LMA Proseal which was reported to be 27 (7.0) cmH_2O but higher than that of Ambu Aura-Gain 24.1 (7.4) cmH_2O [11, 13]. The high OLP can be attributed to the fact that the LMA Protector™ is made of medical grade silicone, with an anatomically shaped airway tube and inflatable cuff that purportedly conforms to the contours of an individual's hypopharynx. In obese patients, the increased adiposity and hypopharyngeal tissue may render it a snugger fit. Obese patients have poor chest compliance due to their thick chest wall, and often require higher peak inspiratory pressures when positive pressure ventilation is instituted [1]. This high OLP of the LMA Protector™ therefore makes it a suitable SGA to be used in obese patients as it is beneficial to mitigate any air leak that may predispose patients to inadequate ventilation, gastric insufflation, and increased risk of aspiration. The insertion of gastric drain tube into the oesophagus was rated easy in 79% and with the tip of the gastric channel aligned with the oesophagus, there was effective venting of gastric content.

On assessment of the anatomical position of the LMA Protector™, we found a clear view of the vocal cords in 93% of the patients. This could be attributed to the anatomically curved tube of the LMA Protector™ enabling insertion to the optimal position. A good anatomical position, in conjunction with high sealing pressures enables obese patients to be ventilated more safely even with higher peak pressures. A good anatomical position also makes it an effective conduit for endotracheal tube insertion in these obese patients, either as a rescue procedure after difficult or failed initial laryngoscopy, or in those individuals who require a conversion from a SAD to tracheal tube for their surgeries or further postoperative ventilation in the ICU.

In two patients, we did not have an entirely clear view of the vocal cords. The vocal cords were partially seen with the posterior epiglottis in one patient, and partial VC with anterior epiglottis sighted in the other patient.

No problems with ventilation were encountered and during maintenance of anaesthesia over a mean surgical duration of 71 min, the LMA Protector™ performed well without the need for airway manipulation to optimize ventilation.

Van Zundert et al. similarly found a high OLP with the LMA protector of 31.7 (2.9) cm H2O as we did. Uniquely, their device insertions were performed under vision of a video laryngoscope using an 'insert-detect-correct-as-you-go' technique with standardized corrective measures, and they achieved a near-optimal fibreoptic position in the LMA-Protector of 94%, similar to our results [14]. This is reassuring as our study showed that simple manual insertion of the LMA Protector in obese patients, without "vision" adjuncts, worked just as well.

We had assessed immediate and delayed postoperative complications associated with the LMA Protector™ in our study. The only complication encountered during the immediate phase was mucosal injury, seen in 14 patients (48%). The incidence was high compared to figures from non-obese patients [7]. The airway of an obese patient is shown on MRI to have deposition of excess adipose tissue into nearly all pharyngeal structures including the uvula, the tonsils, the tonsillar pillars, the tongue, aryepiglottic folds, and most predominantly, the lateral pharyngeal walls. This leads to airway narrowing, which can be exaggerated by external compression from superficial depositions of fat in the neck [15]. Therefore, at insertion of LMA, the pharyngeal structures could be easily abraded especially if there is concomitant tissue congestion. Another possible reason for the increased incidence of mucosal injury could be the larger tip of the LMA Protector that may collide with the arytenoids upon its insertion. Additionally, the bulky posterior curvature of LMA Protector and its slightly larger cuff may contribute to a more challenging insertion in the Asian population with their smaller builts and mouth opening in this study. Ensuring a well lubricated LMA Protector and a completely deflated cuff before insertion is paramount.

The LMA Protector™ pilot balloon has an Integrated Cuff Pilot™ which is used for intraoperative cuff pressure monitoring. The provision of continuous intra-cuff pressure monitoring is ideal as intracuff pressure could change, at a given volume, because of temperature changes, muscular tone or administration of nitrous oxide [16]. The use of the Integrated Cuff Pilot™ can prevent nerve or pressure injuries of the airway especially with prolonged usage. We followed up our patients via phone call after discharge from hospital and found a 27% incidence of postoperative sore throat, which was comparable to a study using Proseal LMA™ in obese patients [17]. It was self-limiting and only lasted for a few hours postoperatively. We found a lower incidence of dysphagia (10%) and dysphonia (20%) compared to Rieger et al. [18] This can perhaps be attributed to the continuous cuff pressure monitoring with the integrated cuff pressure indicator, which is targeted between 40 and 60 mmHg. In addition, the cuff is made of medical grade silicone, which increases its flexibility and hence potentially more pliable and less traumatic to insert into the pharynx [6]. We also did not find any hypoglossal nerve injury with the use of LMA Protector™ as reported by Tham et al. [19]

Most patients did not have a significant increase in heart rate and mean arterial pressure when compared to baseline, except two patients (7%). This is consistent with a previous study reporting stable haemodynamics as LMA insertion is easy and less stimulating to the patients [19].

Our study had a few limitations. Firstly, we evaluated the LMA Protector™ in obese patients with BMI of 30–35, and the results cannot be extrapolated to patients beyond BMI > 35. Secondly, our study sample size was a relatively small cohort number, albeit powered adequately. Thirdly, surgical duration in our study lasted a mean of 71 min, with the longest duration 180 min. Any incidence of dysphonia beyond that is still unknown. But our results are reassuring in support of the LMA Protector's use in the obese.

Conclusion

This evaluation study showed that the LMA Protector™ was associated with easy, expedient first attempt insertion success, demonstrating high oropharyngeal pressures and good anatomical position in the moderately obese population, with relatively low postoperative airway morbidity with good spontaneous recovery.

Abbreviations
LMA: Laryngeal mask airway; SAD: Supraglottic airway device; OLP: Oropharyngeal leak pressure; ASA: American Society of Anaesthesiologist; $ETCO_2$: End tidal carbon dioxide; APL: Adjustable pressure-limiting; IQR: Interquartile range; PVC: Polyvinyl chloride

Acknowledgements
Not applicable.

Authors' contributions
IIS and WHT conceptually conceived the trial, and were both involved in study design, trial protocol, manuscript writing, critical review, and revision. IIS also analysed and interpreted the results. CSH contributed to the writing of the manuscript and revision. NLW, LCH, MFZA and WAWZ carried out the data collection, and critically reviewed the manuscript. The authors read and approved the final manuscript.

Author details
[1]Department of Anesthesiology, Faculty of Medicine, University of Malaya, 50603 Kuala Lumpur, Malaysia. [2]Wendy Teoh Pte.Ltd, Private Anaesthesia Practice, Singapore, Singapore.

References
1. Cook TM, Woodall N, Frerk C. Major complications of airway management in the UK: results of the fourth National Audit Project of the Royal College of Anaesthetists and the difficult airway society. Part 1: anaesthesia. Br J Anaesth. 2011;106(5):617–31.
2. LMA Protector Instruction for use, Teleflex, 2015 [http://www.lmacoifu.com/sites/default/files/node/1928/ifu/revision/3285/pbe2100000b-lma-protector-ifuuk.pdf].
3. Brimacombe J, Berry AJA. A proposed fiber-optic scoring system to standardize the assessment of laryngeal mask airway position. Analgesia. 1993;76(2):457.
4. Sorbello M, Petrini FJTJA. Supraglottic airway devices: the search for the best insertion technique or the time to change our point of view? Reanimation. 2017;45(2):76.
5. Daniel WW, Cross CL. Biostatistics: a foundation for analysis in the health sciences. New York: Wiley; 2018.
6. Moser B, Audige L, Keller C, Brimacombe J, Gasteiger L, Bruppacher HR. A prospective, randomised trial of the Ambu AuraGain laryngeal mask versus the LMA protector airway in paralysed, anaesthetised adult men. Minerva Anestesiol. 2018;84(6):684–92.
7. Sng BL, Ithnin FB, Mathur D, Lew E, Han NL, Sia AT. A preliminary assessment of the LMA protector™ in non-paralysed patients. BMC anesthesiology. 2017;17(1):26.
8. Sorbello M, Gaçonnet C, Skinner MJA. Intrinsic plan B airway for patients undergoing bronchial thermoplasty. Analgesia. 2018;127(5):e83–4.
9. Sorbello M. Evolution of supraglottic airway devices: the Darwinian perspective. Minerva anestesiologica. 2018;84(3):297–300.
10. Asai T, Murao K, Yukawa H, Shingu K. Re-evaluation of appropriate size of the laryngeal mask airway. British journal of anaesthesia. 1999;83(3):478–9.
11. Shariffuddin I, Teoh W, Tang E, Hashim N, Loh PJA. Ambu® AuraGain™ versus LMA supreme™ second seal™: a randomised controlled trial comparing oropharyngeal leak pressures and gastric drain functionality in spontaneously breathing patients. care i. 2017;45(2):244–50.
12. Weber U, Oguz R, Potura LA, Kimberger O, Kober A, Tschernko E. Comparison of the i-gel and the LMA-Unique laryngeal mask airway in patients with mild to moderate obesity during elective short-term surgery. Anaesthesia. 2011;66(6):481–7.
13. Keller C, Brimacombe J, Kleinsasser A, Brimacombe LJA. The laryngeal mask airway ProSeal™ as a temporary ventilatory device in grossly and morbidly obese patients before laryngoscope-guided tracheal intubation. Analgesia. 2002;94(3):737–40.
14. Van Zundert AA, Skinner MW, Van Zundert TC, Luney SR, Pandit JJ. Value of knowing physical characteristics of the airway device before using it. BJA. 2016;117(1):12–6.
15. Leykin Y, Brodsky JB. Controversies in the anesthetic management of the obese surgical patient. Verlag Italia: Springer Science & Business Media; 2012.
16. Sorbello M, Zdravkovic I, Cataldo R, Di Giacinto IJR. Spring recoil and supraglottic airway devices: lessons from the law of conservation of energy. care i. 2018;25(1):7–9.
17. Natalini G, Franceschetti ME, Pantelidi MT, Rosano A, Lanza G, Bernardini A. Comparison of the standard laryngeal mask airway and the ProSeal laryngeal mask airway in obese patients. British journal of anaesthesia. 2003; 90(3):323–6.
18. Rieger A, Brunne B, Hass I, Brummer G, Spies C, Striebel HW, Eyrich K. Laryngo-pharyngeal complaints following laryngeal mask airway and endotracheal intubation. Journal of clinical anesthesia. 1997;9(1):42–7.
19. Tham LY, Beh ZY, Shariffuddin II, Wang CY. Unilateral hypoglossal nerve palsy after the use of laryngeal mask airway (LMA) Protector. Korean journal of anesthesiology. 2019;72(6):606.

Permissions

All chapters in this book were first published by BioMed Central; hereby published with permission under the Creative Commons Attribution License or equivalent. Every chapter published in this book has been scrutinized by our experts. Their significance has been extensively debated. The topics covered herein carry significant findings which will fuel the growth of the discipline. They may even be implemented as practical applications or may be referred to as a beginning point for another development.

The contributors of this book come from diverse backgrounds, making this book a truly international effort. This book will bring forth new frontiers with its revolutionizing research information and detailed analysis of the nascent developments around the world.

We would like to thank all the contributing authors for lending their expertise to make the book truly unique. They have played a crucial role in the development of this book. Without their invaluable contributions this book wouldn't have been possible. They have made vital efforts to compile up to date information on the varied aspects of this subject to make this book a valuable addition to the collection of many professionals and students.

This book was conceptualized with the vision of imparting up-to-date information and advanced data in this field. To ensure the same, a matchless editorial board was set up. Every individual on the board went through rigorous rounds of assessment to prove their worth. After which they invested a large part of their time researching and compiling the most relevant data for our readers.

The editorial board has been involved in producing this book since its inception. They have spent rigorous hours researching and exploring the diverse topics which have resulted in the successful publishing of this book. They have passed on their knowledge of decades through this book. To expedite this challenging task, the publisher supported the team at every step. A small team of assistant editors was also appointed to further simplify the editing procedure and attain best results for the readers.

Apart from the editorial board, the designing team has also invested a significant amount of their time in understanding the subject and creating the most relevant covers. They scrutinized every image to scout for the most suitable representation of the subject and create an appropriate cover for the book.

The publishing team has been an ardent support to the editorial, designing and production team. Their endless efforts to recruit the best for this project, has resulted in the accomplishment of this book. They are a veteran in the field of academics and their pool of knowledge is as vast as their experience in printing. Their expertise and guidance has proved useful at every step. Their uncompromising quality standards have made this book an exceptional effort. Their encouragement from time to time has been an inspiration for everyone.

The publisher and the editorial board hope that this book will prove to be a valuable piece of knowledge for researchers, students, practitioners and scholars across the globe.

List of Contributors

Ashley V. Fritz, Gregory J. Mickus, Michael A. Vega, J. Ross Renew and Sorin J. Brull
Department of Anesthesiology and Perioperative Medicine, Mayo Clinic, 4500 San Pablo Road S, Jacksonville, Florida 32224, USA

Jin Xu and Xiaoming Deng
Department of Anesthesiology, Plastic Surgery Hospital, Chinese Academy of Medical Sciences and Peking Union Medical College, No. 33, Ba Da Chu Road, Shi Jing Shan, Beijing 100144, China

Fuxia Yan
Department of Anesthesiology, Fuwai Hospital, National Center for Cardiovascular Diseases, Chinese Academy of Medical Sciences and Peking Union Medical College, 167 North Lishi Road, XiCheng District, Beijing 100037, China

Sanghee Park, Hyung Gon Lee, Jeong Il Choi, Seongheon Lee, Eun-A Jang, Hong-Beom Bae, Jeeyun Rhee and Seongtae Jeong
Department of Anesthesiology and Pain Medicine, Chonnam National University Medical School, Chonnam National University Hospital, 42 Jebong-ro, Dong-gu, Gwangju 61469, South Korea

Hyung Chae Yang
Department of Otolaryngology-Head and Neck Surgery, Chonnam National University Medical School, Chonnam National University Hospital, Gwangju, South Korea

Jee-Eun Chang, Hyerim Kim, Jung-Man Lee and Dongwook Won
Department of Anesthesiology and Pain Medicine, SMG-SNU Boramae Medical Center, Boramae-ro, Dongjak-gu, Seoul 156-707, Republic of Korea

Jin-Young Hwang
Department of Anesthesiology and Pain Medicine, SMG-SNU Boramae Medical Center, Boramae-ro, Dongjak-gu, Seoul 156-707, Republic of Korea
College of Medicine, Seoul National University, Seoul, Republic of Korea

Kwanghoon Jun
Department of Anesthesiology and Pain Medicine, Seoul National University Hospital, Seoul, Republic of Korea

De-Xing Liu, Ying Ye, Yu-Hang Zhu, Jing Li, Hong-Ying He, Liang Dong and Zhao-Qiong Zhu
Department of Anesthesiology, Affiliated Hospital of Zunyi Medical College, No. 149 Dalian Road, Zunyi 563000, China

Ahmed Hasanin, Hager Tarek, Maha M. A. Mostafa, Amany Arafa, Mona H. Elsherbiny, Osama Hosny, Ahmed A. Gado, Ghada Adel Hamden, Mohamed Mahmoud and Sarah Amin
Department of anesthesia and critical care medicine, Cairo university, Giza, Egypt

Ahmed G. Safina
Department of surgery, Cairo university, Giza, Egypt

Tarek Almenesey
Department of anesthesia and critical care medicine, Beni suef university, Beni suef, Egypt

Go Un Roh, Joon Gwon Kang and Jung Youn Han
Department of Anesthesiology and Pain Medicine, CHA Bundang Medical Center, CHA University School of Medicine, 59 Yatap-ro, Bundang-gu, Seongnami-si, Gyeonggi-do 13496, Korea

Chul Ho Chang
Department of Anesthesiology and Pain Medicine, and Anesthesia and Pain Research Institute, Yonse University College of Medicine, Gangnam Severance Hospital, 211 Eonju-ro, Gangnam-gu, Seoul 06273, Korea

Kurt Ruetzler
Departments of Outcomes Research and General Anesthesia, Cleveland Clinic, Anesthesiology Institute, Cleveland, OH, USA

Jacek Smereka
Department of Emergency Medical Service, Wroclaw Medical University, Wroclaw, Poland

Cristian Abelairas-Gomez
CLINURSID Research Group, University of Santiago de Compostela, Santiago de Compostela, Spain
Faculty of Education, University Santiago de Compostela, Santiago de Compostela, Spain
Institute of Research of Santiago (IDIS) and SAMID-II Network, Santiago de Compostela, Spain

Michael Frass and Oliver Robak
Department of Internal Medicine I, Medical University
of Vienna, Vienna, Austria

Marek Dabrowski
Chair and Department of Medical Education, Poznan
University of Medical Sciences, Poznan, Poland

Szymon Bialka and Hanna Misiolek
Department of Anaesthesiology and Critical Care,
School of Medicine with Division of Dentistry in
Zabrze, Medical University of Silesia, Zabrze, Poland

Tadeusz Plusa
Medical Faculty, Lazarski University, Warsaw, Poland

Olga Aniolek, Damian Gorczyca and Lukasz Szarpak
Polish Society of Disaster Medicine, Swieradowska 43
Str, 02-662 Warsaw, Poland

Jerzy Robert Ladny
Department of Emergency Medicine, Medical
University Bialystok, Bialystok, Poland

Sanchit Ahuja
Department of Anesthesia, Henry Ford Health System,
Detroit, MI, USA

Huafeng Wei
Department of Anesthesiology and Critical Care,
Hospital of the University of Pennsylvania,
Philadelphia, PA 19104, USA

**Yahong Gong, Xiaohan Xu, Jin Wang, Lu Che, Weijia
Wang and Jie Yi**
Department of Anesthesiology, Peking Union Medical
College Hospital (PUMCH), 1 Shuai Fuyuan, Wangfujing
Street, Dongcheng District, Beijing 100730, China

Bon-Wook Koo, Jung-Won Hwang and Hyo-Seok Na
Department of Anesthesiology and Pain Medicine,
Seoul National University Bundang Hospital, 137-82
Gumi-ro, Bundang-gu, Sungnam-si, Gyeonggi-do 463-
707, South Korea

Ah-Young Oh
Department of Anesthesiology and Pain Medicine,
Seoul National University Bundang Hospital, 137-82
Gumi-ro, Bundang-gu, Sungnam-si, Gyeonggi-do 463-
707, South Korea
Department of Anesthesiology and Pain Medicine,
Seoul National University College of Medicine, Seoul,
South Korea

Seong-Won Min
Department of Anesthesiology and Pain Medicine,
Seoul National University College of Medicine, Seoul,
South Korea

Department of Anesthesiology and Pain Medicine,
Boramae Hospital, Seoul, South Korea
Department of Anesthesiology and Pain Medicine,
SMG-SNU Boramae Medical Center, Boramae-ro,
Dongjak-gu, Seoul 156-707, Republic of Korea
College of Medicine, Seoul National University, Seoul,
Republic of Korea

Min Xu, Yue Liu and Jing Yang
Department of Anesthesiology, West China Hospital,
Sichuan University, No.37 Guo Xue Ave, Chengdu,
Sichuan 610041, PR China

Hao Liu and Chen Ding
Department of Orthopedics, West China Hospital,
Sichuan University, No.37 Guo Xue Ave, Chengdu,
Sichuan 610041, PR China

**Robert Ruemmler, Alexander Ziebart, Thomas Ott,
Dagmar Dirvonskis and Erik Kristoffer Hartmann**
Department of Anaesthesiology, Medical Centre of the
Johannes Gutenberg-University, Langenbeckstrasse 1,
55131 Mainz, Germany

**Fredy-Michel Roten, Richard Steffen, Robert Greif
and Lorenz Theiler**
Department of Anesthesiology and Pain Therapy, Bern
University Hospital and University of Bern, CH-3010
Bern, Switzerland

Maren Kleine-Brueggeney
Department of Anesthesiology and Pain Therapy, Bern
University Hospital and University of Bern, CH-3010
Bern, Switzerland
Department of Anaesthesia, Evelina London Children's
Hospital, Guys and St. Thomas' NHS Foundation
Trust, London SE1 7EH, UK

Marius Wipfli
Department of Anaesthesiology and Pain Therapy,
Lindenhofspital, CH-3011 Bern, Switzerland

Andreas Arnold
Department of Otorhinolaryngology, Head and Neck
Surgery, Bern University Hospital and University of
Bern, CH-3010 Bern, Switzerland

Henrik Fischer
Medical School, Sigmund Freud University,
Kelsenstraße 2, A -1030 Vienna, Austria

**Yoko Okumura, Masahiro Okuda, Aiji Sato Boku,
Naoko Tachi, Mayumi Hashimoto, Tomio Yamada,
Masahiro Yamada and Aiji Sato-Boku**
Department of Anesthesiology, Aichi Gakuin
University School of Dentistry, 2-11 Suemori-dori,
Chikusaku, Nagoya 464-8651, Japan

Keiji Nagano
Department of Oral microbiology, School of Dentistry
Health Sciences University of Hokkaido 757 Kanazawa,
Ishikari-Tobetsu, Hokkaido 061-0293, Japan

Yoshiaki Hasegawa
Department of Microbiology, Aichi Gakuin University
School of Dentistry, 1-100 Kusumotocho, Chikusa-ku,
Nagoya 464-8650, Japan

**Yuji Kamimura, Yoshiki Sento, MinHye So, Eisuke
Kako and Kazuya Sobue**
Department of Anesthesiology and Intensive Care
Medicine, Nagoya City University Graduate School of
Medical Sciences, 1 Kawasumi, Mizuho-cho, Mizuho-
ku, Nagoya 467-8601, Japan

Hidekazu Ito
Department of Anesthesiology, Aichi Developmental
Disability Center Central Hospital, 713-8 Kagiya-cho,
Kasugai-city, Aichi 480-0392, Japan

Yushi Adachi
Department of Anesthesiology, Nagoya University
Graduate School of Medicine, 65 Tsurumaicho,
Showaku, Nagoya 466-8550, Japan

Zhi Zhang
Hefei National Laboratory for Physical Sciences
at the Microscale, Department of Biophysics and
Neurobiology, University of Science and Technology
of China, Hefei 230027, People's Republic of China

Junma Yu
Hefei National Laboratory for Physical Sciences
at the Microscale, Department of Biophysics and
Neurobiology, University of Science and Technology
of China, Hefei 230027, People's Republic of China
Department of Anesthesiology, The First People's
Hospital of Hefei, Anhui Medical University, Hefei,
Anhui 230061, People's Republic of China

Rui Hu, Lining Wu and Peng Sun
Department of Anesthesiology, The First People's
Hospital of Hefei, Anhui Medical University, Hefei,
Anhui 230061, People's Republic of China

**Hyung-Been Yhim, Soo-Hyuk Yoon, Young-Eun
Jang, Ji-Hyun Lee and Eun-Hee Kim**
Department of Anesthesiology and Pain Medicine,
Seoul National University Hospital, #101 Daehakno,
Jongnogu, Seoul 03080, Korea

Jin-Tae Kim and Hee-Soo Kim
Department of Anesthesiology and Pain Medicine,
Seoul National University Hospital, #101 Daehakno,
Jongnogu, Seoul 03080, Korea

Department of Anesthesiology and Pain Medicine,
College of Medicine, Seoul National University, #101
Daehak-ro, Jongno-gu, 03080 Seoul, Republic of Korea

**Jeremy Juang, Martha Cordoba, Alex Ciaramella,
Mark Xiao, Jeremy Goldfarb and Alvaro Andres
Macias**
Department of Anesthesiology, Massachusetts Eye
and Ear, 243 Charles St, Boston, MA 02114, USA
Harvard Medical School, Boston, MA 20114, USA

Jorge Enrique Bayter
Clinica El Pinar, Km 2 Anillo vial Floridablanca –
Girón, Ecoparque Empresarial Natura Torre 2 piso 1
y 2, Piedecuesta, Colombia

**Lianxiang Jiang, Peng Zhang, Weidong Yao, Yan
Chang and Zeping Dai**
Department of Anaesthesia, Yijishan Hospital of
Wannan Medical College, No. 2, Zheshan West Road,
Wuhu City, Anhui Province, China

Shulin Qiu
Department of Anaesthesia, Beijing Tiantan Hospital
of Capital Medical University, Beijing, China

Andre Tran
Discipline of Medicine, The University of Adelaide,
Adelaide, South Australia, Australia

**Venkatesan Thiruvenkatarajan, Medhat Wahba,
John Currie, Anand Rajbhoj and Roelof van Wijk**
Department of Anaesthesia, The Queen Elizabeth
Hospital, 28 Woodville Rd, Adelaide, South Australia
5011, Australia

Edward Teo and Mark Lorenzetti
Department of Gastroenterology, The Queen Elizabeth
Hospital, 28 Woodville Rd, Adelaide, South Australia,
Australia

Guy Ludbrook
Discipline of Acute Care Medicine, The University of
Adelaide, Adelaide, South Australia, Australia

Jochen Hinkelbein
Department of Anaesthesiology and Intensive Care
Medicine, University Hospital of Cologne, Kerpener
Str. 62, 50937 Köln, Germany

Ivan Iovino
Department of Anaesthesiology and Intensive Care
Medicine, University Hospital of Cologne, Kerpener
Str. 62, 50937 Köln, Germany
Department of Neurosciences, Reproductive and
Odontostomatological Sciences, University of Naples
"Federico II", Via S. Pansini, 5, 80131 Naples, Italy

Peter Kranke
Department of Anaesthesia and Critical Care, University Hospital of Wuerzburg, Wuerzburg, Germany

Edoardo De Robertis
Department of Neurosciences, Reproductive and Odontostomatological Sciences, University of Naples "Federico II", Via S. Pansini, 5, 80131 Naples, Italy
Department of Surgical and Biomedical Sciences, University of Perugia, Perugia, Italy

Joachim Risse
Center of Emergency Medicine, University Hospital Essen, Hufelandstrasse 55, 45122 Essen, Germany
Department of Anesthesiology and Intensive Care Medicine, Philipps-University Marburg, Baldingerstraße, 35033 Marburg, Germany

Ann-Kristin Schubert, Thomas Wiesmann, Ansgar Huelshoff, David Stay, Michael Zentgraf, Hinnerk Wulf, Carsten Feldmann and Karl Matteo Meggiolaro
Department of Anesthesiology and Intensive Care Medicine, Philipps-University Marburg, Baldingerstraße, 35033 Marburg, Germany

Andreas Kirschbaum
Visceral, Thoracic and Vascular Surgery Clinic, University Hospital Giessen and Marburg GmbH, Baldingerstraße, 35033 Marburg, Germany

Michael St. Pierre, Frederick Krischke, Bjoern Luetcke and Joachim Schmidt
Anästhesiologische Klinik, Universitätsklinikum Erlangen, Krankenhausstrasse 12, 91054 Erlangen, Germany

Hansheng Liang, Yuantao Hou, Liang Sun, Qingyue Li and Yi Feng
Department of Anesthesiology, Peking University People's Hospital, Beijing100044, Beijing, China

Li Zhang, Jian Fei, Jian Jia, Xiaohua Shi, Meimin Qu and Hui Wang
Department of Anesthesiology, Children's Hospital of Nanjing Medical University, Nanjing 210008, Jiangsu Province, China

Yuanyuan Ma, Ping Shi, Xue Cao and Shengjin Ge
Department of Anesthesia, Zhongshan Hospital, Fudan University, No. 180 Fenglin Road, Shanghai 200032, China

Yan Wang
Department of Anesthesia, Zhongshan Hospital, Fudan University, No. 180 Fenglin Road, Shanghai 200032, China
Kashgar Regional Second People's Hospital, Kashi City, Xinjiang Uygur Autonomous Region, China

Uzung Yoon, Jeffrey Mojica, Matthew Wiltshire, Michael Block, Anthony Pantoja, Marc Torjman and Elizabeth Wolo
Department of Anesthesiology, Thomas Jefferson University Hospital, Suite 8290 Gibbon, 111 South 11th Street, Philadelphia PA 19107, USA

Kara Segna
Department of Anesthesiology, Johns Hopkins University Hospital, Baltimore, MD, USA

Ina Ismiarti Shariffuddin, Sook Hui Chaw, Ling Wei Ng, Ching Hooi Lim, Mohd Fitry Zainal Abidin and Wan A. Wan Zakaria
Department of Anesthesiology, Faculty of Medicine, University of Malaya, 50603 Kuala Lumpur, Malaysia

Wendy H. Teoh
Wendy Teoh Pte.Ltd, Private Anaesthesia Practice, Singapore, Singapore

Index

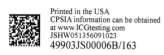

9 781639 897810